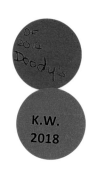

Postpartum Mood Disorders
A Guide for Medical, Mental Health, and Other Support Providers

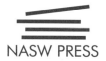

Kimberley Zittel

NASW PRESS

National Association of Social Workers
Washington, DC

James J. Kelly, PhD, ACSW, *President*
Elizabeth J. Clark, PhD, ACSW, MPH, *Executive Director*

Cheryl Y. Bradley, *Publisher*
Lisa M. O'Hearn, *Managing Editor*
Sarah Lowman, *Project Manager*
Sara Jones, *Copyeditor*
Juanita Doswell, *Proofreader*
Bernice Eisen, *Indexer*

Cover by Eye to Eye Design Studio
Interior design by Rick Soldin
Printed and bound by Hamilton Printing Company

Library of Congress Cataloging-in-Publication Data

Zittel, Kimberley.
  Postpartum mood disorders : a guide for medical, mental health, and other support providers / Kimberley Zittel.
     p. ; cm.
  Includes bibliographical references and index.
  ISBN 978-0-87101-399-6
  1. Postpartum depression. 2. Puerperal disorders. I. National Association of Social Workers. II. Title.
  [DNLM: 1. Mood Disorders. 2. Puerperal Disorders. WQ 500]
  RG852.Z58 2010
  618.7'6--dc22

                                     2010028657

Printed in the United States of America

Dedicated to my boys
Joseph and Joshua

To my family
Raymond, Dorothea, Daniel, Janet, Elijah, Jennifer, Mary Ellen, Sarah, Renee, Steven, Mary Rose, and Margit

In memory of
Bertha E. Reiner

To my supportive family
Bonnie Smith, Tosca and Sam Miserendino, Dr. Ramona Santa Maria, Dr. Dian Leoa Wells, Brangwynne Purcell, June Steckler, Dr. Jayne Maugans Swanson, Jessica Markarian, Kristen Mytych Hahn, Sara Kochanowski, Kristen Hillman, Judy McCaffery, Melissa Miszkiewicz, Janet Lawton

To my mentors and strong women
Jane Epstein, LCSW-R, Dr. Nancy Smyth, Sonia Murdock, Dr. Kim Griswold, Kathleen Martin, LCSW, Louann Saine, LCSW, Dr. Barbara Rittner, Dr. Sanna Thompson

Much appreciation to
The Postpartum Resource Center of New York, Inc., The Buffalo Prenatal Perinatal Network, The Niagara Family Health Clinic, maternity nurses at Millard Filmore Gates Suburban and Sisters Hospitals, Tonawanda Pediatrics, Dr. Barbara Segal, Erie County Doulas, Buffalo State College Social Work Department, Buffalo State College Research Foundation, Phi Alpha Social Work Honor Society, State University of New York School of Social Work, Center for the Development of Human Services, Gail Daniels, Thomas Needell, Kevin Garrity, Laurie Rashkin, Julie R. Rockmaker, Sarah A. Cercone, Jodi Hitchcock, Mary Colman, Grethe Gruarin, Dawn Shinn, Dr. Louise Ferretti, Dr. Wendy L. Weinstein, Dr. Maria Cartagena, Dr. William Wieczorek, Sandy Lindaman, and all those working tirelessly to help improve women's mental health

Special mention
Dr. Jerry Gillis and the Reverend Kristen Fishbaugh Looney

Contents

About the Author

Kimberley Zittel, PhD, MSW, is an assistant professor in the social work department at Buffalo State College (BSC). She holds a bachelor's degree in psychology from Houghton College, an MSW from SUNY at Buffalo, and a PhD in social welfare from SUNY at Buffalo. She has extensive clinical experience working in medical settings and research experience with postpartum mood disorders and access to care issues. Dr. Zittel is the principle investigator of the Postpartum Mood Disorders Initiative at BSC, committee member for the Buffalo State College Women's Studies program, and board member of Postpartum Resource Center of New York. She has published nearly 20 peer-reviewed articles, and she has lectured locally, nationally, and internationally. Dr. Zittel has received serveral national and regional awards for her clinical and research accomplishments, including the 2007 NASW WNY Social Worker of the Year Award and honorary membership in Phi Alpha Social Work Honor Society.

About the Contributor

Brangwynne Purcell was born and raised in western New York, where she graduated from Houghton College with concentrations in fine art and creative writing. She has lived in the United States, England, and Canada. She later graduated from the Department of Family Medicine at the University of British Columbia with a bachelor's of midwifery. She currently lives in North Vancouver, British Columbia, with her husband and three children. Brangwynne works as a registered midwife and enjoys a very active midwifery practice.

Chapter 1

Introduction

Postpartum mood disorders (PMDs) include the experience of depression, anxiety, or psychosis typically six weeks after the delivery of a baby. These disorders occur with alarming frequency. Conservatively, one in seven women experience postpartum depression (PPD) (Moses-Kolko & Roth, 2004). Women in the United States had an estimated 4.3 million live births (U.S. Department of Health and Human Services, 2009). Using conservative postpartum depression rates, approximately 430,000 to 645,000 women in the United States experienced postpartum depression; compare this with the estimated 192,280 men who were diagnosed with prostate cancer in 2009 (American Cancer Society, 2009) Although it is certainly important to have education campanions, patient and doctor education, and research dedicated to prostate cancer, it is vital to offer the same for postpartum mood disorders. A woman is more likely to be admitted into a psychiatric hospital during the first postpartum year than during any other time in the life cycle (Kendall et al., 1987). Currently, suicide resulting from PMDs is the leading cause of death for perinatal women in the United States (Lindahl, Pearson, & Colpe, 2005). Failing to assess, diagnose, or treat women with PMDs can have detrimental results on women, children, spousal or partner relationships, and the entire family (Tammentie, Tarkka, Astedt-Kurki, & Paavilainen, 2002). Left untreated, these women often have difficulty developing a strong bond with their baby (Sagami, Kayama, & Senoo, 2004), which can lead to cognitive, behavioral, language, and developmental delays (Deave, Heron, Evans, & Emond, 2008; Poobalan et al., 2007; Sohr-Preston & Scaramella, 2006). Despite the negative effects of PMDs on the family, many women are still not receiving the assistance they need, and few social workers, counselors, psychologists, or doctors ever receive specific training on how to assess, diagnose, or treat these disorders (Oates, 2000).

I first became aware of postpartum mental health through a friend of mine. She was very open with me and others about her experience, due to a strong desire to create change and to help others who may be suffering in silence. She described in vivid detail, that following the birth of her daughter she began to have irrational thoughts like accidentally throwing her newborn over the railing of the stairs or into a fire burning in the fireplace. Paralyzed by these fears, she avoided the stairs and the fireplace. As she spoke, I found it peculiar that she had not had these fears prior to having her baby. This caused me to look into her condition a little further. The more I looked, the more I realized that I, too, had suffered with mental health changes both during and after pregnancy. During my fourth month of pregnancy, I became extremely anxious, depressed, and irritable. Coincidentally, it had been just weeks since my father-in-law passed away from cancer, and I was one month away from completing my PhD coursework. During delivery, my son's heart rate dropped rapidly, the umbilical cord was wrapped around his neck and an emergency cesarean section was imminent. Within minutes, there was a doctor sitting on my gurney, holding my son's head in place to avoid further complications. Doctors and nurses were running everywhere, pulling cords from the walls, throwing them onto the gurney, and I was traveling full-speed down a brightly lit hall. As the gurney turned a corner, I looked up and saw three doctors scrubbing for surgery in a sterile, cold, metallic sink. No sooner had we turned the corner, I was placed on an icy metal table, bright lights on my body, a screen placed between my head and my body, my arms stretched out and I remembered asking, "Where is my husband?" I knew just enough about medicine to know what was happening, but not enough to be secure in the situation. I could feel pressured movements. I could hear the instruments suctioning my blood. When my husband finally arrived, he looked me in the eyes, and I continually asked, "Are they done yet?" He was supportive and reassuring, but I could tell that he was nervous as well. He recalled later that in a matter of seconds the entire birthing room was vacated; he was left standing there with my cousin, a physician's assistant, both of them staring at each other, unsure of what to do, what was happening, or if things would be all right. About 30 minutes after the surgery, , a nurse came in with our son, who was wrapped in warm blankets. She undid my gown, put him in my arms, squeezed my nipple hard, and led my son toward it to encourage him to suckle. I was so "out of it." Then, while he was still in my arms trying to feed, she placed a form on the table in front of me and told me to sign it. The form stated that she had taught me how to breastfeed. Seriously!

When we returned home, I had the baby blues. I remember crying to my mother, "Things will just never be the same again." She comforted me and reassured me. Things were not the same. I was overjoyed with my son, overjoyed by watching my husband hold him, watching everyone enjoy him. However, I was not producing enough milk for him. I started to think, "I am unable to care for him—to keep him alive—to nurture him the right way." This evolved into thinking that I was killing him because I could not feed him right. I stopped nursing and felt better knowing that he was eating, but still felt immense guilt that I was unable to nurse him, to be a good mother. In addition, for about six weeks, I had flashbacks to the events in the hospital, thinking that he could have died, that I could have died. These feelings of guilt, fear, anxiety, and depression only grew. I would lie on the couch and watch others helping him and think, "Thank God someone knows how to care for him, how to love him the right way, to give him what he needs." I became terrified when he slept that he would die from sudden infant death syndrom (SIDS). Therefore, I would place my hand on him while he slept or laid him on me—so in case he stopped breathing I would feel it. I did not sleep very well and felt constantly exhausted.

Why am I explaining this to you? Well, at the time I had my first son, I was a masters-level, practicing, clinical social worker for six years. Mental health and medicine were my specialties. Moreover, if I was not aware that what I was experiencing were postpartum depression, anxiety, and post-traumatic stress symptoms until speaking with my friend three years later, how do untrained mothers, fathers, family members, and friends know? I had no idea that mental health changes during or after pregnancy occurred so frequently. Most of us have heard of the sad story of Andrea Yates, the mother of five from Texas who, in the late 1990s, drowned her children in response to voices in her head telling her "killing them would save them from the devil." In Andrea's mind, she was protecting her children from evil, thereby loving them. I thought that what the Yates family went through was postpartum depression, not what I had experienced.

In fact, in all my years of professional education, up through my PhD, I had never heard postpartum depression mentioned. Research states that many medical professionals will not assess for PMDs because they are unsure of what to do if detected. Therefore, when I started my first position as a college professor, I made it one of my missions to educate students, my peers, and the general community about PMDs.

The effects of PMDs on the family, particularly when not treated, are enormous. Many communities lack PMD treatments, leaving medical professionals with limited alternatives such as medication or hospitalization. Making matters more complicated, many women who silently suffer with PMDs and continue to remain silent out of fear that her children will be removed, that there is "something wrong with her," or have experienced unsupportive remarks from professionals or unwanted treatment options (Hanson-Lynn, 2005; Logsdon, Wisner, Billings, & Shanahan, 2006; Small, Brown, Lumley, & Astbury, 1994; Wood & Meigan, 1997).

Luckily, more people are speaking out about PMDs. Brooke Shields, for example, courageously published *Down Came the Rain: My Journey Through Postpartum Depression* in 2005, where she openheartedly described her postpartum depression experience. She not only provides a well-described picture of postpartum depression, but also supports the need for women to receive education and care.

This text explores theories, epidemiology, risk factors, at-risk populations, and treatment options, to best prepare families, social workers, other counseling professionals, and medical professionals at all system levels to assist women who are experiencing PMDs. Chapter 2 presents biologically, psychologically, and sociologically based theories that propose underlying predictive factors for developing PMDs.

Chapters 3 through 5 cover details of each mental health diagnosis in the PMD spectrum, including: baby blues, depression, general anxiety, panic, posttraumatic stress, obsessive compulsion, and psychosis. Each of these chapters includes a biopsychosocial theoretical support, symptom descriptions, and diagnostic considerations.

Through research projects and by presenting at community seminars, I have learned a lot from others. During question-and-answer moments, several community professionals have also inquired about the postpartum mental health of men, couples who adopt, women who miscarry, women who have abortions, couples with infertility issues, and the effects of postpartum mood changes on children. Therefore, I chose to address these questions in chapters 6 through 10.

I also chose to write this book in a helpful format for medical and mental health professionals, family members, family supports, other paraprofessional support providers, and as an educational self-help guide—an "every-person guide" leading families toward assistance. Chapters 11 through 14 present assistance options from a multidisciplinary, multicultural, and international perspective, with particular emphasis on access to care needs.

It is important to note that some of the terminology used across disciplines and countries varies. A glossary is included at the end of the book to clarify terms. Sometimes, I use the terms interchangeably. Sometimes, I refer to women, but as fathers experience postpartum mood changes, the term "women" can be interchangeable with fathers at times. In addition, I will often refer to couples as mother and father; however, same-sex couples can be considered in these instances as well.

By the end of this text, you will have comprehensive knowledge about the full range of PMDs, how to assess and diagnose these disorders, intervention and treatment options, and the tools and strategies needed to advocate for people with PMDs across disciplines and system levels. You will understand the effect of PMDs on partners, children, other family members, and support systems. You will also understand the need to develop more programs in communities to improve access to care for those experiencing PMDs and for those supporting a loved one with these disorders.

References

American Cancer Society. (2009). *Prostate cancer.* Retrieved from http://www.cancer.org/downloads/PRO/ProstateCancer.pdf

Deave, T., Heron, J., Evans, J., & Emond, A. (2008). The impact of maternal depression in pregnancy on early child development. *BJOG: An International Journal of Obstetrics & Gynaecology, 115,* 1043–1051.

Hanson-Lynn, J. A. (2005). Help-seeking with postpartum depression: A retrospective analysis of women's experiences of PPD and their help-seeking process. *Dissertation Abstracts International: Section B: The Sciences and Engineering, 65*(12-B), 6652.

Kendell, R. E., Chalmers, J. C., & Platz, C. (1987). Epidemiology of puerperal psychoses. *British Journal of Psychiatry, 150,* 662–673.

Lindahl, V., Pearson, J. L., & Colpe, L. (2005). Prevalence of suicidality during pregnancy and the postpartum. *Archives of Women's Mental Health, 8*(2), 77–87.

Logsdon, M. C., Wisner, K., Billings, D. M., & Shanahan, B. (2006). Raising the awareness of primary care providers about postpartum depression. *Issues in Mental Health Nursing, 27* (1), 59–73.

Moses-Kolko, E. L., & Roth, E. K. (2004). Antepartum and postpartum depression: Healthy mom, healthy baby. *Journal of the American Medical Women's Association, 59*(3), 181–191.

Oates, M. (2000). *Perinatal maternal mental health services.* London, England: Royal College of Psychiatrists.

Poobalan, A. S., Aucott, L. S., Ross, L., Smith, W.C.S., Helms, P. J., & Williams, J.H.G. (2007). Effects of treating postnatal depression on mother–infant interaction and child development: Systematic review. *British Journal of Psychiatry, 191,* 378–386.

Sagami, A., Kayama, M., & Senoo, E. (2004). The relationship between postpartum depression and abusive parenting behavior of Japanese mothers:

A survey of mothers with a child less than one year old. *Bulletin of the Menninger Clinic, 68*(2), 174–187.

Shields, B. (2005). *Down came the rain: My journey through postpartum depression.* New York: Hyperion.

Small, R., Brown, S., Lumley, J., & Astbury, J. (1994). Missing voices: What women say and do about depression after childbirth. *Journal of Reproductive and Infant Psychology, 12,* 19–22.

Sohr-Preston, S. L., & Scaramella, L. V. (2006). Implications of timing of maternal depressive symptoms for early cognitive and language development. *Clinical Child & Family Psychology Review, 9*(1), 65–83.

Tammentie, T., Tarkka, M. T., Astedt-Kurki, P., & Paavilainen, E. (2002). Sociodemographic factors of families related to postnatal depressive symptoms of mothers. *International Journal of Nursing Practice, 8,* 240–246.

U.S. Department of Health and Human Services. (2009). *Women's Health USA 2009.* Health Resources and Services Administration, Maternal and Child Health Bureau. Rockville, Maryland: U.S. Department of Health and Human Services.

Wood, A. F., & Meigan, M. (1997). The downward spiral of postpartum depression. *American Journal of Maternal/Child Nursing, 22,* 308–316.

Chapter 2

Postpartum Mood Disorder Theories

Introduction

In the 6th century BCE, women's mental health symptoms were termed "hysteria," a derivative of a word meaning womb, and what is sometimes referred to today as anxiety, nervousness, or being out of control of one's emotions. Centuries later, people believed the womb actually moved throughout the female body. When this movement was at its peak, the "wandering womb" was thought to be the source of health and mental health problems (Klein, 2009). In the 1800s, women who expressed symptoms of postpartum psychological change were said to have diseased reproductive organs and, sometimes, identified as rebelling against motherhood (Taylor, 1995). As a result, many women did not discuss mood or thought changes after delivery.

By the 1900s, psychiatric thought excluded the idea of diseased reproductive organs, yet other medical specialties continued to understand female mental health conditions based on earlier Hippocratic traditions that viewed reproductive syndromes and raging hormones as the cause of women's depression, anxiety, sexual performance, and suicide (Dalton, 1964; Ussher, 1992). It was not until the 1970s that the postpartum support group movement materialized from the larger women's health movement. This movement challenged the medically defined concepts of motherhood in society (Taylor, 1995). This chapter discusses the most current biological, psychological, sociological, and environmental theories that propose reasons why women experience postpartum mood disorders (PMDs).

Biologically Based Theories

Between the onset of puberty and menopause, women are two times more likely to experience major depression than are men, even when racial and socioeconomic factors are controlled (Kessler, McGonagle, Swartz, Blazer, & Nelson, 1993; Nolen-Hoeksema, 1990; Weissman & Klerman, 1997). Given this trend, the primary way medical professionals understand PMDs is a reaction to hormones, particularly the role of estrogen, during reproductive changes throughout the lifecycle. Specifically, as estrogen levels decrease, depression symptoms appear to increase (refer to Figure 1) (Ahokas, Aito, & Rimon, 2000; Pearlstein, 1995).

Figure 2-1   Estrogen levels' effects on neurotransmitters and mood (modified from Douma et al., 2005)

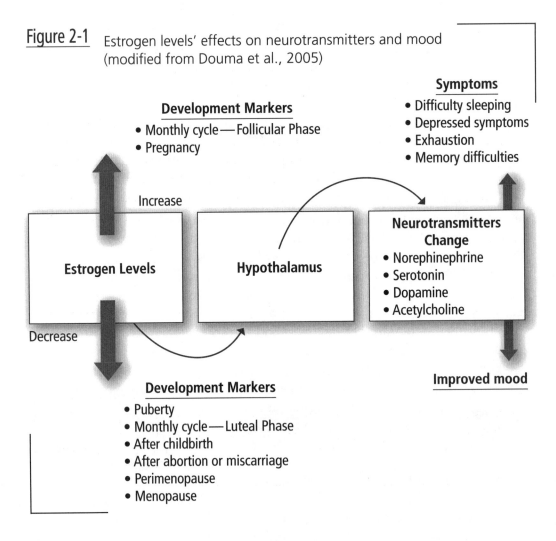

Hypothalamic–Pituitary–Adrenal (HPA) Axis

One physiological model used to understand PMDs is imbalance in the HPA axis. The hypothalamus is a part of the brain that produces and releases neurohormones. Neurohormones communicate with the pituitary gland, telling the pituitary to allow or not allow the release of pituitary hormones. Pituitary hormones travel as messengers to the adrenal glands, which are located above the kidneys. The adrenal glands create corticosteroids and catecholamines—the most common are cortisol and adrenaline—to regulate the body's reaction to stress. The detection of stress triggers the hippocampal release of corticotropin hormone. In response, the pituitary gland discharges adrenocorticotropic hormone (ACTH). ACTH signals the adrenal cortex to discharge glucocorticoids, which triggers stress responses throughout the body. Any increase or decrease in HPA axis functioning results in mental health or physical problems such as hyperarousal, changes in thought processes, sleep disturbances, immune system functioning, inflammatory conditions, increased body fat, and hypertension (refer to Figure 2) (Haefner et al., 2008; McEwen, 2008; Shalev et al., 2009).

Genetic links (such as the glucocorticoid receptor gene, GABRA6 gene, and mu-opioid receptor gene) and gender differences have been identified in HPA axis reactions to stress (Chong et al., 2006; Shalev et al., 2009; Uhart, McCaul, Oswald, Choi, & Wand, 2004; Wust et al., 2004). This genetic link may increase the understanding between increased risks for developing postpartum mood conditions and having a relative who has also experienced postpartum mood disturbances.

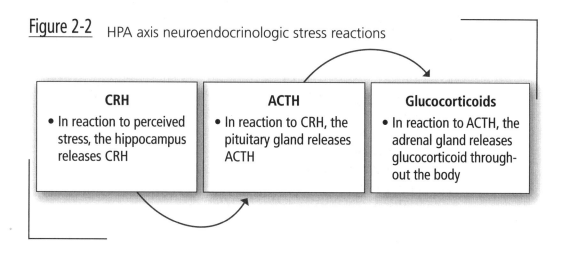

Figure 2-2   HPA axis neuroendocrinologic stress reactions

CRH	ACTH	Glucocorticoids
• In reaction to perceived stress, the hippocampus releases CRH	• In reaction to CRH, the pituitary gland releases ACTH	• In reaction to ACTH, the adrenal gland releases glucocorticoid throughout the body

Hypothalamic–Pituitary–Gonadal (HPG) Axis

The HPG axis functions to regulate the reproductive and immune systems in the body. In this axis, the hypothalamus discharges luteinizing hormone releasing hormone (LHRH). The pituitary gland receives the LHRH and responds by releasing follicle-stimulating hormone (FSH) and luteinizing hormone (LH). FSH is responsible for the development of ovarian follicles in preparation for ovulation and LH activates ovulation and the release of estrogen.

The HPA axis has a relationship with the HPG axis where information passes back and forth between the two axes. Dysfunctions in the communication between the HPA axis and the HPG axis can influence the development of mental health and physical conditions. The recent work of Luecken, Kraft, and Hagan (2009) found difficult and abusive childhood family environments and abuse experiences linked to health and mental health difficulties throughout the life cycle. The low-level detection of cortisol, a major hormone associated with the HPA axis, was found in women who grew up in these difficult family situations. This suggests a developmental influence on healthy HPA-axis reactions to stressors (Gunnar & Quevedo, 2007). Given this, it is not surprising that risk factors for the development of PMDs include relationship difficulties, poor familial support, the experience of negative events, family-of-origin mental health history, and exposure to abuse. In addition, adults who grew up in dysfunctional family environments often experience other HPA-axis dysfunction-related symptoms that are also risk factors for PMDs such as difficulty sleeping, somatic symptoms, and autoimmune disorders (Luecken et al., 2009).

Hormonal Fluctuation

Statistically, women are more susceptible to depression once menstruation starts and on through menopause, referred to as reproductive mental health. Prior to menstruation and after menopause, some suggest that girls and women are less likely than boys and men to have a depression diagnosis (Rosenbaum & Covino, 2006). A key denominator across this timeline is hormone and sex-steroid fluctuations. Sex-steroids are reproduction-related hormones in the female body that fluctuate monthly and include estrogens, progesterone, and androgens. These hormones are able to manipulate neurotransmitter levels in the brain commonly associated with mental health symptoms: dopamine, norepinephrine, and serotonin (Joffe & Cohen, 1998). Estrogen, in particular, is a mood booster and is able to influence serotonergic and opioid neurons, thereby increasing serotonin concentrations (Carretti et al., 2005; Joffe & Cohen, 1998; McEwen & Alves, 1999; Serrano & Warnock,

2007). When estrogen levels are elevated, serotonin, norepinephrine, opiates, and dopamine are able to travel more easily, thereby improving mood. However, if estrogen levels are low, the result can be depression symptoms exhibited during the postpartum period as well as during premenstruation and perimenopause (Douma, Husband, O'Donnell, Barwin, & Woodend, 2005). At times, the influence of estrogen on neurotransmitter regulation can result in schizophrenic symptoms, body temperature changes, and alterations in memory (particularly verbal memory), concentration, and sleeping patterns (Carretti et al., 2005; Douma et al., 2005). Women who experience PMDs report some, if not all, of these symptoms as well.

According to the hormone-based model, *postpartum blues* is the experience of mild depression symptoms that last no more than two weeks and results from the sudden, extreme hormonal changes that occur after the baby is born. Levels of estradiol, an estrogen-based hormone, can increase up to 50 times their normal levels during pregnancy and then drop to regular menstruation cycle levels by the third day after delivery (Rosenbaum & Covino, 2006). It is suggested that the sudden decrease in postpartum estrogen levels creates a reaction to dopamine receptors (Wieck et al., 1991). When these dramatic hormonal changes occur in conjunction with other biopsychosocial risk factors, the woman is susceptible to developing PMDs.

Hormonal changes also serve positive purposes. Oxytocin levels dramatically change after delivery and appear to be linked to the development of strong mother–baby attachment postpartum (L. Miller, 1996). Therefore, the body is naturally changing—assimilating—to no longer *carrying* a baby but toward *caring* for a baby. When compromised, this naturally occurring homeostasis may result in mental health symptoms.

Psychosocially Based Theories

Bonding Theory

One of the common results of PMDs is difficulty bonding with the baby, which usually starts to develop shortly after delivery and continues to evolve over the first postpartum year. Typical bonding behaviors between mother and baby include cooing, facial recognition, response to facial cues, holding and cuddling, nurturing touch, and sometimes breastfeeding. When a strong bond fails to grow, the mother will start to focus more on herself rather than her baby. Statistically, women with this kind of inward focus report experiencing more pain, discomfort, anxiety, and depression six weeks after delivery (Besser, Vliegen, Luyten, & Blatt, 2008; Ferber & Feldman, 2005).

Difficulty bonding can result in long-term attachment disorders (Crouch & Manderson, 1996). Attachment, different from bonding, is emotional connectedness that develops and matures over time (Karl, Beal, O'Hara, & Rissmiller, 2006; Zauderer, 2008). Attachment difficulties can compromise the baby's growth and development, resulting in emotional and cognitive difficulties (Armstrong, Fraser, Dadds, & Morris, 2000; Essex, Klein, Miech, & Smider, 2001; Zauderer, 2008).

Historically, the medical profession conceptualizes maternal–infant bonding as a natural, biologically based process. One assumption in the medical model of bonding is that the desire for emotional attachment to the baby has biological underpinnings. According to this model, mothers who are unable to naturally bond with the child are labeled pathological (Crouch & Manderson, 1996; Margison, 1982). It is assumed that the mother's thought process must be altered if healthy bonding to her child is unsuccessful, resulting in faulty beliefs. The mother then starts to say things herself such as, "I have failed," "there is no hope for this relationship," "I am a bad mother," "I can't do this right," or "I am a failure." Reminiscent thoughts of childhood can also emerge like, "I am just as bad as my mother was," or "I will never be a good mother like my mother was." These thoughts become self-reinforcing and the mother stops trying to bond, causing the feelings of guilt, shame, depression, or anxiety to become stronger. In addition, popular books have buttressed the presumption that bonding is a natural and healthy process for new mothers. Although the intention of these books is to instruct and prepare mothers and to optimize the mother–baby relationship, for a mother who has difficulty bonding with her child, these books can further highlight her feelings of inadequacy as a mother.

As many mothers need to return to work shortly after delivery, bonding difficulties due to reliance on others (such as day care) can further add to the feelings of guilt. This economic, cognitive, and physiological desire (or lack thereof) to bond and be a "good mom" can be *ego dystonic* (a source of internal turmoil and conflict) for the mother and ultimately expressed through depression or anxiety symptoms. For example, societal and economic pressures might make it necessary for a woman to put her child in day care, despite the fact that, internally, she feels and thinks that she "should" be with her baby. This creates an internal conflict without an adequate outcome for either option (do not return to work and take care of the baby, resulting in financial disparity or return to work, do not take care of the baby full-time, and feel like the baby's needs have been neglected). Another conflict can arise when the mother enjoys working, finds herself depressed by staying at home, but feels guilt for returning to work, thereby perceiving that she has put her needs over her child's bonding needs. Again, these conflicts can create inner turmoil, resulting in depression or anxiety.

Psychoanalytic Theory of Personality Development

A hierarchical development of the self examines the interactions between the evolving understanding of self and the evolving aptitude to relate with others (Besser, Priel, Flett, & Wiznizer, 2007; Blatt, 2006, 2008; Blatt & Blass, 1990, 1996). Healthy self-understanding occurs when a person is able to realistically, and positively, accept their unique characteristics and roles. An ability to create interpersonal relationships that increases in maturity and that are mutually satisfying undergirds a healthy aptitude to relate with others. When the two dynamics of self-understanding and interpersonal aptitude are balanced, the person is able to develop self-sufficiency. When one of these two dynamics is not balanced, the person develops symptoms of depression (refer to Figure 2-3 on page 14).

It is interesting that women who lean more toward self-criticism based on her understanding of self are more predisposed to postpartum depression (Priel & Besser, 2000). These women are more apt to try to meet an idealized definition of motherhood. When the idealized expectation remains unachieved, these women become overly critical of themselves in the mother role and undermine their concept of self. In addition, a self-critical woman can interpret support from others as revealing her failure in the role of mother and as a restriction on her autonomy (Besser et al., 2008). Women who lean more toward dependency are less likely to experience postpartum depression as the need for social support and excessive closeness may act as a buffer (Priel & Besser, 2000).

Psychodynamic and Developmental Theories

A key lifetime developmental phase for many women is the transition to motherhood. Pregnancy and the transition to motherhood is one of the most powerful and life-changing experiences for women (Besser et al., 2008; Cohen & Slade, 2000). One aspect of this developmental phase is the process of redefining self and other (Besser et al., 2008), as women need to reconceptualize their relationships to spouses or partners, friends, family members, and themselves. Furthermore, women must deal with physical changes, employment opportunities, and child care options. Some women in this phase identify themselves as the "vessel that brought parents grandchildren." Such a statement clearly indicates a perceived role change in the family.

As discussed by Besser et al. (2008), the transition to motherhood contains four themes: life-growth, primary relatedness, supporting matrix, and identity reorganization (Stern, 1995) (refer to Chart 2-1). Another way to conceptualize these themes is the mother's self-efficacy in these four areas;

Figure 2-3 Interactions between Self-Identity and Interpersonal Relationships (based on Besser et al., 2008)

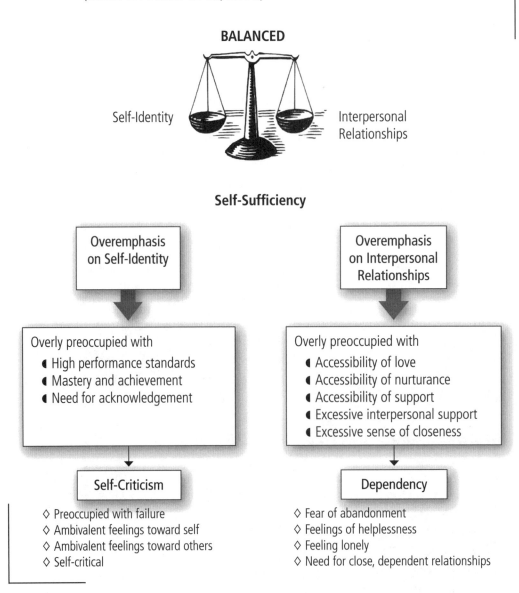

BALANCED

Self-Identity — Interpersonal Relationships

Self-Sufficiency

Overemphasis on Self-Identity	Overemphasis on Interpersonal Relationships
Overly preoccupied with ◀ High performance standards ◀ Mastery and achievement ◀ Need for acknowledgement	Overly preoccupied with ◀ Accessibility of love ◀ Accessibility of nurturance ◀ Accessibility of support ◀ Excessive interpersonal support ◀ Excessive sense of closeness
Self-Criticism ◇ Preoccupied with failure ◇ Ambivalent feelings toward self ◇ Ambivalent feelings toward others ◇ Self-critical	**Dependency** ◇ Fear of abandonment ◇ Feelings of helplessness ◇ Feeling lonely ◇ Need for close, dependent relationships

the greater the mother's self-efficacy, or belief that she is able to successfully achieve the thematic goal, the more likely it is that she will have an easier transition into motherhood; the less self-efficacy the mother has, the more likely it is that she will have a difficult transition into motherhood. The latter can result in symptoms of depression or anxiety.

Chart 2-1 Transition to Motherhood Themes in Relation to the Development of Postpartum Mood Disorder Symptoms (based on the themes presented by Stern, 1995).

Transition to Motherhood Themes	Theme Characteristics	Successful Theme Integration	Unsuccessful Theme Integration
Life–Growth	The belief that the mother is able to sustain life and physical growth of the baby	• Baby's primary basic physiological needs are met • Mother cognitively identifies as successfully fulfilling her mother role	• Withdraw or overly protective of the baby • Mother cognitively identifies as a "bad mother" and incapable of taking care of her child
Primary Relatedness	The belief that the mother is able to emotionally interact with the baby naturally and support the baby's psychologically based development (such as attachment, emotional well-being, environmental reactions)	• Baby's bonding and attachment needs are met • Mother cognitively identifies as successfully fulfilling her mother role	• Mother–baby bonding and attachment becomes compromised • Reinforces the mother's perception of herself as a "bad mother"
Supporting Matrix	The mother's belief that her support network will enable her to support her baby's physical and psychological development	• The mother is replenished physically and psychologically to contine providing for the baby • Externally reinforces her role as mother • Reinforces her ability to continue providing for the baby's basic physiological and emotional needs	• The mother feels overwhelmed by and unable to meet the baby's needs • She may feel guilt and shame about this and not seek out assistance • Reinforces her perception of herself as a bad mother compromising the mother–baby relationship, the baby's needs being met, and the mother's mental health
Identity Reorganization	The mother's belief that she can retain her sense of self (internally & externally) while attending to the baby's physical and psychological development and while she is depending on her support networks to enable her	• The transition into motherhood is eased by retaining core concepts of self in relation to others, her baby, and her own needs • Reinforces attachment, bonding, and provision of other care needs for the baby	• The transition into motherhood is difficult • Anxiety, depression, and role confusion increase • Social supports and interpersonal relationships are strained or nonexistent • The baby's needs are not met

Schemas

Do you recall the phrase, "seeing the world through rose colored glasses"? This is an analogy for schemas: how individuals interpret situations and experiences. For example, whereas one person may interpret the question, "How is your baby doing?" as a general question, another person may interpret the same question as, "they know that I am a bad mother and are checking up on me." The development of schemas often starts in childhood. Negative schemas, seeing the world through "depressed," "anxious," or "the world is unpredictable" glasses, can drastically influence a woman's transition into motherhood (Besser et al., 2008). Past negative childhood events, dysfunctional family relationships, and preexisting mental health conditions can flood a woman's thoughts and interfere with her interpretations of her newborn's cry, her perception of herself as being able to take care of the baby's needs, her interactions with support networks, and the incorporation of her new role as mother with previous, prepregnancy roles. So, rather than interpreting a baby's cry as a communication tool, a woman with negative schemas may interpret the cry as an indication of her failure as a mother or getting in the way of her ability to perform previous roles. Rather than finding support and encouragement when offered help, a woman with negative schemas may believe that her friends and family know that she really is a "bad" mom and therefore want to "save" her baby from her inability to care for it. Therefore, rather than face this, she might alienate herself from those most important in her and her baby's lives. In another scenario, the mother may simply give the baby to others to be cared for and thereby alienate herself from the baby and significant others out of shame.

Grief and Loss

Although for many, motherhood is a blissful, exhilarating experience, it also represents a huge change in roles. While pregnant women may turn to a book, friend, or elder to consult on how best to prepare for these role changes, often times, it is impossible to foresee and accommodate fully. This concept is similar to a person who is experiencing the death of a loved one, let us say a spouse, from cancer. The person is aware and well informed of the diagnosis, has discussed the diagnosis with the spouse, has attended support groups, and consulted with others in a similar situation and with those who have recently lost a loved one to cancer. The person believes that they understand what will happen and are expecting it to happen. Yet, despite all of that knowledge, when it does finally happen, the person is overwhelmed with grief and loss all the same; even though, intellectually the person may also feel a sense of relief for the spouse and for himself or herself. In that same vein, a woman may have gone through all the intellectual steps of preparing for pregnancy and birth; yet when it happens, she may experience a whole range of emotions for which she was not prepared. In their discussions with postpartum, depressed, Swedish women, Edhborg, Friberg, Lundh, and Widstrom (2005) revealed that several women reported a sense of loss, unmet expectations for herself, identity confusion, and loss of personal space.

My discussions with other women reveal that other factors can cause feelings of loss as well, including time spent away from the child because of work obligations or an overall feeling of loss regarding the ability to pursue personal or professional goals. Some women may have obtained high educational degrees and make more money than their partners but may still feel that it is their responsibility to stay at home with the child. Although these women may enjoy staying at home with their child, they may also mourn the loss of past roles in the workplace and in the family as a financial provider. They may experience grief over the perceived loss of educational and professional achievements. Therefore, these role transitions can be bittersweet for some.

Beyond
~ Brangwynne Purcell

Did the quiet age of poverty strike you
force you upward
make you weep
or was it your own tenacity?
None of my own has crept back into me yet
I am still a bit of nowhere
and coupled with impossibility and
a man who spells his love out with
his fingers on my palm.

I am glad for weeping and arms of a man
and eyes that are salty.
I have more to say in weeping
than I have already said

I am down
not upward
not here
I am gone
I am finding gladness never in cracks
or holes or secret places
only in the arms

I am selfish and a bit gloomy
with suicide and iniquity
unable to worship the ground
or take myself beyond homelessness

Socioculturally Based Theories

The Myth of Motherhood Model

According to the social causation model, PMDs result from an idealized perception of motherhood, termed the "myth of motherhood" (Weaver & Ussher, 1997). The myth of motherhood portrays the ideal mother figure as being ever-caring, loving, patient, and self-sacrificing (Johnstone & Swanson, 2003). Passed down from generation to generation, these myths are supported through the media and are nearly constant in every culture (Knudson-Martin & Silverstein, 2009). Women cannot possibly live up to these ideals and in turn report feeling overwhelmed, devalued by society, and plagued by a sense of loss and limited freedom. When women are unable to meet the expectation of being a "superwoman," they express feelings of inadequacy, self-blame, and isolation and begin to use repression to cope with life stressors (Ussher, 2002, 2003).

Another facet of the "myth of motherhood" is the belief that all children are capable of being improved upon and that it is the mother's responsibility to "sculpt" the perfect being (Swigart, 1991). Women who believe that they are incompetent or unable to meet culturally supported expectations of motherhood feel judged by others as a "bad" mother because of the behavior, successes, and failures of their children (Knudson-Martin & Silverstein, 2009).

African American women express another take on the "myth of motherhood." African American women report the need to be "a strong black woman" with an ability to take care of children, home, employment, extended family, spouses, and themselves without complaint of pain or discomfort after delivery, making reference to those who have delivered a baby and remained working "in the field" (Amankwaa, 2003). Although similar to the general myth of motherhood, African American women face a double bind. They face this developmental transition while simultaneously struggling against racism and discrimination. African American women have resiliently fought against racism and discrimination by taking on the role of "strong black woman." Although tremendously successful, this strategy may make it even more difficult for an African American woman to reach out for assistance if she is struggling.

Postpartum Mood Disorders

Relational–Cultural Theory

The relational-cultural theory (RCT) takes the stance that social status and social structures benefit dominant groups in society. Dominant-group members of a society define nondominant-group members of that society as "lacking something," resulting in marginalization and treatment as a "second class citizen" (Jordan, Walker, & Hartling, 2004). These social inequities contribute to feelings of disconnection from others and an increase of personal and group suffering. All of which further alienates members of the nondominant group, and reaffirms the dominant groups' definition of the nondominant group as "lacking" (Stiver, Rosen, Surrey, & Miller, 2008). Some examples of dominant group standards in society are behavioral expectations and fashion and beauty ideals that can only be met by a privileged few. Typically, white, male, heterosexual values and principles lay the foundation for standards, which are hierarchical in nature with clearly defined dominant and subordinate roles (Jordan, Walker, & Hartling, 2004). RCT presumes that nondominant-group responses to these unachievable standards results in shame, and in feeling and being treated as unworthy, humiliated, and vulnerable (Hoffnung, 2005). Conversely, the ability for nondominant-group individuals to create new connections with others can result in changed self-perception within the larger societal construct (Stiver et al., 2008). This change in perception of self, then, changes feelings of "being stuck" and converts this to vitality. In other words, women can find their inner voice. By thinking about who she is and who she would like to become, a woman can create ways to fulfill these hopes, thereby becoming "unstuck."

The interpersonal framework of equality and mutuality are essential to understanding women's mental health and for the treatment of these conditions according to RCT. Established developmental theories describe transitions from dependence on others into independence. RCT does not view psychological development in a hierarchical sense, but as the ability to be interdependent on self and others throughout every stage in the life cycle (Comstock, 2005; Comstock et al., 2008; Jordan, 2000; Penzerro, 2006). According to RCT, the self develops through relationship differentiation. This dynamic process continually evolves and matures. Simultaneously, one maintains emotional connectedness and closeness to others (Freedberg, 2007).

Self-identity begins with the mother–baby empathetic relationship— or the bonding and attachment period. The self-identity then grows and matures by adapting and redefining relationships throughout a lifetime, with attention to environmental constraints (Kaplan, Klein, & Gleason, 1991). How important in this model, then, is the bonding and attachment that a woman can provide to her baby?

For growth and maturity to occur, mutual empowerment and mutual empathy—or allowing the self to relate to another person by focusing on the other person, attempting to understand the other person's perspective, recognizing emotional availability, and responding to the other person in suit—are imperative (Freedberg, 2007; Jordan, 1986, 2008). If, however, a person experiences themselves as nondominant in the relationship (feeling invalidated, humiliated, or the subject of violence); they will resort to self-protection and disconnection (Jordan, 2008). This state of disconnection is expressed through six symptoms: decreased energy, clarity, and productivity; lack of self worth, decreased interaction in all relationships, and an increase in confusion—all symptoms of depression.

Women with PMDs may experience a double bind according to RCT. First, these women may have developed their self-identity without the influence of healthy mutual empathy. We see this through such PMD risk factors as traumatic childhood experiences, minimal social support, and minimal spousal or partner support, a family history of mental health conditions, alcohol or substance abuse, and other cognitive factors. Second, once a baby is born, these women face the task of initiating a healthy, mutually empathetic relationship with the baby. Without these kinds of healthy relationships in a mother's life, it is nearly impossible to create one with a newborn that demands the mutually empathetic interaction that the mother herself needs, for her own sense of identity and self-esteem.

Societal Perspective

During the human rights movement of the 1970s, women publically vocalized their discontent about female roles within the family and in the realms of politics and business. The mental health care system was criticized regarding the hierarchical counselor and client model that encouraged women to remain in their "place" in society (West, 2005; Zerbe Enns, 1993). A lasting remnant from this criticism sprung into the mental health literature through Jean Baker Miller's 1976 book, *Toward a New Psychology of Women,* resulting in the RCT (Jordan, 2008).

It was also during this time that women's social experiences and expressions of mental health symptoms were labeled as illnesses and, in 1968, the term "postnatal depression" was coined (Lee, 2006). Maternal anxiety and mood imbalance, experienced by approximately 65 percent of women, fall somewhere between the postpartum blues and postpartum depression and are present where anxiety levels are high in the mother (Lee, 2006). In this light, some medical and mental health professionals view pregnancy and the prospect of becoming a parent as a risk factor for a mental health diagnosis.

Meanwhile, society maintains a generally unsupportive and judgmental stance toward these mental health conditions (Lee, 2006). Mental health problems remain stigmatized and are perceived to be something the person can control or prevent (Pinto-Foltz & Logsdon, 2008)—even though 20 percent of all Americans experience mental health conditions (Satcher, n.d.). Furthermore, these mental health symptoms may lead to passivity, or the perception that one will "always" have these symptoms because she or he is "ill" and become preoccupied by postpartum mood symptoms (Lee, 2006).

In her discourses on premenstrual symptoms, Jane Ussher (2003, 2004) described the female monthly experience as not simply a biological reaction within the woman, but the interaction among hormones, stress, cultural definitions of feminine and reproduction, self-expectations, the ability to reflect and accommodate to change, and defense mechanisms. In other words, an internal discussion with the external, and vice versa. Ussher (2004) referred to the resulting expressions of anger and depression during the premenstrual period as self-policing strategies within the context of a patriarchal society. Therefore, women will internalize societal expectations of "idealized femininity" and will impose these expectations on themselves rather than externalize pressures in the form of social or authoritative control. Examples of idealized femininity include providing nurturance to children and men; being dependable, capable of handling stressful situations, and able to control emotions; and physically embodying feminine beauty (Ussher, 2004). The result of idealized femininity and self-policing is becoming judgmental. Women wind up judging themselves as "good" or "bad," mentally healthy or not. Therefore, a woman whose experience contradicts the notion of idealized femininity will often withdraw from others and think of herself as a "bad mom."

Knudson-Martin and Silverstein's (2009) meta-analysis of qualitative postpartum depression research findings revealed a relational environment where snowballing negative feelings are unexpressed within the context of the social definitions of motherhood. They labeled this the "silencing process." Women who experience the silencing process feel inept to perform the expected motherhood roles while simultaneously finding it difficult to maintain connection and interaction with others. This results in isolation that fuels the cycle of depression symptoms. As women experience isolation, resulting from the belief that negative feelings about being a mother are unspeakable, they start to physically separate from the baby, friends, family, and significant others. This separation reinforces feeling of alienation and disconnection to others who misunderstand them. Knudson-Martin and Silverstein (2009) provided examples of women who "describe a progression from fatigue and difficulties in soothing and caring for the baby to a debilitating sense of incompetence that results in deep despair and detachment from others." (p. 150). Women caught in a downward spiral of despair begin to experience thoughts of harming themselves or their baby, viewing suicide or infanticide as the only way out (Knudson-Martin & Silverstein, 2009).

In summary, there are several theoretical ways to understand PMDs. It is probable that these theoretical underpinnings interact and overlap. Therefore, the interplay between biopsychosocial and cultural influences provides the best understanding of PMDs.

References

Ahokas, A., Aito, M., & Rimon, R. (2000). Positive treatment effect of estradiol in postpartum psychosis: A pilot study. *Journal of Clinical Psychiatry, 61,* 166–169.

Amankwaa, L. C. (2003). Postpartum depression among African-American women. *Issues in Mental Health Nursing, 24,* 297–316.

Armstrong, K. L., Fraser, J. A., Dadds, M. R., & Morris, J. (2000). Promoting secure attachment, maternal mood and child health in a vulnerable population: A randomized controlled trial. *Journal of Pediatric and Child Health, 36,* 555–562.

Besser, A., Priel, B., Flett, G. L., & Wiznizer, A. (2007). Linear and nonlinear models of vulnerability to depression: Personality and postpartum depression in a high risk population. *Individual Differences Research, 5,* 1–29.

Besser, A., Vliegen, N., Luyten, P., & Blatt, S. J. (2008). Systematic empirical investigation of vulnerability to postpartum depression from a psychodynamic perspective: Commentary on issues raised by Blum (2007). *Psychoanalytic Psychology, 25,* 392–410.

Blatt, S. J. (2006). A fundamental polarity in psychoanalysis: Implications for personality development, psychopathology, and the therapeutic process. *Psychoanalytic Inquiry, 26,* 492–518.

Blatt, S. J. (2008). *Polarity of experience: Relatedness and self-definition in personality development, psychopathology and the therapeutic process.* Washington, DC: American Psychological Association.

Blatt, S. J., & Blass, R. (1990). Attachment and separateness: A dialectic model of the products and processes of psychological development. *Psychoanalytic Study of the Child, 45,* 107–127.

Blatt, S. J., & Blass, R. (1996). Relatedness and self definition: A dialectic model of personality development. In G. G. Noam & K. W. Fischer

(Eds.), *Development and vulnerabilities in close relationships* (pp. 309–338). Hillsdale, NJ: Lawrence Erlbaum.

Carretti, N., Florio, P., Bertonlin, A., Costa, C.V.L., Allegri, G., & Zilli, G. (2005). Serum fluctuations of total and free tryptophan levels during the menstrual cycle are related to gonadotrophins and reflect brain serotonin utilization. *Human Reproduction, 20,* 1548–1553.

Chong, R.Y., Oswald, L., Yang, X., Uhart, M., Lin, P. I., & Wand, G. S. (2006). The micro-opioid receptor polymorphism A118G predicts cortisol responses to naloxone and stress. *Neuropsychopharmacology, 31*(1), 204–211.

Cohen, L. J., & Slade, A. (2000). The psychology and the psychopathology of pregnancy: Reorganization and transformation. In C. H. Zeanah (Ed.), *Handbook of infant mental health* (2nd ed., pp. 20–36). New York: Guilford Press.

Comstock, D. (Ed). (2005). *Diversity and development: Critical contexts that shape our lives and relationships.* Belmont, CA: Thompson Brooks/Cole.

Comstock, D. L., Hammer, T. R., Strentzsch, J., Cannon, K., Parsons, J., & Salazar II, G. (2008). Relational-cultural theory: A framework for bridging relational, multicultural, and social justice competencies. *Journal of Counseling & Development, 86,* 279–287.

Crouch, M., & Manderson, L. (1995). The social life of bonding theory. *Social Science & Medicine, 41,* 837–844.

Dalton, K. (1964). *The premenstrual syndrome.* Springfield, IL: Charles C. Thomas.

Douma, S. L., Husband, C., O'Connell, M. E., Barwin, B. N., & Woodend, A. K. (2005). Estrogen-related mood disorders: Reproductive life cycle factors. *Advances in Nursing Science, 28,* 364–375.

Edhborg, M., Friberg, M., Lundh, W., & Widstrom, A. M. (2005). "Struggling with life": Narratives from women with signs of postpartum depression. *Scandinavian Journal of Public Health, 33,* 261–267.

Essex, M. J., Klein, M. H., Miech, R., & Smider, N. A. (2001). Timing of initial exposure to maternal major depression and children's mental health symptoms in kindergarten. *British Journal of Psychiatry, 179,* 151–156.

Ferber, S., & Feldman, R. (2005). Delivery pain and the development of mother–infant interaction. *Infancy, 8,* 43–62.

Freedberg, S. (2007). Re-examining empathy: A relational–feminist point of view. *Social Work, 52,* 251–259.

Gunnar, M. R., & Quevedo, K. (2007). The neurobiology of stress and development. *Annual Review of Psychology, 58,* 145–173.

Haefner, S., Baghai, T. C., Schule, C., Eser, D., Spraul, M., Zill, P., et al. (2008). Impact of gene–gender effects of adrenergic polymorphisms on hypothalamic-pituitary–adrenal axis activity in depressed patients. *Neuropsychobiology, 58,* 154–162.

Hoffnung, M. (2005). No more blaming the victim: Therapy in the interest of social justice. *Psychology of Women Quarterly, 29,* 454–455.

Joffe, H., & Cohen, L. S. (1998). Estrogen, serotonin, and mood disturbance: Where is the therapeutic bridge? *Biological Psychiatry, 44,* 798–811.

Johnstone, D. D., & Swanson, D. H. (2003). Invisible mothers: A content analysis of motherhood ideologies and myths in magazines. *Sex Roles, 49*(1–2), 21–33.

Jordan, J.V. (1986). *The meaning of mutuality.* (Working Paper Series, Work in progress, No. 23). Wellesley, MA: Stone Center.

Jordan, J. V. (2000). A relational–cultural model: Healing through mutual empathy. *Bulletin of the Menninger Clinic, 65*(1), 92–103.

Jordan, J. V. (2008). Recent developments in relational–cultural theory. *Women & Therapy, 31*(2–4), 1–4.

Jordan, J.V., Walker, M., & Hartling, L. M. (2004). *The complexity of connection: Writings from the Stone Center's Jean Baker Miller Training Institute.* New York: Guilford Press.

Kaplan, A., Klein, R., & Gleason, N. (1991). Women's self-development in late adolescence. In J.V. Jordan, A. G. Kaplan, J. B. Miller, I. P. Stiver, & J. L. Surrey (Eds.), *Women's growth in connection: Writings from the Stone Center* (pp. 122–143). New York: Guilford Press.

Karl, D. J., Beal, J. A., O'Hara, C. M., & Rissmiller, P. N. (2006). Reconceptualizing the nurse's role in the newborn period as an "attacher." *American Journal of Maternal/Child Nursing, 31,* 257–262.

Kessler, R.C., McGonagle, K. A., Swartz, M., Blazer, D. G., & Nelson, C. B. (1993). Sex and depression in the National Comorbidity Survey. I: Lifetime prevalence, chronicity and recurrence. *Journal of Affective Disorders, 29,* 85–96.

Klein, J. E. (2009). *Ancient gynecology.* Retrieved from http://www.hsl.virginia.edu/historical/artifacts/antiqua/gynecology.cfm

Knudson-Martin, C., & Silverstein, R. (2009). Suffering in silence: A qualitative meta-data-analysis of postpartum depression. *Journal of Marital and Family Therapy, 35,* 145–158.

Lee, E. (2006). Medicalizing motherhood. *Society, 43*(6), 47–50.

Luecken, L. J., Kraft, A., & Hagan, M. J. (2009). Negative relationships in the family-of-origin predict attenuated cortisol in emerging adults. *Hormones and Behavior, 55,* 412–417.

Margison, F. (1982). The pathology of the mother–child relationship. In I. F. Brockington & R. Kumar (Eds.), *Motherhood and mental illness* (pp. 191–219). Academic Press: London.

McEwen, B. S. (2008). Central effects of stress hormones in health and disease: Understanding the protective and damaging effects of stress and stress mediators. *European Journal of Pharmacology, 583,* 174–185.

McEwen, B. S., & Alves, S. E. (1999). Estrogen actions in the central nervous system. *Endocrine Reviews, 20,* 279–307.

Miller, J. B. (1976). *Toward a new psychology of women.* Boston: Beacon Press.

Miller, L. (1996). Beyond "the blues": Postpartum reactivity and the biology of attachment. *Primary Psychiatry, 3,* 35–39.

Nolen-Hoeksema, S. (1990). *Sex differences in depression.* Stanford, CA: Stanford University Press.

Pearlstein, T. B. (1995). Hormones and depression: What are the facts about premenstrual syndrome, menopause, and hormone replacement therapy? *American Journal of Obstetrics & Gynecology, 173,* 646–653.

Penzerro, R. M. (2006). Diversity and development: Critical contexts that shape our lives and relationships [Book review]. *Journal of Ethnic & Cultural Diversity in Social Work, 15*(3/4), 173–175.

Pinto-Folz, M. D., & Logsdon, M. C. (2008). Stigma towards mental illness: A concept analysis using postpartum depression as an exemplar. *Issues in Mental Health Nursing, 29,* 21–36.

Priel, B., & Besser, A. (2000). Dependency and self-criticism among first-time mothers: The roles of global and specific support. *Journal of Social and Clinical Psychology, 19,* 437–450.

Rosenbaum, J. F., & Covino, J. (2006). *Depression and women's health.* Paper presented at Medscape Perspectives on the American Psychiatric Association 2006 Annual Meeting, May 20–25, 2006, Toronto, Ontario.

Satcher, D. (n.d.). *Mental health: A report of the surgeon general.* Retrieved from http://www.surgeongeneral.gov/library/mentalhealth/home.html

Serrano, E., & Warnock, J. K. (2007). Depressive disorders related to female reproductive transitions. *Journal of Pharmacy Practice, 20,* 385–391.

Shalev, I., Lerer, E., Israel, S., Uzefovsky, F., Gritsenko, I., Mankuta, D., Ebstein, R. P., & Kaitz, M. (2009). BDNF Val66Met polymorphism is associated with HPA axis reactivity to psychological stress characterized by genotype and gender interactions. *Psychoneuroendocrinology, 34,* 382–388.

Stern, D. (1995). *The motherhood constellation: A unified view of parent–infant psychotherapy.* New York: Basic Books.

Stiver, I. P., Rosen, W., Surrey, J., & Miller, J. M. (2008). Creative moments in relational–cultural therapy. *Women & Therapy, 31*(2–4), 7–29.

Swigart, J. (1991). *The myth of the bad mother.* New York: Random House, Knopf Doubleday Publishing Group.

Taylor, V. (1995). Self-labeling and women's mental health: Postpartum illness and the reconstruction of motherhood. *Sociological Focus, 28*(1), 23–47.

Uhart, M., McCaul, M. E., Oswald, L. M., Choi, L., & Wand, G. S. (2004). GABRA6 gene polymorphism and an attenuated stress response. *Molecular Psychiatry, 9,* 998–1006.

Ussher, J. M. (1992). Research and theory related to female reproduction: Implications for clinical psychology. *British Journal of Clinical Psychology, 31,* 129–151.

Ussher, J. M. (2002). Processes of appraisal and coping in the development and maintenance of premenstrual dysphoric disorder. *Journal of Community and Applied Social Psychology, 12,* 1–14.

Ussher, J. M. (2003). The ongoing silencing of women in families: An analysis and rethinking of premenstrual syndrome and therapy. *Journal of Family Therapy, 25,* 388–406.

Ussher, J. M. (2004). Premenstrual syndrome and self-policing: Ruptures in self-silencing leading to increased self-surveillance and blaming of the body. *Social Theory & Health, 2,* 254–272.

Weaver, J. J., & Ussher, J. M. (1997). How motherhood changes life: A discourse analytic study with mothers of young children. *Journal of Reproduction and Infant Psychology, 15*(1), 51–68.

Weissman, M. M., & Klerman, G. L. (1997). Sex differences and the epidemiology of depression. *Archives of General Psychiatry, 34,* 98–111.

West, C. K. (2005). The map of relational–cultural theory. *Women & Therapy, 28*(4), 93–110.

Wieck, A., Kumar, R., Hirst, A. D., Marks, M. N., Campbell, I. C., & Checkley, S. A. (1991). Increased sensitivity of dopamine receptors and recurrence of affective psychosis after childbirth. *British Medical Journal, 303,* 613–616.

Wust, S., Van Rossum, E. F., Federenko, I. S., Koper, J. W., Kumsta, R., & Hellhammer, D. H. (2004). Common polymorphisms in the glucocorticoid receptor gene are associated with adrenocortical responses to psychosocial stress. *Journal of Clinical Endocrinology, 89,* 565–573.

Zauderer, C. R. (2008). A case study of postpartum depression and altered maternal–newborn attachment. *American Journal of Maternal/Child Nursing, 33,* 173–178.

Zerbe Enns, C. (1993). Twenty years of feminist counseling and therapy: From naming biases to implementing multifaceted practice. *Counseling Psychologist, 21*(1), 3–87.

Chapter 3

Baby Blues and Postpartum Depression

The Baby Blues

Between 20 percent and 80 percent of all women worldwide experience the postpartum blues (Gonidakis, Rabavalis, Varsou, Kreatsas, & Christoudoulou, 2007; Hau & Levi, 2003; Lanczik et al., 1992; Nagata et al., 2000). Symptoms of the baby blues include depressed mood, confusion, physical and mental exhaustion, irritability, anxiety, sleeping difficulties, and tearfulness (Koshchavtsev, Mul'tanovskaya, & Lorer, 2008; Newport, Hostetter, Arnold, & Stowe, 2002). Medical or mental health practitioners may clinically identify the baby blues as a mild depressive episode, neurotic depression, postnatal disturbance, or an adaptation or adjustment disorder, distinct from a postpartum major depressive episode (Kennerley & Gath, 1989; Koshchavtsev et al., 2008). Although some new millennium publications define the baby blues as a disorder, those that do are typically referring to postpartum depression—moderate to severe depression symptoms that last longer than two weeks to six weeks after delivery.

Physiological Factors

Many researchers view the baby blues as the female body's way of regaining physiological balance and, therefore, not a disorder, but a normal response that develops a few hours up to two weeks following childbirth (Beck, 2002b; Brockington, 1996; Martinez, Johnston-Robledo, Ulsh & Chrisler,

2000; National Women's Health Information Center, 2005; O'Hara, 1987; Pit, 1973; Teissedre & Chabroi, 2004; Welberg, 2008). This realignment of hormonal levels is also a way for the body to prepare for breastfeeding. During the realignment process, some hormone levels are temporarily "off," which can result in transient, mild depression symptoms. For example, women who have the baby blues are more likely to have higher cortisol levels in the morning—particularly on days when baby blues symptoms are at their highest (Ehlert, Patalla, Kirschbaum, Piedmont, & Hellhammer, 1990).

One of the hormones promoting lactation is prolactin, which can increase tear production (Lutz, 2001). As prolactin, T3 (thyroid-released hormone), and other hormones are found in tears, some postulate that tears assist women in regulating hormonal levels (Fooladi, 2006; Glomaud & Liotet, 1987; Lutz, 2001). In other words, increased tearfulness may not be symptomatic of depression, but, rather, a normative physiological reaction to feed the newborn and to regain inner physiological, psychological, and spiritual (holistic) balance (Bagby, 1999; Fooladi, 2005). It is interesting that women have neurotransmitters that respond to prolactin in their tear ducts (lachrymal glands), which may make women more tearful, in general, than men (nearly four times more frequently per month) (Becht, Poortinga, & Vingerhoets, 2001). These neurotransmitters aid the body in its effort to help regulate the female reproductive hormones, which fluctuate monthly, during pregnancy, and after delivery (Fooladi, 2006). In fact, testosterone appears to decrease tearfulness (Lutz, 2001). So, ladies, cry freely—it helps female bodies to maintain balance.

Women who release higher levels of prolactin (hyperprolactinemia) have a tendency to behave aggressively and irritably, report higher levels of anxiety and anger, and experience depression symptoms (Broer & Turanli, 1996; Fooladi, 2006; Lutz, 2001). Doctors sometimes refer to these women as having "hormone sensitivity." Following delivery, the heightened prolactin levels can also increase these hyperprolactinemia symptoms (irritability, increased anger, and feelings of depression).

Neurotransmitters

Neurotransmitter imbalances influence mental health symptoms. During pregnancy and following childbirth, the production, release, and metabolism of serotonin (5-HT) (one of the neurotransmitters implicated in depression) for maternal use decreases due to tryptophan, the precursor to serotonin. Rather, during pregnancy, placental development takes precedence and tryptophan is available for that process instead (Munn et al., 1998; Schrocksnadel, Baier-Bitterlich, Dapunt, Wachter, & Fuchs, 1996). Several studies show the link between decreased tryptophan availability and the development of the baby blues (Bailara et al., 2006; Doornbos, Fekkes, Tanke, de Jonge, & Korf, 2008; Kohl et al., 2005; Maes, Lin, et al., 2000; Maes, Verkerk, et al., 2002; Maurer-Spurej, Pittendreigh, & Misri, 2007).

Psychosocial Factors

Some researchers and professionals consider the baby blues to be a transient experience of mild depression symptoms, similar to an adaptation or adjustment disorder (Koshchavtsev et al., 2008; Suri, Burt, Altschuler, Zuckerbrow-Miller, & Fairbanks, 2001). These professionals indicate that although there is substance to the hormonal readjusting theory, this alone cannot account for all cases of women who experience the baby blues, as not all women experience it; and comparison studies on hormonal levels between those who had the baby blues and those who did not are inconsistent (Bloch, Daly, & Rubinow, 2003; Hendrick, Altshuler, & Suri, 1998). Yet women who have the baby blues more likely experience a combination of hormonal readjustments with other risk factors. The risk factors examined in the empirical literature include having a traumatic delivery, a history of anxiety prior to the pregnancy, difficulty with initial bonding with the baby, and limited supports.

Traumatic Delivery

It is common to have a cesarean section delivery in the United States. However, unless the woman has preplanned this type of delivery, the procedure is typically an emergency. Several of the postpartum mood disorders (PMDs) are linked to the experience of having an emergency C-section. Although not clearly understood yet, some women successfully have the emergency C-section and are fine; some experience the baby blues, while others experience more severe mental health symptoms. Typically, those women who have the baby blues following a C-section exhibit symptoms three to five days postpartum (Hannah, Adams, Lee, Glover, & Sandler, 1992).

Preexistent Anxiety/Stress

Several researchers have implicated the state of pre-existent anxiety in the development of the baby blues (Ehlert, Patalla, Kirschbaum, Piedmont, & Hellhammer, 1990, Gonidakis et al., 2007). Women who tend to cope with stress and anxiety in a passive manner, coupled with marital relationship difficulties, and who express difficulty adjusting to her new mother role are more likely to experience the baby blues (Ehlert et al., 1990).

Early Mother–Baby Interaction and Bonding

During pregnancy, women and couples may dream of feeling overwhelming bliss when they are finally able to hold their newborn. Imagine the discouragement a woman feels when she is unable to produce enough milk to feed her child, or the baby has colic and cries for long periods of time. When these conditions co-occur with other risk factors, the woman may withdraw from the baby, feeling overwhelmed or depressed. Picture a couple who thought they were unable to have children. After years of infertility treatments and several miscarriages, they finally conceive. Throughout the pregnancy, they emotionally prepare themselves—just in case there is another miscarriage. This emotional buffering does not simply "turn off" after delivery. Although feeling overjoyed, the couple may still be hesitant to bond emotionally with the child.

One study hypothesizes that the baby blues is an indicator of an adaptation problem in the mother–child bonding process (Koshavtsev et al., 2008). Adaptation problems occur through mother–child interactive behaviors, such as ambivalence from the mother when interacting with the baby or the baby refusing to nurse. Koshavtsev et al. (2008) referred to the baby blues under these conditions as "egotistical adaptation" to the new mother–child system. In other words, the mother is focused on herself rather than on the baby or the new family unit, thereby hindering the development of a strong and nurturing bonding process between herself and the baby.

Limited Support

In the United States, family and long-term friends tend to relocate for education or employment. Because of this relocation, the multigenerational communities that used to exist are no longer available to new mothers (Priest, 1983). These multigenerational communities played a pivotal role for women during pregnancy and the first year following delivery by creating a support system, providing an outlet for emotions and stress, mentoring, and assisting in the transition into motherhood. A risk factor for developing the baby blues (as well as postpartum depression) is the lack or limited availability of this supportive community (Ahmad & Munaf, 2006). It is interesting that studies done in countries where multigenerational communities endure show a reduced frequency of the baby blues and postpartum depression (Kendall-Tackett, 1994; Kottler, 1996; Lutz, 2001). Those women in community-focused societies that do exhibit depression symptoms are more likely to have a difficult relationship with their mothers-in-law and limited financial or other support from their husbands (Chandran, Tharyan, Muliyil, & Abraham, 2002; Ghani, 2000).

Postpartum Depression

The World Health Organization (WHO) projects depression to be one of the three leading causes of death worldwide by the year 2030 (Mathers & Loncar, 2006). In 2005, suicide due to depression was the leading cause of death for pregnant or postpartum women in the United States (Lindahl, Pearson, & Colpe, 2005). Of women who experience postpartum depression, nearly half will experience symptoms again; recurrent postpartum depression symptoms are often more severe (Nonacs & Cohen, 2000).

It is estimated that, around the world, 7 percent to nearly 57 percent of women experience depression symptoms after childbirth (Austin, Hadzi-Pvalovic, Saint, & Parker, 2005; Beeghly et al., 2003; Black et al., 2007; Boynce, 2003; Declercq, Sakala, Corry, & Applebaum, 2008; Gavin et al., 2005; Howell, Mora, & Leventhal, 2006; Husain, Creed, & Tomenson, 2000; Kazi et al., 2006; Milgrom, Negri, Ericksen, & Gemmill, 2005; Milgrom et al., 2008; Wolf, DeAndraca, & Lozoff, 2002; Zayas, Cunningham, McKee, & Jankowski, 2002). The most commonly accepted prevalence rate for postpartum depression in the United States and most other industrialized nations is between 7 percent and 20 percent (Beck, 2002a; Dennis, 2004; Dennis & Creedy, 2004; Gaynes et al., 2005; Robertson, Grace, Wallington, & Stewart, 2004; Stowe, Hostetter & Newport, 2005; Verkerk, Pop, Van Son, & Van Heck, 2003).

Clinically, there is no "official" *Diagnostic and Statistical Manual of Mental Disorders* (4th ed., text rev.) (DSM-IV-TR) (American Psychiatric Association, 2000) diagnosis for postpartum depression. Rather, it is a subcharacterization of major depression, with a postpartum onset. Symptoms of postpartum depression include sadness, tearfulness, anxiety, feeling hopeless or helpless, guilt, short temper, irritability, decreased desire to eat, difficulty concentrating, changes in sleep, little to no interest in the baby or life in general, and suicidal thoughts (WHO, 2003). The two main differences between the baby blues and postpartum depression are the duration and intensity of symptoms. Women with the baby blues can expect symptoms to decrease and subside within two weeks. Women with postpartum depression experience a worsening of symptoms between two to six weeks after delivery. In one large U.S. study, 67 percent of women, from delivery up to six months postpartum reported depression symptoms (Declercq et al., 2008). This frequency dropped slightly over time to 62 percent between seven and nine months after delivery and down to 59 percent between 10 months to one year after delivery. This is similar to findings in other research projects where 30 percent to 50 percent of women continued to experience postpartum depression one year after delivery (Beeghly et al., 2003; Mayberry, Horowitz, & Declecq, 2007; Whiffen & Gotlib, 1993). One study even found one in three women still exhibiting depression symptoms two years postpartum (Horowitz & Goodman, 2004). In addition, this change in mental health status created much more difficultly for single women, who often lack adequate child care support (Declercq et al., 2008).

Ethnicity

In the United States, some studies indicate higher rates of postpartum depression in women who identify as not white (Beeghly et al., 2003; Yonkers, Ramin, Rush, Navarrete, & Carmody, 2001). However, when controlling for socioeconomic status in statistical analysis, rate of prevalence becomes more similar across races, indicating that socioeconomic status is more predictive of postpartum depression than is race (Howell et al., 2006; Rich-Edwards et al., 2006). However, some studies have found racial differences in their samples. Wei and colleagues (2008) found that, in a sample of 586 women, Native Americans experienced postpartum depression most frequently (nearly 20 percent), followed by white Americans (nearly 18 percent), African Americans (nearly 15 percent), and Hispanics (nearly 3 percent). A large, Iowa-based sample found that African Americans and Native Americans reported postpartum depression more often than white women (Segre, O'Hara, & Losch, 2006). Yet when other risk factors for developing postpartum depression were included in the statistical analysis, African American women with less than a college education, with an income less than $30,000 per year, and who had to leave their infant in the hospital after delivery were most likely to develop postpartum depression. Similar to other studies, Hispanic women were the least likely to report postpartum depression.

All over the world, minority racial and ethnic groups appear to be more susceptible to postpartum depression than the majority population in the respective country. Several factors are proposed to explain this phenomenon, including language or cultural value differences, feeling like an "outsider" in the country, exposure to racism, unresponsiveness from legal and social services organizations, and socioeconomic status (Commission for Racial Equality, 1993; Templeton, Velleman, Persaud, & Milner, 2003). Individuals from minority ethnic or racial groups may seek out assistance from within minority communities and traditional customs as a result.

African American Mothers

Amankwaa (2000, 2003) has done a significant amount of research that describes the experience of African American women with postpartum depression. African American women identified postpartum depression with pessimistic beliefs about depression being a sign of personal weakness. Similar to the "myths of motherhood" where there is an unrealistic attempt to be the "perfect mom," African American women developed feelings of guilt when unable to be a "good mother," "a superwoman," or a "strong black woman" (Amankwaa, 2000, 2003). African American women indicated a distrust of the U.S. health and mental health systems. This distrust has been linked to community and family conversations and attitudes regarding the stigma attached to programs such as Child Protective Services (CPS) and Aid to Families with Dependent Children (now referred to as Temporary Assistance for Needy Families) and historical maltreatment of minorities (Amankwaa, 2000). Rather than risking the removal of the child from the home through CPS or having to face the stigma surrounding the social service programs, many African American women will silently suffer with postpartum depression symptoms.

Risk Factors for Postpartum Depression

Literally, hundreds of studies discuss risk factors for postpartum depression with or without co-occurring anxiety symptoms. Despite an extensive list of risk factors, a limited studies create predictive models using these risk factors. Mayberry and colleagues (2007) reported the following significant risk factors for postpartum depression in a sample of over 1,000 women in the United States: lower educational achievement, less than full-time employment, younger age, lower socioeconomic status, and having two or more children. Other studies point to six key risk factors (Beck, 1996, 2001; O'Hara & Swain, 1996):

1. Having had at least one depressive episode prior to pregnancy

2. Having depression during pregnancy

3. Having anxiety during pregnancy

4. Experiencing major life-stressing events during pregnancy

5. Having poor social supports

6. Having low self-esteem

Milgrom et al. (2007) further researched these predictive factors with pregnant women in Australia. They found that having had at least one depressive episode prior to pregnancy, depression during pregnancy, anxiety during pregnancy, and minimal support from a spouse or partner was the best predictor of postpartum depression.

Although similar in nature, cultural settings do alter the risk factors slightly. For example, in Pakistan, risk factors include women with a history of depression prior to becoming pregnant, difficult life stressors one year prior to the third trimester of pregnancy, lower socioeconomic standing, husband with low educational achievement, limited social support, and having five or more children (Rahman & Creed, 2007).

Risk factors for postpartum depression are physical, psychological, sociological, relational, and cultural in nature. After an examination of approximately 800 research articles, I have summarized the current knowledge about each in the remaining sections of this chapter.

Physically Based Risk Factors

Autoimmune System

During pregnancy, the immune system activates to protect the developing fetus (Hunt, McIntire, & Petroff, 2006). Over the past 20 years, researchers have been finding a link between depression, anxiety, behavior, and immune system activation (Anisman & Merli, 2003; Dantzer, 2004, 2006; Irwin & Miller, 2007; Leonard & Song, 1999). Through blood and cerebrospinal fluid samples, cytokine analysis revealed activation of the immune system (Boufidou et al., 2009). This activation was associated with women who exhibited depression symptoms six weeks after delivery.

Nutrition

Healthy nutritional intake is imperative during and after pregnancy. As this is the case, several studies examine possible links between nutritional intake and mental health symptoms. These studies looked at calcium, vitamin Bs, folate, minerals, and omega 3-fatty acids; yet none could predict postpartum depression based on these factors alone (Derbyshire & Costarelli, 2008). One small study found that women with low folate levels were more likely than women with higher levels to develop postpartum depression symptoms (Abou-Saleh, Ghubash, Karim, Krymski, & Anderson, 1999). However, two studies were unable to replicate this link (Livingston, MacLeod, & Applegarth, 1978; Miyake et al., 2006).

Minerals

Copper influences the expression of psychological disorders when found in high concentration levels. At these higher levels, copper changes the amount of dopamine and norepinephrine in the brain (Pfeiffer, 1975). Dopamine and norepinephrine are important neurotransmitters linked to depression, anxiety, bipolar disorder, and psychosis. In 2007, Crayton and Walsh found that women who had postpartum depression also had copper serum levels 15 percent higher than women who had depression (but who never had postpartum depression), and 19 percent higher than women without depressive histories.

Calcium

Preliminary results of calcium intake suggest that calcium may have a protective function against postpartum depression (Derbyshire & Costarelli, 2008). In 1997, Levine, Hauth, Curet, Sibai, and colleagues found that women with higher calcium intake buffered postpartum depression symptoms three months after delivery. In 2001, another project showed that women who did not take calcium carbonate in tablet form were more likely to develop postpartum depression as compared with women who did take the supplement (Harrison-Hohner et al., 2001).

Carbohydrates

Attempts have been made to examine women who consume large amounts of carbohydrates and sugars, with the implication being that the drastic drop in insulin postpartum may induce the onset of depression symptoms. However, there is no current evidence to support high-glycemic diets as a predictor for postpartum depression (Derbyshire & Costarelli, 2008).

Sleep Disturbances

Sleep disturbances are common for pregnant women and mothers of newborns, especially during the first six weeks after delivery (Karacan, Williams, Hursch, McCaulley, & Heine, 1969; Nishihara & Horiuchi, 1998). This is due to physiological changes, particularly in hormone levels, as well as an increased need to go to the bathroom during the later stages of pregnancy, positioning of the fetus, feeding schedules, and infant temperament after delivery (Gay, Lee, & Lee, 2004; Kennedy, Gardiner, Gay, & Lee, 2007).

During pregnancy, the nature of sleep begins to change. One study found that eight out of 10 women experienced changes in their dreams (Kennedy et al., 2007). Dreams shifted into dramatic experiences involving their baby, often in dangerous situations. These types of dreams remain after delivery for some women. Common symptoms reported by those who frequently suffer interrupted sleep include poor short-term memory and delayed reactions (Harrison & Horne, 2000).

Women of newborns will have disrupted sleep, particularly if breastfeeding. This sleep deprivation can make it more difficult to recover and heal from delivery. Most often, newborns start to sleep longer after four to six weeks, but this can last up to a year and a half (Kennedy et al., 2007; Lee, Zaffke, & McEnany,

2000; Romito, Saurel-Cubizolles, & Cuttini, 1994; Wolfson, Crowley, Anwer, & Bassett, 2003). Quality of life and mood changes occur when sleep is interrupted for a length of time (Kennedy et al., 2007). Kennedy and colleagues (2007) found that eight in 10 women had a hard time adjusting to waking up in the hospital to feed their newborn. This study also found that during the first three months postpartum, women found sleep deprivation to accentuate the feelings of fatigue overtime, with women who had surgical deliveries feeling exhausted even prior to returning home. One unfortunate consequence of feeling exhausted was feeling irritated and having limited patience, and often times the recipient of these behaviors was the significant other (Kennedy et al., 2007). Goyal, Gay, and Lee (2007) found that pregnant and postpartum women who scored highest for depression also experienced more disrupted sleep, including duration of sleep, difficulty falling asleep, and feeling tired during the day; yet these symptoms could not predict postpartum depression.

Spontaneous and Elective Abortions

Women who have experienced miscarriages or who have elected to have abortions seem to be more prone to developing postpartum depression (Pope, 2000; Robertson, Grace, Wallington, & Stewart, 2004), and there is a higher risk for women who have had a miscarriage compared with those who opt to terminate the pregnancy. In contrast, women who have elective abortions experience high anxiety and depression symptoms prior to the procedure, with these symptoms diminishing significantly afterward.

Negative Birthing Experiences

Having a difficult pregnancy or a difficult birthing experience are other risk factors for developing postpartum depression and anxiety (Tuohy & McVey, 2008; Waldenström, Hildingsson, Rubertsson, & Rådestad, 2004). Examples include unanticipated medical complications or procedures during labor, feeling out of control or extreme pain during labor, and limited support from significant others during the delivery process (Waldenström et al., 2004). The negative effect on women's mental health due to these experiences may result in depression, anxiety, or posttraumatic stress.

PMS History

Women who experience severe to very severe premenstrual syndrome are four times more likely to develop postpartum depression than are women who do not (Kendall-Tackett, 2007). A Turkish-based study found the combination of premenstrual irritability and past episodes of depression to be risk factors for the onset of postpartum depression symptoms (Kara, Ünalan, Çifçili, Cebeci, & Sarper, 2008).

Thyroid Dysfunction

The most common thyroid problem that leads to postpartum depression is hypothyroidism (low-functioning thyroid, resulting in low thyroid hormone production) (Parry, 1995). Thyroid-related imbalances may be the culprit when a mother exhibits delayed onset of postpartum depression symptoms (Edwards et al., 2006; Harris et al., 1994).

Psychologically Based Risks

Abuse History and Current Exposure

Women who experience abuse at any time in life are more predisposed to developing PMDs than women without these experiences (Kendall-Tackett, 2005, 2007). Childhood trauma affects the development of brain networks and structures that control reactions to emotional and stressful events (McEwen, 1999). These developmental changes are often permanent unless there is some kind of intervention, such as medication to correct brain circuits, counseling, or EMDR (eye movement desensitization reprocessing). Because of these structural changes in childhood; psychosocial and cognitive development changes often lead to depression and anxiety (Heim, Meinlschmidt, & Nemeroff, 2003).

The experience of childbirth may trigger several biopsychosocial responses such as stimulating altered brain circuits, neurochemical imbalances, fight–flight response, irrational thoughts, sudden recall of past traumatic events (emotional issues, body memories, and pictorial memories), leading a woman into a depressed or anxious state. Given the strong neuro–emotional interconnection and reactivity among abuse survivors, it is not surprising that the experience of childbirth can trigger mental health symptoms, particularly in women who have been sexually abused (Romano, Zoccolillo, & Paquette, 2006). Nearly one in three women with a history of childhood sexual abuse experienced her first mental health diagnosis following delivery. In 2005, a Canadian study of 332 postpartum depressed women found that 14 percent had experienced childhood sexual abuse and 7 percent had suffered childhood physical abuse (Ansara, Cohen, Gallop, Kung, & Schei, 2005). Buist (1998) found that women who experienced childhood physical or sexual abuse had longer mother–child hospital-based treatment and had more difficulty interacting with their baby than did mothers without a child abuse history. Mothers with a history of childhood sexual abuse report more depression and anxiety symptoms than women with other types of childhood abuse. These women also experience more severe postpartum depression, anxiety, and life stressors and less mental health progress long term, when compared with women without a childhood sexual abuse history (Buist & Janson, 2001).

Regrettably, not only do some women experience abuse as children, but it can happen in adult relationships as well. It is not surprising that there appears to be a link between these adult abusive experiences and the development of postpartum depression. Ansara et al. (2005) found that 30 percent of postpartum depressed women experienced emotional abuse as an adult, and 7 percent experienced physical abuse. Women exposed to emotional abuse as an adult are approximately three and a half times more at risk of developing postpartum depression than women without this exposure (Cohen et al., 2002).

Unfortunately, globally, many women experience domestic violence, and often, pregnancy offers no protection (Kendall-Tackett, 2005, 2007). Domestic violence during pregnancy occurs in 3.9 percent to 8.3 percent of relationships, internationally (Gazmarian et al., 1996) and increases the likelihood of attempted or completed female murders threefold (McFarlane, Campbell, Sharps, & Watson, 2002). In one Chinese study, just under 4 percent of women were physically abused while pregnant (Guo, Wu, Qu, & Yan, 2004). In the United Kingdom, one project revealed that one in 20 women experienced physical abuse during pregnancy (Bowen et al., 2005). Furthermore, a project in the United States found that nearly 6 percent of women were physically abused while pregnant (Martine, Mackie, Kupper, Buescher, & Moracco, 2001).

Sadly, abuse during pregnancy often continues postpartum. Nearly three in four women who are physically abused during pregnancy are still being abused two years after delivery (Harrykissoon, Rickert, & Wiemann, 2002; Lutz, 2005). In 1999, Nayak and Al-Yattama found that women with histories of domestic violence were more likely to develop postpartum depression symptoms than women without this history.

In addition to suffering abuse, women who witness others being abused can also influence the onset of postpartum mood changes. In a recent study of South African women, the most predictive factor for developing postpartum depression was having seen a violent crime or being put in a situation where their lives were in danger (Ramchandani, Richter, Stein, & Norris, 2009). The second leading predictor was interpersonal difficulties with significant others.

Mental Health History

Women with the baby blues are 20 percent to 50 percent more likely to develop postpartum depression or anxiety during the first year after delivery (Brockington, 1996; Crotty & Sheehan, 2004; Lanczik et al., 1992; O'Hara, Schlechte, Lewis, & Wright, 1991; Teissedre & Chabrol, 2004). In one study, women who experienced the baby blues were nearly 3.8 times as likely to develop postpartum depression and 3.9 times as likely to develop postpartum anxiety (Reck, Stehle, Reinig, & Mundt, 2009).

There is significant comorbidity of postpartum depression and anxiety disorders. Postpartum anxiety disorders include general anxiety, panic, post-traumatic stress, and obsessive–compulsive disorder. These conditions are explained in greater detail in chapter 5.

Personality Traits

Just as early attachment to the mother can have deleterious effects on the baby's development, early attachment for mothers when they were babies also affects their susceptibility to PMDs. Mothers with negative attachment history, difficulty attaching to their partners, and perceptions of less support from their partners appear to have a greater likelihood of experiencing PMDs after delivery (Besser, Priel, & Wiznizer, 2002; McMahon, Barnett, Kowalenko, & Tennant, 2005). Fonagy, Gergely, and Target (2007) have suggested that this early attachment history correlates to the new mother's learned exposure of what motherhood entails—modeled from her experiences with her own mother and other primary caregivers. If this concept is integrated into the transition to motherhood, then it is almost as if the new mother is predisposed to a "self-fulfilling prophecy" of being a "bad mother" because that is what has been modeled to her, despite the fact that she may be "fighting" against these feelings, or lacks the capacity to create other models of attachment to her baby. Conversely, having strong supports and a strong, trusting relationship with her partner appears to buffer against these primitively learned attachment patterns.

Josefsson, Larsson, Sydsjö, and Nylander (2007) examined other personality traits characteristic of women who experience postpartum depression. Their study found that women who had postpartum depression were more likely to have expressed the following traits or characteristics: "harm avoidance," "anticipatory worry," "fear of uncertainty," shyness, find strength in spirituality, and complain of exhaustion. These postpartum depressed women reported low ability to self-direct, less cooperativeness, less tolerance, low empathy levels, limited ability for helpfulness, and poor impulse control. In addition, they were less purposive, resourceful, and self-accepting when compared with women without postpartum depression. These characteristics are similar to the findings of Akman, Uguz, and Kaya (2007), whose analysis showed that avoidant, obsessive–compulsive, and dependent personality disorders were independent predictors of postpartum depression.

Role Changes

The idealized mother, as described by Weaver and Ussher (1997) creates an internalized conflict whereby some moms feel as if they are unable to achieve the standards they have set for themselves and the standards they perceive that others may have for them. The perception of being unable to perform multiple roles—including being a mother, wife, daughter, sister, employee, and active member of community organizations—can lead to a self-defeating thought process, resulting in immobilization, depression, and anxiety. Serrano and Warnock (2007) described these multiple role conflicts as "traditional expectations of women, current financial demands, and societal changes that significantly and uniquely influence women" (p. 386). They further reported that women often struggle to find support for competing child-rearing demands in the workplace.

Although the transition into motherhood encompasses several positive emotional responses such as nurturance, love, and joy, there can also be a sense of loss, grief, resentment, anger, irritability, ambivalence, guilt, depression, and anxiety (Besser et al., 2007; Knudson-Martin & Silverstein, 2009). These latter feelings are usually overlooked by others, including the mother, which can result in "uncontrollable anger" outbursts, "anger turned inward" (depression symptoms), and delays in the newborn's development (Besser et al., 2007).

Social Supports

A growing body of literature discusses the key role social supports play in the development of PMDs. Examining social supports through the lens of relational–cultural theory (discussed in chapter 2), mutual respect and empathy are important factors for women's mental health generally. More specifically, for postpartum women, the quality of these relationships, as well as interactions with other mothers, can significantly affect the psychoemotional adjustment during pregnancy and after childbirth (Mauthner, 1994). Positive interactions between mothers (in a support group setting) have, at times, been shown to prevent or remit postpartum depression symptoms (Elliott, Sanjack, & Leverton, 1988). Social supports in the form of other mothers and friends can act as a buffer within the larger context of a predominantly patriarchal society and the traditional medical model that pathologizes women's bodies (hormonal imbalances). Such supports allow a nonjudgmental venue for women to find consolation, value, and empowerment during the experience of mental health changes (Gilligan, 1982; Mauthner, 1995; Ussher, 1991). In contrast, women who are isolated or remove themselves from supports are more likely to feel depressed or anxious (Mauthner, 1995). Such is the case of Ruth. Ruth and her husband did not plan to get pregnant, they were waiting, but despite their contracptive efforts, she became pregnant sooner than planned. The first five months of pregnancy she spent alone with her dog, as her husband had recently joined the military and was at boot camp. For about three months, she was so sick from a migraine that she did not eat, losing nearly 30 pounds as a result. She felt lonely, bored, and sad. She also felt angry that she was so alone—living in a new town with no friends, no family, and no husband. Following the birth of the baby, her anger intensified—this time focused on the medical staff. She was very dissatisfied by the care she and her baby received throughout delivery and in maternity. Over the next few weeks, her frustration grew as did her tearfulness and sadness. She was happy to be a mother, but she felt guilt about needing assistance from others. The crying became worse, her sex drive decreased, communication deteriorated with her husband, and she felt useless and unproductive. She also started to think that she was damaging her daughter—a thought reinforced by unsupportive parents. For social support, she went to a local chain restaurant to talk to the waitress. Unfortunately, there are fewer centralized locations where mothers can simply meet up with one another than there were in the past (Mauthner, 1995; O'Connor, 1992). In earlier years, women would take their children to the park or take walks down a main street and engage in casual conversations. Due to the fragmentation of our communities, as well as the trend for individuals to relocate long distances for school or employment, these happenstance meetings with neighbors, family members, and childhood friends occur infrequently, furthering the feelings of isolation reported by many women with PMD (Amankwaa, 2003). One place that women may find an intact community setting is religious institutions. Along these lines, a recent study by Cathy St. Pierre (2007) found that a lack of strength in religion or spirituality predicted postpartum depression.

Despite the benefits of social supports, women may find it difficult to retain these relationships after having a baby, particularly if many of their friends do not have children or if the mothers work. Mauthner (1995) found that mothers with babies wanted to socialize more frequently with other mothers but found a limited number of meetings or meeting locations. When a location was found, many gatherings took place during working hours. In addition, not all mothers suffer with mental health changes after delivery. Women who experience depressed or anxious feelings following delivery report feeling disconnected from other moms who are not enduring these symptoms (Mauthner, 1995). Instead, women with postpartum mental health changes pretended to be a "happy mom" around these other mothers to "fit in," but left the gatherings feeling more isolated and inadequate. This can lead to further withdrawal from future group activities or restricted communication during group gatherings. Women with mental health changes want to have a friend to talk to who understands these changes, can normalize these changes, and can offer hope that these uncertain and uncomfortable feelings will not last forever (Scrandis, 2005).

Logsdon, Birkimer, and Usui (2000) reported on social supports that are important to women, particularly African American women, including the following:

- giving time to the mom for herself

- giving time to the mom to rest

- making sure that the mom has enough emotional and financial support

- assuring her that accepting assistance is healthy to her and to her baby

- assuring her that her concerns are legitimate

- pointing out ways that the mom is responsible with her baby and her household

- checking in with the mom to make sure that she has contact with others

The issue of social support leads into a discussion about cultural norms and customs regarding pregnancy and child rearing. In many non-Westernized countries, specific people in the family, extended family, friends, and the general community have predetermined roles in the life of the antenatal and postpartum woman (Cox, 1988, 1996). The presence of these predetermined roles and individuals may prevent postpartum depression (Ugarriza, 1992). Early research suggests that PMDs are less prevalent in these cultures, with the community's designated roles preventing the onset of mental health symptoms (Bina, 2008; Heh, Coombes, & Bartlett, 2004; Jones & Dougherty, 1982; Kim & Buist, 2005; Lee, 2001; Seel, 1986; Stern & Kruckman, 1983; Yoshida, Yamashita, Ueda, & Tashiro, 2001). More specifically, women who live in cultures that provide limited social structures, minimal acknowledgment of role changes by society, and little everyday child care or housekeeping assistance are more likely to develop postpartum depression (Stern & Kruckman, 1983).

More recent findings suggest that postpartum depression occurs in all cultures. However, not all cultures identify symptoms similarly to United States definitions, nor do all cultures view depression symptoms as an indicator for treatment outside of the community and familial helping roles (Amankwaa, 2003; Oates et al., 2004). For example, in a rural area of India, approximately one in ten women reported symptoms commensurate with postpartum depression; however, risk factors were somewhat different from those in traditional westernized countries (Chandran, Tharyan, Muliyil, & Abraham, 2002). These risk factors included low socioeconomic status, an estranged relationship with the mother-in-law, giving birth to a daughter (where a son was preferred), difficult events during the pregnancy, and limited provisional assistance. Limited in-law support has been found to be a risk factor for the development of postpartum depression in other places as well, such as Hong Kong, Japan, and Turkey (Bashiri & Spielvogel, 1999; Chan, Levy, Chung, & Lee, 2002; Danaci, Dinc, Deveci, Sen, & Icelli, 2002; Leung, 2002; Yoshida et al., 2001). The aforementioned risk factor of having a daughter instead of a son is supported by other culture-based postpartum depression research, such as in Lebanon (Nahas, Hillege, & Amasheh, 1999). It is proposed that in cultures that promote the birth of boys over girls, a woman who has a daughter faces a status change within the family and in her community, resulting in postpartum depression symptoms (Patel, Rodrigues, & De Souza, 2002; Saravanan, 2002). In the United States, however, the community has a minimal role, and the primary focus in on the individual. This can make it difficult for pregnant or postpartum women to ask for assistance or general support (Logsdon, 2005).

Socioculturally Based Risks

Low-Income Levels

Experiencing financial difficulties or living in poverty increases general stress levels and negatively influences the entire family in several ways. These include living in high-risk neighborhood environments and having limited access to transportation, food stores, and health and mental health care (Segre, O'Hara, Arndt, & Stuart, 2007; Zittel-Palamara, Rockmaker, Schwabel, Weinstein, & Thompson, 2008). These stressors are shown to increase interrelational conflicts between partners and to exacerbate stress levels in women who do not live with a significant other or receive financial support from the child's father, which in turn, increases the development of depression symptoms (Dearing, Taylor, & McCartney, 2004; Evans & English, 2002; Lorant et al.,

2003; Pearlin, 1989). Studies that examine the interplay between postpartum depression and financial difficulties show that low socioeconomic status, low income, and one's reputation in the workplace predict the development of depression after delivery (Beck, 2001; O'Hara & Swain, 1996; Patel et al., 2002; Segre et al., 2007). In addition, individuals who have not obtained high levels of education appear more susceptible to postpartum depression (Tammentie, Tarkka, Astedt-Kurki, & Paavilainen, 2002). However, it is not yet clear how lower education attainment, low socioeconomic status, status in the workplace, and postpartum depression interact and influence one another.

Residency Location

Bilszta and his research team (2008) conducted a very interesting project in Australia, examining risk factors for developing postpartum depression based on living in a rural or urban setting. This study of nearly 2,000 women found different risk factors based on residency location. Predictors for developing postpartum depression in women who lived in rural areas included moderate to severe depression during pregnancy, mental health history, and socioeconomic status. The only predictor for developing postpartum depression in women who lived in urban areas was experiencing moderate to severe depression during pregnancy.

References

Abou-Saleh, M. T., Ghubash, R., Karim, L., Krymski, M., & Anderson, D. N. (1999). The role of pterins and related factors in the biology of early postpartum depression. *European Neuropsychopharmacology, 9,* 295–300.

Ahmad, R., & Munaf, S. (2006). Nuclear family system as an important risk factor for the development of the baby blues. *Pakistan Journal of Social and Clinical Psychology, 4*(1), 67–74.

Akman, C., Uguz, F., & Kaya, N. (2007). Postpartum-onset major depression is associated with personality disorders. *Comprehensive Psychiatry, 48,* 343–347.

Amankwaa, L. C. (2000). Enduring: A grounded theory investigation of postpartum depression among African-American women (Doctoral dissertation, Georgia State University, 2000). *Dissertation Abstracts International, 60,* 03B.

Amankwaa, L. C. (2003). Postpartum depression, culture, and African-American women. *Journal of Cultural Diversity, 10*(1), 23–29.

American Psychiatric Association. (2000). *Diagnostic and statistical manual of mental disorders* (4th ed., text rev.). Washington, DC: Author.

Anisman, H., & Merli, Z. (2003). Cytokines, stress and depressive illness: Brain-immune interactions. *Annals of Medicine, 35,* 2–11.

Ansara, D., Cohen, M. M., Gallop, R., Kung, R., & Schei, B. (2005). Predictors of women's physical health problems after childbirth. *Journal of Psychosomatic Obstetrics & Gynecology, 26,* 115–125.

Austin, M-P., Hadzi-Pvalovic, D., Saint, K., & Parker, G. (2005). Antenatal screening for the prediction of postnatal depression: Validation of a psychosocial Pregnancy Risk Questionnaire. *Acta Psychiatrica Scandinavica, 122,* 310–317.

Bagby, D. G. (1999). *Seeing through our tears: Why we cry, how we heal.* Philadelphia: Augsburg Fortress.

Bailara, K. M., Henry, C., Lestage, J., Launay, J. M., Parrot, F., Swendsen, J., et al. (2006). Decreased brain tryptophan availability as a partial determinant of post-partum blues. *Psychoneuroendocrinology, 31,* 407–413.

Bashiri, N., & Spielvogel, A. M. (1999). Postpartum depression: A cross-cultural perspective. *Primary Care Update for OB/GYNS, 6*(3), 82–87.

Becht, M. C., Poortinga, Y. H., & Vingerhoets, A.J.J.M. (2001). Crying across countries. In A. J. J. M. Vingerhoets & R. R. Cornelius (Eds.), *Adult crying: A biopsychosocial approach.* Hove, England: Brunner-Routledge.

Beck, C. T. (1996). A meta-analysis of predictors of postpartum depression. *Nursing Research, 50,* 275–285.

Beck, C. T. (2001). Predictors of postpartum depression: An update. *Nursing Research, 50,* 275–285.

Beck, C. T. (2002a). Postpartum depression: A metasynthesis. *Qualitative Health Research, 12,* 453–472.

Beck, C.T. (2002b). Revision of the postpartum depression predictors inventory. *Journal of Obstetric, Gynecologic, & Neonatal Nursing, 31,* 394–402.

Beeghly, M., Olson, K. L., Weinberg, M. K., Pierre, S. C., Downey, N., & Tronick, E. Z. (2003). Prevalence, stability, and socio-demographic correlates of depressive symptoms in black mothers during the first 18 months postpartum. *Maternal Child Health Journal, 7,* 157–168.

Besser, A., Priel, B., & Wiznizer, A. (2002). Childbearing depressive symptomatology in high-risk pregnancies: The roles of working models and perceived spouse support. *Personal Relationships, 9,* 395–413.

Besser, A., Priel, B., Flett, L. G., & Wiznitzer, A. (2007). Linear and nonlinear models in vulnerability to depression: Personality and postpartum depression in a high risk population. *Individual Differences Research, 5,* 1-29.

Bilszta, J.L.C., Gu, Y. Z., Meyer, D., & Buist, A. E. (2008). A geographic comparison of the prevalence and risk factors for postnatal depression in an

Australian population. *Australian & New Zealand Journal of Public Health, 32,* 424–430.

Bina, R. (2008). The impact of cultural factors upon postpartum depression: A literature review. *Health Care for Women International, 29,* 568–592.

Black, M. M., Baqui, A. H., Zaman, K., McNary, S. W., Le, K., Arifeen, S. E., Hamadani, J. D., Parveen, M., & Yunus, M. (2007). Depressive symptoms among rural Bangladeshi mothers: Implications for infant development. *Journal of Child Psychology and Psychiatry, 48,* 764–772.

Bloch, M., Daly, R. C., & Rubinow, D. R. (2003). Endocrine factors in the etiology of postpartum depression. *Comprehensive Psychiatry, 44,* 234–246.

Boufidou, F., Lambrinoudaki, I., Argeitis, J., Zervas, I. M., Pliatsika, P., Leonardou, A. A., Petropoulos, G., Hasiakos, D., Papadias, K., & Nikolaou, C. (2009). CFS and plasma cytokines at delivery and postpartum mood disturbances. *Journal of Affective Disorders, 115,* 287–292.

Bowen, E., Heron, J., Waylen, A., Wolke, D., & ALSPAC Study Team. (2005). Domestic violence risk during and after pregnancy: Findings from a British longitudinal study. *British Journal of Obstetrics & Gynecology, 112,* 1083–1089.

Boynce, P. (2003). Risk factors for postnatal depression: A review and risk factors in Australian population. *Archives of Women's Mental Health, 6*(Suppl. 2), 43–50.

Brockington, I. F. (1996). *Motherhood and mental health.* Oxford, England: Oxford University Press.

Broer, K. H., & Turanli, I. (1996). *New trends in reproductive medicine.* Berlin, Germany: Springer.

Buist, A. (1998). Childhood abuse, parenting, and postpartum depression. *Australian and New Zealand Journal of Psychiatry, 32,* 479–487.

Buist, A., & Janson, H. (2001). Childhood sexual abuse, parenting, and postpartum depression: A 3-year follow-up study. *Child Abuse & Neglect, 25,* 909–921.

Chan, S. W. C., Levy, V., Chung, T. K. H., & Lee, D. (2002). A qualitative study of the experiences of a group of Hong Kong Chinese women diagnosed with postnatal depression. *Journal of Advanced Nursing, 39,* 571–579.

Chandran, M., Tharyan, P., Muliyil, J., & Abraham, S. (2002). Post-partum depression in a cohort of women from a rural area of Tamil Nadu, India: Incidence and risk factors. *British Journal of Psychiatry, 181,* 499–504.

Cohen, M. M., Schei, B., Ansara, D., Gallop, R., Stuckless, N., & Stewart, D. E. (2002). A history of personal violence and postpartum depression: Is there a link? *Archives of Women's Mental Health, 4,* 83–92.

Commission for Racial Equality. (1993). *The sorrow in my heart: Sixteen Asian women speak about depression.* London: Commission for Racial Equality.

Cox, J. L. (1988). Childbirth as a life event: Sociocultural aspects of postnatal depression. *Acta Psychiatrica Scandinavica, 344*(Suppl.), 75–83.

Cox, J. L. (1996). Perinatal mental disorders: A cultural approach. *International Review of Psychiatry, 8,* 9–16.

Crayton, J. W., & Walsh, W. J. (2007). Elevated serum copper levels in women with a history of post-partum depression. *Journal of Trace Elements in Medicine and Biology, 21,* 17–21.

Crotty, F., & Sheehan, J. (2004). Prevalence and detection of postnatal depression in an Irish community sample. *Irish Journal of Psychological Medicine, 21*(4), 117–121.

Danaci, A. E., Dinc, G., Deveci, A., Sen, F. S., & Icelli, I. (2002). Postnatal depression in Turkey: Epidemiological and cultural aspects. *Social Psychiatry and Psychiatric Epidemiology, 37*(3), 125–129.

Dantzer, R. (2004). Cytokine-induced sickness behaviour: A neuroimmune response to activation of innate immunity. *European Journal of Pharmacology, 500,* 399–411.

Dantzer, R. (2006). Cytokine, sickness behaviour, and depression. *Neurologic Clinics, 24,* 441–460.

Dearing, E., Taylor, B. A., & McCartney, K. (2004). Implications of family income dynamics for women's depressive symptoms during the first 3 years after childbirth. *American Journal of Public Health, 94,* 1372–1377.

Declercq, E. R., Sakala, C., Corry, M. P., & Applebaum, S. (2008). *New mothers speak out: National survey results highlight women's postpartum experiences.* New York: Childbirth Connection.

Dennis, C. L. (2004). Preventing postpartum depression part II: A critical review of nonbiological interventions. *Canadian Journal of Psychiatry, 49,* 525–538.

Dennis, C. L., & Creedy, D. (2004). Psychosocial and psychological interventions for preventing postpartum depression. *Cochrane Database of Systematic Reviews, 2004*(4), CD001134.

Derbyshire, E., & Costarelli, V. (2008). Dietary factors in the aetiology of postnatal depression. *Nutrition Bulletin, 33,* 163–168.

Doornbos, B., Fekkes, D., Tanke, M.A.C., de Jonge, P., & Korf, J. (2008). Sequential serotonin and noradrenalin associated processes involved in postpartum blues. *Progress in Neuro-Psychopharmacology & Biological Psychiatry, 32,* 1320–1325.

Edwards, G. D., Shinfuku, N., Gittelman, M., Ghozali, E. W., Haniman, F., Wibisono, S., et al. (2006). Postnatal depression in Surabaya, Indonesia. *International Journal of Mental Health, 35*(1), 62–74.

Ehlert, U., Patalla, U., Kirschbaum, C., Piedmont, E., & Hellhammer, D. H. (1990). Postpartum blues: Salivary cortisol and psychological factors. *Journal of Psychosomatic Research, 34,* 319–325.

Elliott, S. A., Sanjack, M., & Leverton, T. J. (1988). Parent groups in pregnancy: A preventive intervention for postnatal depression. In B. H. Gottlieb (Ed.), *Marshalling social support: Formats, processes and effects.* Thousand Oaks, CA: Sage Publications.

Evans, G. W., & English, K. (2002). The environment of poverty: Multiple stressor exposure, psychophysiological stress, and socioemotional adjustment. *Child Development, 73,* 1238–1248.

Fonagy, P., Gergely, G., & Target, M. (2007). The parent–infant dyad and the construction of the subjective self. *Journal of Child Psychology & Psychiatry, 48*(3/4), 288–328.

Fooladi, M. M. (2005). The therapeutic effects of crying. *Journal of Holistic Nursing Practice, 19*(6), 248–255.

Fooladi, M. M. (2006). Therapeutic tears and postpartum blues. *Holistic Nursing Practice, 20* (4), 204–211.

Gavin, N. I., Gaynes, B. N., Lohr, K., Meltzer-Brody, S., Gartlehner, G., & Swinson, T. (2005). Perinatal depression: A systematic review of prevalence and incidence. *Obstetrics and Gynecology, 106,* 1071–1083.

Gay, C. L., Lee, K. A., & Lee, S. Y. (2004). Sleep patterns and fatigue in new mothers and fathers. *Biological Research for Nursing, 5,* 311–318.

Gaynes, B. N., Gavin, N., Lohr, K. N., Meltzer-Brody, S., Gartlehner, G., & Swinson, T. (2005). Perinatal depression: A systematic review of prevalence and incidence. *Obstetrics & Gynecology, 106*(5, Pt. 1), 1071–1083.

Gazmarian, J. A., Lazorick, S., Spitz, A. M., Ballard, T. J., Saltzman, L. E., & Marks, J. S. (1996). Prevalence of violence against pregnant women. *JAMA, 275,* 1915–1920.

Ghani, S. (2000). *Sociology of family and community.* Islamabad, Pakistan: University Grants Commision.

Gilligan, C. (1982). *In a different voice: Psychological theory and women's development.* Cambridge, MA: Harvard University Press.

Glomaud, J., & Liotet, S. (1987). Importance of the assay of T3 and T4 in tears and plasma for the diagnosis of endocrine exophthalmos. *Journal of French Ophthalmology, 10,* 639–645.

Gonidakis, F., Rabavalis, A. D., Varsou, E., Kreatsas, G., & Christoudoulou, G. N. (2007). Maternity blues in Athens, Greece: A study during the first 3 days after delivery. *Journal of Affective Disorders, 99,* 107–115.

Goyal, D., Gay, C. L., & Lee, K. A. (2007). Patterns of sleep disruption and depressive symptoms in new mothers. *Journal of Perinatal and Neonatal Nursing, 21*(2), 123–129.

Guo, S. F., Wu, J. L., Qu, C. Y., & Yan, R. Y. (2004). Physical and sexual abuse of women before, during, and after pregnancy. *International Journal of Gynaecology and Obstetrics, 84,* 281–286.

Hannah, P., Adams, D., Lee, A., Glover, V., & Sandler, M. (1992). Links between early post-partum mood and post-natal depression. *British Journal of Psychiatry, 160,* 777–780.

Harris, B., Lovett, L., Newcombe, R. G., Read, G. F., Walter, R., & Riad-Fahmy, D. (1994). Maternity blues and major endocrine changes: Cardiff puerperal mood and hormone study II. *British Medical Journal, 208,* 949–952.

Harrison, Y., & Horne, J. A. (2000). The impact of sleep deprivation on decision making: A review. *Journal of Experimental Psychology: Applied, 6,* 236–249.

Harrison-Hohner, J., Coste, S., Dorato, V., Curet, L. B., McCarron, D., & Hatton, D. (2001). Prenatal calcium supplementation and postpartum depression: An ancillary study to a randomised trial of calcium for prevention of preeclampsia. *Archives of Women's Mental Health, 3,* 141–146.

Harrykissoon, S. D., Rickert, V. I., & Wiemann, C. M. (2002). Prevalence and patterns of intimate partner violence among adolescent mothers during the postpartum period. *Archives of Pediatric and Adolescent Medicine, 156,* 325–330.

Hau, F. W., & Levy, V. A. (2003). The maternity blues in Hong Kong Chinese women: An exploratory study. *Journal of Affective Disorders, 2,* 197–203.

Heh, S., Coombes, L., & Bartlett, H. (2004). The association between depressive symptoms and social support in Taiwanese women during the month. *International Journal of Nursing Studies, 41,* 573–579.

Heim, C., Meinlschmidt, G., & Nemeroff, C. B. (2003). Neurobiology of early-life stress. *Psychiatric Annals, 33*(1), 18–26.

Hendrick, V., Altshuler, L. L., & Suri, R. (1998). Hormonal changes in the postpartum and implications for postpartum depression. *Psychosomatics, 39,* 93–101.

Horowitz, J. A., & Goodman, J. (2004). A longitudinal study of maternal depression symptoms. *Research and Theory for Nursing Practice: An International Journal, 18,* 149–163.

Howell, E. A., Mora, P., & Leventhal, H. (2006). Correlates of early postpartum depressive symptoms. *Maternal and Child Health Journal, 10*(2), 149–157.

Hunt, J. S., McIntire, R. H., & Petroff, M. G. (2006). Immunobiology of human pregnancy. In J. D. Neill (Ed.-in-Chief), *Knobil and Neill's physiology of reproduction* (3rd ed., pp. 2759–2785). St. Louis: Academic Press.

Husain, N., Creed, F., & Tomenson, B. (2000). Depression and social stress in Pakistan. *Psychological Medicine, 30,* 395–402.

Irwin, M. R., & Miller, A. H. (2007). Depressive disorders and immunity: 20 years of progress and discovery. *Brain Behavior and Immunity, 4,* 374–383.

Jones, A. D., & Dougherty, C. (1982). Childbirth in a scientific and industrial society. In C. P. MacCormack (Ed.), *Ethnography of fertility and birth* (pp. 259–280). London: Academic Press.

Josefsson, A., Larsson, C., Sydsjö, G., & Nylander, P. O. (2007). Temperament and character in women with postpartum depression. *Archives of Women's Mental Health, 10,* 3–7.

Kara, B., Ünalan, P., Çifçili, S., Cebeci, D. S., & Sarper, N. (2008). Is there a role for the family and close community to help reduce the risk of postpartum depression in new mothers? A cross-sectional study of Turkish women. *Maternal and Child Health Journal, 12,* 155–161.

Karacan, I., Williams, R. L., Hursch, C. J., McCaulley, M., & Heine, M. W. (1969). Some implications of the sleep patterns of pregnancy for postpartum emotional disturbances. *British Journal of Psychiatry, 115,* 929–935.

Kazi, A., Fatmi, Z., Hatcher, J., Kadir, M. M., Niaz, U., & Wasserman, G. A. (2006). Social environment and depression among pregnant women in urban areas of Pakistan: Importance of social relations. *Social Science Medicine, 63,* 1466–1476.

Kendall-Tackett, K. (1994). Postpartum rituals and prevention of postpartum depression: A cross-cultural perspective. *Newsletter of the Boston Institute for the Development of Infants and Parents, 13*(1), 3–6.

Kendall-Tackett, K. A. (2005). *Depression in new mothers: Causes, consequences, and treatment options.* Binghamton, NY: Haworth Press.

Kendall-Tackett, K. A. (2007). Violence against women and the perinatal period: The impact of lifetime violence and abuse on pregnancy, postpartum, and breastfeeding. *Trauma, Violence, & Abuse, 8,* 344–353.

Kennedy, H. P., Gardiner, A., Gay, C., & Lee, K. A. (2007). Negotiating sleep: A qualitative study of new mothers. *Journal of Perinatal & Neonatal Nursing, 21*(2), 114–122.

Kennerley, H., & Gath, D. (1989). Maternity blues: I. Detection and measurement by questionnaire. *British Journal of Psychiatry, 155,* 356–362.

Kim, J., & Buist, A. (2005). Postnatal depression: A Korean perspective. *Australasian Psychiatry, 13*(1), 68–71.

Knudson-Martin, C., & Silverstein, R. (2009). Suffering in silence: A qualitative meta-data-analysis of postpartum depression. *Journal of Marital and Family Therapy, 35*(2), 145–158.

Kohl, C., Walch, T., Huber, R., Kemmler, G., Neurauter, G., Fuchs, D., et al. (2005). Measurement of tryptophan, kynurenine and neopterin in women with and without postpartum blues. *Journal of Affective Disorders, 86,* 135–142.

Koshchavtsev, A. G., Mul'tanovskaya, V. N., & Lorer, V. V. (2008). Baby blues syndrome as an adaptation disorder in the early stages of formation of the mother–child system. *Neuroscience and Behavioral Physiology, 38,* 439–442.

Kottler, J. A. (1996). *The language of tears.* San Francisco: Jossey-Bass.

Lanczik, M., Spingler, H., Heidrich, A., Becker, T., Kretzer, B., Albert, P., & Fritze, K. (1992). Postpartum blues: Depressive disease or pseudoneuroasthenic syndrome. *Journal of Affective Disorders, 25,* 47–52.

Lee, D.T.S. (2001). Postnatal depression in Hong Kong Chinese. *Dissertation Abstracts International: Section B: The Sciences and Engineering, 61*(8-B), 4076.

Lee, K. A., Zaffke, M. E., & McEnany, G. (2000). Parity and sleep patterns during and after pregnancy. *Obstetrics & Gynecology, 95,* 14–18.

Leonard, B. E., & Song, C. (1999). Stress, depression, and the role of cytokines. In R. Dantzer, E. E. Wollman, & R. Yirmiya (Eds.), *Cytokines, stress, and depression* (pp. 251–266). New York: Kluwer Academic/Plenum Publishers.

Leung, S.S.K. (2002). Postpartum depression: Perceived social support and stress among Hong Kong Chinese women. *Dissertation Abstracts International: Section B: The Sciences and Engineering, 62*(10-B), 4469.

Levine, R. J., Hauth, J. C., Curet, L. B., Sibai, B. M., Catalano, P. M., Morris, C. D., et al. (1997). Trial of calcium to prevent preeclampsia. *New England Journal of Medicine, 337,* 69–76.

Lindahl, V., Pearson, J. L., & Colpe, L. (2005). Prevalence of suicidality during pregnancy and the postpartum. *Archives of Women's Mental Health, 8,* 77–87.

Livingston, J. E., MacLeod, P. M., & Applegarth, D. A. (1978). Vitamin B6 status in women with postpartum depression. *American Journal of Clinical Nutrition, 31,* 886–891.

Logsdon, M. C. (2005). Social support to childbearing women: What are the rules? [Commentary]. *Journal of Obstetric, Gynecologic, & Neonatal Nursing, 34,* 754.

Logsdon, M. C., Birkimer, J. C., & Usui, W. M. (2000). The link of social support and postpartum depressive symptoms in African-American women with low incomes. *American Journal of Maternal/Child Nursing, 25,* 262–266.

Lorant, V., Deliege, D., Eaton, W., Robert, A., Phillippot, P., & Ansseau, M. (2003). Socioeconomic inequalities in depression: A meta-analysis. *American Journal of Epidemiology, 157,* 98–112.

Lutz, K. F. (2005). Abuse experiences, perceptions, and associated decisions during the childbearing cycle. *Western Journal of Nursing Research, 27,* 802–824.

Lutz, T. (2001). *Crying: A natural and cultural history of tears.* New York: W. W. Norton.

Maes, M., Lin, A. H., Ombelet, W., Stevens, K., Kenis, G., de Jongh, R., Cox, J., & Bosmans, E. (2000). Immune activation in the early puerperium is related to postpartum anxiety and depressive symptoms. *Psychoneuroendocrinology, 25,* 121–137.

Maes, M., Verkerk, R., Bonaccorso, S., Ombelet, W., Bosmans, E., & Scharpe, S. (2002). Depressive and anxiety symptoms in the early puerperium are related to increased degradation of tryptophan into kynurenine, a phenomenon which is related to immune activation. *Life Science, 71,* 1837–1848.

Martine, S. L., Mackie, L., Kupper, L. L., Buescher, P. A., & Moracco, K. E. (2001). Physical abuse of women before, during, and after pregnancy. *JAMA, 285,* 1581–1584.

Martinez, R., Johnston-Robledo, I., Ulsh, H. M., & Chrisler, J. C. (2000). Singing 'The Baby Blues': A content analysis of popular press articles about postpartum affective disturbances. *Women & Health, 31*(2/3), 37–56.

Mathers, D. C., & Loncar, D. (2006). Projections of global morality and burden of disease from 2002 to 2030. *PLoS Medicine, 3*(11), e442. doi:10.137/journal.pmed.0030442.

Maurer-Spurej, E., Pittendreigh, C., & Misri, S. (2007). Platelet serotonin levels support depression scores for women with postpartum depression. *Journal of Psychiatric Neuroscience, 32,* 23–29.

Mauthner, N. S. (1994). *Postnatal depression: A relational perspective.* Unpublished doctoral thesis, University of Cambridge.

Mauthner, N. S. (1995). Postnatal depression: The significance of social contacts between mothers. *Women's Studies International Forum, 18,* 311–323.

Mayberry, L. J., Horowitz, J. A., & Declercq, E. (2007). Depression symptom prevalence and demographic risk factors among U. S. women during the first 2 years postpartum. *Journal of Obstetric, Gynecologic, & Neonatal Nursing, 36,* 542–549.

McFarlane, J., Campbell, J. C., Sharps, P., & Watson, K. (2002). Abuse during pregnancy and femicide: Urgent implications for women's health. *Obstetrics and Gynecology, 100,* 27–36.

McMahon, C., Barnett, B., Kowalenko, N., & Tennant, C. (2005). Psychological factors associated with persistent postnatal depression: Past and current relationships, defense styles and the mediating role of insecure attachment style. *Journal of Affective Disorders, 84,* 15–24.

Milgrom, J., Gemmill, A. W., Bilszta, J. L., Hayes, B., Barnett, B., Brooks, J., et al. (2008). Antenatal risk factors for postnatal depression: A large prospective study. *Journal of Affective Disorders, 108,* 147–157.

Milgrom, J., Negri, L., Ericksen, J. E., & Gemmill, A. W. (2005). Screening for postnatal depression in routine primary care: Properties of the Edinburgh Postnatal Depression Scale in an Australian community. *Australian and New Zealand Journal of Psychiatry, 398,* 745–751.

Miyake, Y., Sasaki, S., Tanaka, K., Yokoyama, T., Ohya, Y., Fukushima, W., et al. (2006). Dietary folate and vitamins B12, B6, and B2 intake and the risk of postpartum depression in Japan: The Osaka Maternal and Child Health Study. *Journal of Affective Disorders, 96,* 133–138.

Munn, D. H., Zhou, M., Attwood, J. T., Bondarev, I., Conway, S. J., Marshall, B., et al. (1998). Prevention of allogeneic fetal rejection by tryptophan catabolism. *Science, 281,* 1191–1193.

Nagata, M., Nagai, Y., Sobajima, H., Ando, T., Nishide, Y., & Honjo, S. (2000). Maternity blues and attachment of children in mothers of full term normal infants. *Acta Psychiatrica Scandinavica, 101*(3), 209–217.

Nahas, V. L., Hillege, S., & Amasheh, N. (1999). Postpartum depression: The lived experiences of Middle Eastern migrant women in Australia. *Journal of Nurse Midwifery, 44,* 65–74.

National Women's Health Information Center. (2005). *Depression during and after pregnancy.* Retrieved from http://www.womenshealth.gov/faq/depression-pregnancy.cfm

Nayak, M. B., & Al-Yattama, M. (1999). Assault victim history as a factor in depression during pregnancy. *Obstetrics & Gynecology, 94,* 204–208.

Newport, D. J., Hostetter, A., Arnold, A., & Stowe, Z. N. (2002). The treatment of postpartum depression: Minimizing infant exposures. *Journal of Clinical Psychiatry, 63,* 31–44.

Nishihara, K., & Horiuchi, S. (1998). Changes in sleep of young women from late pregnancy to postpartum: Relationships to their infant's movements. *Perceptual & Motor Skills, 87,* 1043–1056.

Nonacs, R., & Cohen, L. S. (2000). Postpartum psychiatric syndromes. In B. Sadock & V. Sadock (Eds.), *Comprehensive textbook of psychiatry* (7th ed., pp. 1276–1283). Philadelphia: Lippincott, Williams & Wilkins.

Oates, M. R., Cox, J. L., Neema, S., Asten, P., Glangeaud-Freudenthal, N., Figueiredo, B., et al. (2004). Postnatal depression across countries and cultures: A qualitative study. *British Journal of Psychiatry, 184*(Suppl. 46), s10–s16.

O'Connor, P. (1992). *Friendships between women: A critical review.* Hemel Hempstead, England: Harvester Wheatsheaf.

O'Hara, M. W. (1987). Post-partum "blues," depression, and psychosis: A review. *Journal of Psychosomatic Obstetrics and Gynecology, 7,* 205–227.

O'Hara, M. W., Schlechte, J. A., Lewis, D. A., & Wright, E. J. (1991). Prospective study on postpartum blues: Biologic and psychosocial factors. *Archives of General Psychiatry, 48,* 801–806.

O'Hara, M. W., & Swain, A. (1996). Rates and risk of postpartum depression: A meta-analysis. *International Review of Psychiatry, 8,* 37–54.

Parry, B. (1995). Postpartum psychiatric syndromes. In H. I. Kaplan & B. J. Sadock (Eds.), *Comprehensive textbook of psychiatry* (6th ed., pp. 1059–1066). Baltimore: Williams & Wilkins.

Patel, V., Rodrigues, M., & DeSouza, N. (2002). Gender, poverty, and post-natal depression: A study of mothers in Goa, India. *American Journal of Psychiatry, 159,* 43–47.

Pearlin, L. I. (1989). The sociological study of stress. *Journal of Health and Social Behavior, 30,* 241–256.

Pfeiffer, C. C. (1975). *Mental and elemental nutrients: A physician's guide to nutrition and health care.* New Canaan, CT: Keats Publishing.

Pit, B. (1973). Maternity blues. *British Journal of Psychiatry, 122,* 431–433.

Pope, S. (2000). *Postnatal depression: A systematic review of published scientific literature to 1999.* Canberra, Australia: National Health and Medical Research Council.

Priest, R. G. (1983). *Anxiety and depression: A practical guide to recovery.* Singapore: P. G. Publishing.

Rahman, A., & Creed, F. (2007). Outcome of prenatal depression and risk factors associated with persistence in the first postnatal year: Prospective study from Rawalpindi, Pakistan. *Journal of Affective Disorders, 100,* 115–121.

Ramchandani, P. G., Richter, L. M., Stein, A., & Norris, S. A. (2009). Predictors of postnatal depression in an urban South African cohort. *Journal of Affective Disorders, 113,* 279–284.

Reck, C., Stehle, E., Reinig, K., & Mundt, C. (2009). Maternity blues as a predictor of DSM-IV depression and anxiety disorders in the first three months postpartum. *Journal of Affective Disorders, 113,* 77–87.

Rich-Edwards, J. W., Kleinman, K., Abrams, A., Harlow, B. L., McLaughlin, T. J., Joffe, H., & Gillman, M. W. (2006). Sociodemographic predictors of antenatal and postpartum depressive symptoms among women in a medical group practice. *Journal of Epidemiology and Community Health, 60,* 221–227.

Robertson, E., Grace, S., Wallington, T., & Stewart, D. E. (2004). Antenatal risk factors for postpartum depression: A synthesis of recent literature. *General Hospital Psychiatry, 26,* 289–295.

Romano, E., Zoccolillo, M., & Paquette, D. (2006). Histories of child maltreatment and psychiatric disorder in pregnant adolescents. *Journal of the American Academy of Child & Adolescent Psychiatry, 45,* 329–336.

Romito, P., Saurel-Cubizolles, M. J., & Cuttini, M. (1994). Mothers' health after the birth of the first child: The case of employed women in an Italian city. *Women's Health, 21,* 1–23.

Saravanan, B. (2002). Postnatal depression in India. *American Journal of Psychiatry, 159,* 1437–1438.

Scrandis, D. A. (2005). Normalizing postpartum depressive symptoms with social support. *Journal of the American Psychiatric Nurses Association, 11,* 223–230.

Seel, R. M. (1986). Birth rite. *Health Visitor, 59,* 11–22.

Segre, L. S., O'Hara, M. W., Arndt, S., & Stuart, S. (2007). The prevalence of postpartum depression: The relative significance of three social status indices. *Social Psychiatry & Psychiatric Epidemiology, 42,* 316–321.

Segre, L. S., O'Hara, M. W., & Losch, M. (2006). Race/ethnicity and perinatal depressed mood. *Journal of Reproductive and Infant Psychology, 24,* 99–106.

Schrocksnadel, H., Baier-Bitterlich, G., Dapunt, O., Wachter, H., & Fuchs, D. (1996). Decreased plasma tryptophan in pregnancy. *Obstetrics and Gynecology, 88,* 47–50.

St. Pierre, C. M. (2007). The taboo of motherhood: Postpartum depression. *International Journal for Human Caring, 11*(2), 22–31.

Stern, G., & Kruckman, L. (1983). Multidisciplinary perspectives on postpartum depression: An anthropological critique. *Social Science and Medicine, 17,* 1027–1041.

Stowe, Z. N., Hostetter, A. L., & Newport, D. J. (2005). The onset of postpartum depression: Implications for clinical screening in obstetrical and primary care. *American Journal of Obstetrics and Gynecology, 192,* 522–526.

Suri, R., Burt, V. K., Altschuler, L. L., Zuckerbrow-Miller, J., & Fairbanks, L. (2001). Fluvoxamine for postpartum depression. *American Journal of Psychiatry, 158,* 1739–1740.

Tammentie, T., Tarkka, M., Astedt-Kurki, P., & Paavilainen, E. (2002). Sociodemographic factors of families related to postnatal depressive symptoms of mothers. *International Journal of Nursing Practice, 8,* 240–246.

Taylor, V. (1995). Self-labeling and women's mental health: Postpartum illness and the reconstruction of motherhood. Sociological Focus, 28 (1), 23-47.

Teissedre, F., & Chabrol, H. (2004). Detecting women at risk for postnatal depression using the Edinburgh Postnatal Depression Scale at 2 to 3 days postpartum. *Canadian Journal of Psychiatry, 49*(1), 51–54.

Templeton, L., Velleman, R., Persaud, A., & Milner, P. (2003). The experiences of postnatal depression in women from black and minority ethnic communities in Wiltshire, UK. *Ethnicity & Health, 8*(3), 207–221.

Tuohy, A., & McVey, C. (2008). Experience of pregnancy and delivery as predictors of postpartum depression. *Psychology, Health & Medicine, 13*(1), 43–47.

Ugarriza, D. (1992). Postpartum affective disorders: Incidence and treatment. *Journal of Psychosocial Nursing, 30*(5), 29–32.

Ussher, J. M. (1991). *Women's madness: Misogyny or mental illness?* Hemel Hempstead, England: Harvester Wheatsheaf.

Verkerk, G. J., Pop, V. J., Van Son, M. J., & Van Heck, G. L. (2003). Prediction of depression in the postpartum period: A longitudinal follow-up study in high-risk and low-risk women. *Journal of Affective Disorders, 77,* 159–166.

Waldenström, L., Hildingsson, I., Rubertsson, C., & Rådestad, I. (2004). A negative birth experience: Prevalence and risk factors in a national sample. *Birth, 1,* 17–27.

Wei, G., Greaver, L. B., Marson, S. M., Herndon, C. H., Rogers, J., & Roheson Healthcare Corporation. (2008). Postpartum depression: Racial differences and ethnic disparities in a tri-racial and bi-ethnic population. *Maternal and Child Health Journal, 12,* 699–707.

Welberg, L. (2008). Affective disorders: Baby blues. *Nature Reviews Neuroscience, 9,* 657.

Whiffen, V. E., & Gotlib, I. H. (1993). Comparison of postpartum and nonpostpartum depression: Clinical presentation, psychiatric history, and psychosocial functioning. *Journal of Consulting and Clinical Psychology, 61,* 485–494.

Wolf, A. W., DeAndraca, I., & Lozoff, B. (2002). Maternal depression in three Latin American samples. *Social Psychiatry and Psychiatric Epidemiology, 37,* 169–176.

Wolfson, A. R., Crowley, S. J., Anwer, U., & Bassett, J. L. (2003). Changes in sleep patterns and depressive symptoms in first-time mothers: Last trimester to 1-year postpartum. *Behavioral Sleep Medicine, 1,* 54–67.

World Health Organization (WHO). (2003). Managing complications in pregnancy and childbirth: A guide for midwives and doctors. Retrieved from the Department of Reproductive Health and Research, World Health Organization Web site: http://www.who.int/reproductive-health/impac/Clinical_Principles/Emotional_support_C7_C14.html

Yonkers, K. A., Ramin, S. M., Rush, A. J., Navarrete, C. A., & Carmody, T. (2001). Onset and persistence of postpartum depression in an inner-city maternal health clinic system. *American Journal of Psychiatry, 158,* 1856–1863.

Yoshida, K., Yamashita, H., Ueda, M., & Tashiro, N. (2001). Postnatal depression in Japanese mothers and the reconsideration of "Satogaeri bunben." *Pediatrics International, 43*(2), 189–193.

Zayas, L. H., Cunningham, M., McKee, M. D., & Jankowski, K. R. (2002). Depression and negative life events among pregnant African-American and Hispanic women. *Women's Health Issues, 12,* 16–21.

Zittel-Palamara, K., Rockmaker, J. R., Schwabel, K. M., Weinstein, W. L., & Thompson, S. J. (2008). Desired assistance versus care received for postpartum depression: Access to care differences by race. *Archives of Women's Mental Health, 11,* 81–92.

_____ Chapter 4 _____

Postpartum Anxiety Disorders

Introduction

Women suffer from anxiety twice as frequently as men do; this difference can be detected as early as age six (Lewinsohn, Gotlib, Lewinsohn, Seeley, & Allen, 1998). Nearly half of those diagnosed with an anxiety disorder also have major depression (Regier, Rae, Narrow, Kaelber, & Schatzberg, 1998). When broken down by gender, women are more likely than men to be diagnosed with both conditions (Simonds & Whiffen, 2003). Of women who have postpartum anxiety, approximately 23 percent will also have postpartum depression (Field et al., 2003). The comorbidity of postpartum anxiety and depression increases the negative effect on the woman, baby, and family members (Dion, 2002; Lydiard & Brawman-Mintzer, 1998).

During the first year postpartum, women are adjusting to multiple life changes. Logically, anxiety can increase during these changes. For this reason, women who are more prone to anxiety will express feeling overwhelmed while accommodating to competing time demands, changing roles, diminished sleep, and financial changes (Wenzel, Haugen, Jackson, & Brendle, 2005). According to Holmes and Rahe's (1967) Life Stress Scale, women undergo a minimum of six major life stressors during pregnancy and the postpartum period: pregnancy and physical appearance, family structure, finances, employment or work, personal habits, and sleep. According to the Life Stress Scale, women experiencing these changes score 183; any score above 150 indicates a 50 percent increase in likelihood that the individual will develop a mental disorder. Clearly, pregnancy and postpartum are times of high mental health risks for women and the family.

Perinatal Anxiety

It is estimated that 10 percent to 50 percent of women experience post-partum anxiety annually (Wenzel, Haugen, Jackson, & Brendle, 2005), with symptoms typically beginning during pregnancy or at any time during the first year after delivery. Typically, women experience heightened anxiety during pregnancy, which tapers off after delivery when there is an increase in family, friend, and professional support. However, anxiety symptoms begin to reappear and increase over time (between three to seven months post-partum) when these supports start to wane (Breitkopf et al., 2006; Stuart, Couser, Schilder, O'Hara, & Gorman, 1998).

Although the *Diagnostic and Statistical Manual of Mental Disorders* (4th ed., text rev.) (DSM-IV-TR) (American Psychiatry Association (APA), 2000) does not specify postpartum anxiety as a disorder, for the purpose of this discussion, *postpartum anxiety* is defined as generalized anxiety symptoms; with other postpartum anxiety disorders: panic, posttraumatic stress disorder (PTSD) and obsessive–compulsive disorder, discussed as separate syndromes under the auspices of anxiety disorders. Generalized anxiety disorder is described in the DSM-IV-TR as extreme worry that is difficult to control (APA, 2000). This worry focuses on several events or activities and lasts for the majority of days within a six-month (or more) period. The extreme worry results in at least three of the following six activities: (1) feeling "on edge," restless, or "keyed up"; (2) feeling exhausted; (3) having a difficult time concentrating or feeling like one's mind has "gone blank"; (4) feeling irritable; (5) experiencing muscle tension; (6) having a difficult time falling asleep, staying asleep, or not feeling rested upon waking from sleep. Because of feeling intensely worried, the person finds it difficult to maintain her optimal level of functioning socially, at work, or in other important situations, such as handling household responsibilities.

Perinatal anxiety symptoms are associated with motherhood-specific events, situations, environments, or people. Some examples include fear of labor, pain associated with labor, and the baby's health (Areskog, Kjessler, & Uddenberg, 1981; Beck et al., 1980; Burstein, Kinch, & Stern, 1974; Elliott, Rugg, Watson, & Brough, 1983; Huizink, Mulder, Robles De Medina, Visser, & Buitelaar, 2004; Leifer, 1977; Rizzardo et al., 1985; Sjogren, 1997; Standley, Soule, & Copans, 1979; van Bussel, Spitz, & Demyttenaere, 2009). Women who fear that pregnancy and motherhood will deter their personal goals, tremendously change their lifestyle, or cause them to lose their identity are more predisposed to postpartum anxiety than women who do not have these perceptions (Raphael-Leff, 2005; Sharp & Bramwell, 2004; van Bussel et al., 2009). Women with these fears experience a decreased sense of control during pregnancy; they also tend to fear changes in the relationship with their partner and view the birthing process as a "painful medical event" (Raphael-Leff, 2005; van Bussel et al., 2009). Consequently, these women may detach from the baby during pregnancy and postpartum, with some self-medicating with alcohol (Breitkopf et al., 2006).

When balanced, healthy detachment from the baby can decrease stress levels and allow the mother to address other needs such as bathing and sleeping. Yet many women who perceive their role as the baby's primary caregiver will suffer anxiety when allowing their partner, family members, trusted friends, or day care provider to watch their child (Raphael-Leff, 2005; van Bussel et al., 2009). Women with this "separation anxiety" tend to view feminine identity in terms of their ability to take care of the baby. In contrast to the women described earlier, these women will strongly bond with the baby during pregnancy and during the postpartum period. This strong attachment can evolve into the false belief that the mother is responsible for 100 percent of the baby's needs; the inability to do this is perceived as her failure as a woman. These women will experience an increased fear about the ability to take care of their child and increased feelings of depression when unable to do so.

Anxiety during pregnancy can negatively affect both the woman and the growing fetus physically. Women are more likely to develop uterine artery resistance, high blood pressure, meconium staining, premature rupture of membranes, and may need a cesarean section delivery. The fetus is at an increased risk for congenital abnormalities and low APGAR scores. The infant is more likely to have lower levels of the neurotransmitters dopamine and serotonin, lower vagal tone, decreased alertness, and increased time sleeping (Bhagwanani, Seagraves, Dierker, & Lax, 1997; Breitkopf et al., 2006; Kurki, Hiilesmaa, Raitasalo, Mattila, & Ylikorkala, 2000; Rizzardo et al., 1985; Teixeira, Fisk, & Glover, 1999)

Postpartum Panic

Beck (1996), in her article "A Concept Analysis of Panic," described the idea of panic as originating from the Greek mythological story of Pan, the Greek god of nature. In this story, Pan—a short, goat-legged, and unsightly creature—is in charge of forests, rivers, and animals that live in the countryside. People who passed by a road next to the cave where Pan slept, would be frightened—literally to death—by Pan, who would shriek out a terrifying cry. The word *panic,* through this depiction, describes this abrupt and forceful fear.

Panic disorder occurs twice as often in women than in men. Most frequently, the onset of panic disorder symptoms in women occurs during the reproductive years, particularly in the mid-twenties (Kessler, McGonagle, &

Zhao, 1994). The prevalence rate of mild to severe postpartum panic is about one in five women annually (Wenzel et al., 2005). In one study, approximately 11 percent of women experienced their first panic attacks following childbirth (Bandelow et al., 2006). Interestingly, some studies report that women who have a preexisting panic disorder diagnosis find that their panic symptoms decrease during pregnancy and return after delivery (Cowley & Roy-Byrne, 1989; Fisch, 1989; George, Ladenheim, & Nutt, 1987; Hendrick & Altshuler, 1997; Klein, Skrobala, & Garfinkel, 1994; Kraus, 1989; Metz, Sichel, & Goff, 1988; Northcott & Stein, 1994; Villeponteaux, Lydiard, Laraia, Stuart, & Ballenger, 1992). Panic attacks experienced after delivery tend to be worse than they were prior to pregnancy (Ross & McLean, 2006). Others find that panic attacks remain constant or increase during pregnancy, particularly in the second and third trimesters (Cohen, Sichel, Dimmock, & Rosenbaum, 1994; Cohen et al., 1996; Griez, Hauzer, & Meijer, 1995; Verburg, Griez, & Maijer, 1994; Wisner, Peindl, & Hanusa, 1996). One factor that remains consistent is that panic attacks increase during the postpartum time period (Bandelow et al., 2006). Between 12 percent and 50 percent of these women will also experience postpartum depression (APA, 1994; Bandelow et al., 2006; Ross & McLean, 2006).

Having a panic attack is frightening, particularly when a person has never had one before. However, having panic attacks while attempting to adjust to the responsibilities and role changes related to becoming a mother can limit a woman's ability to respond appropriately to her baby. Attacks may seem to come without warning. Therefore, panic can also limit the extent to which she engages in activities such as shopping or interacting with friends or family, to avoid another attack (Dion, 2002). These women are likely to suffer lower self-esteem and self-confidence, guilt, failure, and dissatisfaction in their ability to parent the child (Beck, 1998).

Panic disorder is differentiated by the DSM-IV-TR (APA, 2000) into two categories: panic with or without agoraphobia. Generally, panic is a distinct period in which a person feels extreme fear that starts immediately. To be diagnosed with panic disorder without agoraphobia, the person needs to experience more than one panic attack followed by at least one of the following for a minimum of one month:

◀ ruminating about the possibility of having more panic attacks in the future;

◀ being bothered by the possible repercussions of having another panic attack such as "losing control," "having a heart attack," or "going crazy";

◀ altering previous behavior in reaction to the panic attacks (for example, avoiding triggers of the panic attack).

Also, those who avoid and fear being in circumstances or locations where there is the potential for embarrassment, or from which escape is difficult, are diagnosed with panic disorder with agoraphobia. Common examples of agoraphobic fears are a fear of going over a bridge, fear of leaving the home, fear of being in a crowd, fear of standing in line, fear of taking public transport, or fear of having a panic attack while in public.

Perinatal panic is different from panic during other life phases in that the primary focus is on the mother–child relationship. For instance, should a woman have a panic attack during pregnancy, she is likely to perceive the symptoms of the attack as something wrong with the fetus (Ross & McLean, 2005; Weisberg & Paquette, 2002). Should the panic attacks occur after delivery, the fear of having a panic attack in public with her child is heightened. The mother may then feel that, if she is seen having a panic attack in public, her child will be removed from her care, and she will be judged as a "bad" mom. Subsequently, these women prefer to stay at home, thereby isolating themselves and their children (Beck, 1998; Ross & McLean, 2006).

Women who breastfeed appear more protected from postpartum panic than women who do not. However, when weaning the child, this protection decreases and the onset of panic symptom begins to increase (Klein, Skrobala, & Garfinkel, 1994; Northcott & Stein, 1994).

Other risk factors for developing postpartum panic disorder include psychosocial stress, partner or family difficulties, health problems, financial stress, employment difficulties, and having an unwanted pregnancy (Bandelow et al., 2006).

Postpartum Posttraumatic Stress

The *New Mothers Speak Out* national survey found mild to severe postpartum posttraumatic stress rates to affect 18 percent of women annually in the United States (Declercq, Sakala, Corry, & Applebaum, 2008). Globally, an estimated 1.7 percent to 6.9 percent of women suffer with postpartum posttraumatic stress (Ayers & Pickering, 2001; Creedy, Shochet, & Horsfall, 2000; Czarnocka & Slade, 2000; Soet, Brack, & Dilorio, 2003; White, Matthey, Boyd, & Barnett, 2006; Wijma, Soderquist, & Wijma, 1997). Women who experience depression during pregnancy are nineteen times more likely to develop postpartum posttraumatic stress (Cohen et al., 2004).

Most postpartum posttraumatic stress symptoms resolve within two months, indicating a more acute PTSD reaction; however, some women have chronic posttraumatic symptoms that last years after delivery (Beech

& Robinson, 1985; Ryding, Wijma, & Wijma, 1997; Zaers et al., 2008). For diagnosis, six categories of posttraumatic stress symptoms must be met:

1. Experiencing or witnessing a traumatic event (the possibility of death, severe injury, or the possibility of physical harm to self or other). Response to the event is extreme fear, a feeling of helplessness or shock.

2. Reexperiencing the traumatic event through repeated thoughts, images, perceptions, or dreams that are invasive; behaving or emotionally reacting as if reliving the event (may be triggered by something in the environment or within the person's mind).

3. Avoiding the source of the traumatic event, avoiding other environmental "triggers" that may symbolize the event, and feeling "numb" in response to the event in three or more of the following ways: thinking, feeling, or talking about the event, locations, activities, people; difficulty remembering details about the event; feeling disconnected or alienated from others due to the event; difficulty expressing a range of feelings, or having a "sense of a foreshortened future."

4. Increased arousal responses in at least two of the following ways: difficulty falling or staying asleep, irritable responses, unexpected angry responses, difficulty concentrating or focusing, or exaggerated reactions to others or to environmental stimuli as if perceiving a threat to one's safety.

5. Symptoms lasting for more than one month.

6. Symptoms resulting in difficulty interacting socially, working, or performing other responsibilities as able to prior to the event (APA, 2000)

Risk Factors

Trauma during Childbirth

Postpartum posttraumatic stress often results from medical and surgical procedures during pregnancy, labor, or immediately following delivery. Cohen, Ansara, Schei, Stuckless, and Stewart (2004) found that women who had two or more maternal complications were four times more likely than women without these complications to develop PTSD symptoms postpartum. According to the American Pregnancy Association (2009), 875,000 women annually will have one or more complications during pregnancy, placing many women at risk for postpartum PTSD. Because of traumatic events, the mother may avoid the baby, other babies and new mothers (Beck, 2004). For some women, the avoidance of her child lasts for years after delivery (Ross & McLean, 2006), affecting interpersonal relationships, the ability to make appropriate care decisions for her baby, increased sleep disturbances, and exaggerated responses to the baby's behaviors (Creedy et al., 2000). Other women request a planned C-section in future pregnancies or opt for abortion procedures should she again become pregnant. These women may also avoid future pregnancies by requesting sterilizing procedures or avoiding sexual activity altogether, which can further strain the woman's relationship with her partner (Ross & McLean, 2006).

Cesarean Sections and Other Medical Procedures

Women who display posttraumatic stress symptoms are more likely to have undergone the following medical procedures: emergency cesarean sections, delivery via forceps, delivery via vacuum, and the extent of pain management medications after delivery (Creedy et al., 2000). These events typically involve pain (anesthesia malfunction or poor pain management), an emergency C-section, unplanned C-section, assisted delivery (for example, forceps or vacuum), hemorrhage, or a near-death experience for the mother or baby (Creedy et al., 2000; Fisch & Tadmor, 1989; MacLean, McDermott, & May, 2000; Mayou & Smith, 1997; Menage, 1993; Ross & McLean, 2006; Shalev, Schreiber, Galai, & Melmed, 1993; Zaers, Waschke, & Ehlert, 2008).

In the United States, approximately 25 percent of all births are now done by cesarean section (Hill, 2000). Given this large number, what causes some women to get PTSD after a C-section and not others? Ryding, Wijma, and Wijma's (2000) qualitative study on 25 women's emergency C-section experiences categorizes four types of emergency C-section reactions:

1. Women were confident in whatever happened during the delivery.
2. Women initially felt confident in the birthing process, but this confidence turned into disappointment when they had the emergency C-section.
3. Women were nervous about the birthing process prior to delivery and perceived the emergency C-section as "their fears coming true."
4. Women felt confused and experienced amnesia about the delivery.

Women in the first category reported feeling safe and happy upon arrival to the hospital and felt confident in themselves and their medical team. The doctors were forthright in discussing a cesarean section as a possible procedure for delivery and included the women in the decision-making process. Following delivery, there were no indications of feeling as if the delivery was traumatic. These women had a greater sense of control over the delivery compared with the other situational categories—even when a C-section was unavoidable from a medical perspective—because their medical team involved them in the decision-making process and encouraged open communication.

Women in the second category had similar feelings upon arrival to the hospital, yet they became suspicious during labor, thinking that they or the baby were having difficulties during the delivery and that they might need to have a C-section. Their emotional reactions to this suspicion was nervousness, displeasure, anguish, and anger. These women reported feeling relieved about the decision made to proceed with the procedure, yet the prior feelings of anxiety remained and the delivery was viewed as traumatic. Women in this category experienced the most difficulty with PTSD symptoms six weeks postpartum compared with women in the other categories. In Ryding, Wijma, and Wijma's (1997) pilot study, 19 out of 25 women (76 percent) felt that the emergency C-section was a traumatic event days after delivery. It is hypothesized that women in the "positive expectations turning into disappointment" category perceived a customary vaginal delivery as "good." When this did not occur, these women expressed feeling offended, upset, and angry with the maternity staff. When the "perfect" birth was unrealized, the event was internalized as evidence of being an unsuccessful mother.

Women in the third category were worried that there was something amiss. When the decision to proceed with an emergency C-section was made, the women felt fear and relief simultaneously. This fear lingered throughout the procedure, and it was reported that the delivery was experienced as traumatic. However, unlike the other categories, the fear-filled potential for surgical intervention may have been worse in their minds than the actual experience turned out to be. This may explain why the majority of women in this category showed fewer signs of PTSD at six weeks follow-up than did the women in the "positive expectations turning into disappointment" category.

Women in the fourth category were in poor physical health related to the pregnancy (for example, high blood pressure, heavy bleeding, and preterm membrane rupture). Once the baby was delivered, these women could not recall any initial thoughts or feelings upon seeing their baby, which possibly points to dissociating during the medical procedure that was perceived to be traumatic.

Women who have an emergency cesarean section are more likely to experience the procedure as traumatic if they feel terror about the baby's or their own life or are fearful that the baby will be born with a serious disability or sickly (Ryding, Wijma, & Wijma, 1998). Having prenatal anxiety or a sensitivity to anxiety during pregnancy may predict posttraumatic stress reactions following a C-section more than the fear experienced during delivery or during the procedure (Fairbrother & Woody, 2007). In addition to posttraumatic stress symptoms, emergency cesarean sections have also been linked to low self-esteem and depression in women postpartum (Boyce & Todd, 1992; Enkin, Keirse, Renfrew, & Neilson, 1995; Fisher, Astbury, & Smith, 1997).

Women who have had traumatic deliveries in the past or have previously had a cesarean section may plan to repeat the procedure for subsequent deliveries. Although women plan C-sections for these reasons, it does not guarantee that trauma during delivery of the next child will not occur. In fact, some women who have had a previous C-section experience increased anxiety about reexperiencing the pain and discomfort of recovery (Creedy et al., 2000).

Quality of Professional Care

Communication between women and their care providers during the delivery and recovery period is crucial for psychological and emotional adjustment. The most often cited communication concerns include: inadequate information provided during the birthing process, facing unsympathetic attitudes from medical and paramedical professionals, misunderstanding informed consent about procedures, and questioning the skills of the medical professionals during the delivery (Creedy et al., 2000; Menage, 1993; Wijma, Soderquist, & Wijma, 1997). When communication is impaired or not supportive, anxiety levels and distrust increase in women. Other risk factors for the development of postpartum PTSD include professionals who do not explain the status of the baby, the mother, or tests or procedures (Beck, 2004; Keogh, Ayers, & Francis, 2002; Menage, 1993). In fact, the more medically based procedures that a woman endures during delivery, the less satisfied she is with the received care (Creedy et al., 2000). These women believe that they had minimal options available during the delivery and minimal choice or control about procedures to assist with the delivery (DiMatteo, Kahn, & Berry, 1993).

Anxiety about the Baby

Fears about the health of the baby have been linked to the development of posttraumatic stress symptoms following childbirth. One study found that a fear of childbirth was the best predictor for the development of PTSD after delivery (Wijma, Ryding, & Wijma, 2002). This result was supported by Söderquist, Wijma, Thorbert, and Wijma (2009), who found that women who feared childbirth were six times more likely to develop postpartum PTSD than women who did not have this fear. This is particularly salient when the mother perceives a threat to the baby's life or risk of serious injury to the baby, such as a sudden drop in the baby's heart rate, the cord being wrapped around the baby's neck, the baby appearing blue or having difficulty initiating breathing, or the baby appearing limp or dead after birth.

In some cases, the mother's (and other partner's) fears are realized. The baby is indeed experiencing a serious life-threatening health problem and winds up in the Pediatric Intensive Care Unit (PICU). In these situations, the prevalence rate of posttraumatic stress increases in parents to between 15 percent and 48 percent (Balluffi et al., 2004; Bronner, Knoester, Bos, Last, & Grootenhuis, 2008; Colville & Gracey, 2006; Judge, Nadel, Vergnaud, & Garralda, 2002; Rees, Gledhill, Garralda, & Nadel, 2004; Shears, Nadel, Gledhill, & Garralda, 2005).

Bronner et al. (2008), found that 41 percent of mothers and 22 percent of fathers experienced two or more hyperarousal symptoms associated with posttraumatic stress one month after a PICU follow-up visit. In this same study, intrusive thoughts about the PICU experience were reported by 84 percent of the mothers and 73 percent of the fathers, and 16 percent of mothers and 12 percent of fathers reported having three or more avoidance symptoms associated with PTSD. Approximately 470,000 babies are born prematurely in the United States every year (American Pregnancy Association, 2009). In some cases, these preemies need additional care in the Neonatal Intensive Care Unit (NICU). This increases the mother's fears about the baby's health and likelihood of survival. Mothers with a baby in the NICU also report difficulty with the separation from their baby, a sense of loss over the expected maternal role with the baby immediately after delivery, and feeling guilt for not being able to carry the baby to full term (Holditch-Davis, Bartlett, Blickman, & Miles, 2003; Holditch-Davis & Miles, 2000). Undoubtedly, these women also feel anxious, depressed, helpless, and emotionally anguished over the baby's condition. When the baby is allowed to go home with the parents, many mothers have difficulty emotionally bonding with the baby—often up to six months after the baby is home (Miles, Holditch-Davis, Burchinal, & Nelson, 1999; Reichman, Miller, Gordon, & Hendricks-Munoz, 2000). From the day the baby leaves the hospital until three years following NICU care, women continue to report symptoms of posttraumatic stress about the ordeal (Affleck, Tennen, Rowe, & Higgins, 1990; Miles & Holditch-Davis, 1995). Due to posttraumatic stress symptoms, some mothers (and parents) may avoid taking the baby to the doctor or may become overprotective of the premature baby (Huber, Holditch-Davis, & Brandon, 1993; Miles & Holditch-Davis, 1995; O'Mara & Johnston, 1989; Perrin, West, & Culley, 1989). The Holditch-Davis et al. (2003) small study found PTSD symptoms six months after the baby was returned home (refer to Table 1). These symptoms were present regardless of the severity of the baby's health, and more likely, were related to childbirth and to the hospitalization of the baby.

Table 4-1   PTSD Symptoms of Women Whose Baby Needed NICU Care
(Based on Holditch-Davis et al. [2003] findings)

PTSD Symptoms and Percent
Increased arousal (overprotective, fear that child might die or become sick, difficulty sleeping, anxiety), 87%
Avoidance (Trying to forget experience, numbing to reminders)/ Re-experiencing (Intrusive thoughts), 80%
Three PTSD symptoms, 53%
Two PTSD symptoms, 40%

Partner Support

The Creedy et al. (2000) study on the development of posttraumatic stress symptoms during and after childbirth showed that the mother's perception of partner support during delivery was significantly predictive of posttraumatic symptoms. Partners who seemed disappointed or did not wish to discuss the birthing process are commonly associated with women who have posttraumatic symptoms. For male partners in particular, feeling distracted in the medical environment, distressed, and alarmed by the female partner's pain and suffering during childbirth can make it difficult for him to tangibly support his partner afterward (DiMatteo et al., 1993). Therefore, postdelivery debriefing from medical and paraprofessional staff could greatly improve this risk factor for both partners.

Traumatic History

As discussed in chapter 3, woman who have a history of traumatic events are more susceptible to PMDs. This is particularly the case for posttraumatic stress, as women may have a pre-pregnancy PTSD diagnosis. Women who have preexisting PTSD are at increased risk for miscarriage, ectopic pregnancy, excessive vomiting, preterm contractions, and excessive fetal growth (Kendall–Tackett, 2007; Seng et al., 2001).

Women who have had two or more traumatic experiences prenatally appear to be more likely to experience postpartum posttraumatic stress than are other women (Cohen et al., 2004; Loveland-Cook et al., 2004). In particular, having a history of sexual abuse predisposes women to posttraumatic stress perinatally. The physical sensations of the baby in utero can trigger body memories and feeling "not in control" of one's body. Perinatal care is invasive during and after pregnancy, with numerous internal examinations.

Women's bodies are examined, poked, probed, and exposed in front of several professionals; the woman knows only some of these professionals. This can increase the feeling of physical vulnerability and even cause some women to avoid prenatal care (Ross & McLean, 2006).

One study found a relationship between experiencing emotional abuse as an adult and the development of postpartum PTSD symptoms (White et al., 2004). In this same study, women who were exposed to two or more traumatic life events including sexual, physical, or emotional abuse as a child or as an adult were three times more likely to develop PTSD after delivery than those without a history of these events. In the Soet et al. (2003) study, women who had a history of sexual abuse and poor social support, combined with several birthing events such as severe pain, feeling of powerlessness, poor communication with medical professionals, and need for a medically assisted birth (C-section, epidural, induced labor) predicted the onset of PTSD following childbirth.

Postpartum Obsessive–Compulsive Disorder

The lifetime pervasiveness of obsessive–compulsive disorder (OCD) is approximately 2 percent of individuals in the general population (Kessler, Berglund et al., 2005). Prevalence rates of postpartum OCD ranges from 2.6 percent to 48 percent worldwide (Neziroglu, Anemone, & Yaryura-Tobias, 1992; Vulink, Denys, Bus, & Westenberg, 2006; Wisner, Peindl, Gigliotti, & Hanusa, 1999). One research project found that the diagnosis of postpartum OCD was twice that of the annual prevalence rate for the general U.S. population (Kessler, Chiu, Demler, & Walters, 2005). During pregnancy, slightly fewer than one in five women had obsessive–compulsive symptoms (Uguz et al., 2007). Of women who showed signs of OCD during or after pregnancy, only 15 percent had a previous OCD diagnosis, making the onset of OCD during the perinatal period a high-risk period. Some have even gone so far as to say that the perinatal period poses the highest risk in the life cycle for women to develop OCD (Abramowitz, Schwartz, Moore, & Luenzmann, 2003; Buttolph & Holland, 1990; Labad et al., 2005; Maina, Albert, Bogetto, Vaschetto, & Ravizza, 1999; Neziroglu, Anemone, & Yaryura-Tobias, 1992).

An estimated two in three women with postpartum OCD also experience postpartum depression (Sichel, Cohen, Dimmock, & Rosenbaum, 1993; Wisner et al., 1999); and approximately one in two women with postpartum OCD have a history of anxiety disorders (Sichel, Cohen, Rosenbaum, &

Driscoll, 1993). However, there is some indication that postpartum depression manifests two to three weeks following the visibility of postpartum OCD (Sichel, Cohen, Rosenbaum, & Driscoll, 1993).

Similar to postpartum panic, some women with a pre-pregnancy OCD diagnosis find that symptoms decrease during pregnancy but return in increased severity following delivery (Labad et al., 2005; Ross & McLean, 2006; Sichel, Cohen, Rosenbaum, & Driscoll, 1993; Vulink, Denys, Bus, & Westenberg, 2006; Williams & Koran, 1997). Approximately one-third of women with pre-pregnancy OCD history experience this pattern: pre-pregnancy symptoms, decreased symptoms during pregnancy, and more severe symptoms postpartum (Williams & Koran, 1997). Roughly two-thirds of women with pre-pregnancy OCD experience a decrease in postpartum OCD (Uguz et al., 2007).

There is general consensus that, when left untreated, postpartum OCD symptoms remain during the entire first postpartum year, negatively affecting family interaction and functioning (Brandes, Soares, & Cohen, 2004). Unfortunately, many women with postpartum OCD will not seek out treatment, unlike the general population of individuals who have OCD symptoms (Fireman, Koran, Leventhal, & Jacobson, 2001; Uguz, Akman, Kaya, Sahingoz, & Cilli, 2008).

To meet the criteria DSM-IV-TR (American Psychiatric Association, 2000) for OCD, obsessions or compulsions must be present *and* the person must be able to distinguish that his or her thoughts or behaviors are over-indulgent or irrational. Obsessions include all of the following, according to the DSM-IV-TR:

1. Repeatedly ruminating about certain "thoughts, impulses, or images," the person wants the ruminations to stop but feels unable to stop them, thereby causing the person to feel a heightened sense of anxiety or anguish.

2. Repeated ruminations are not focused on "real-life problems."

3. To stop ruminations, the person tries to disregard the thoughts or performs an action.

4. The person is able to identify the ruminations as something from his or her own mind.

Compulsions are characterized as feeling pressured to perform specific behaviors or "mental acts" over and over, often in a meticulous manner. The purpose of performing these behaviors or "mental acts" is to decrease anxiety or distress or to avoid an event or situation, but these behaviors and mental acts are impractically linked to the distress, event, or situation that the person is trying to defuse. The obsessions and compulsions interfere with the person's life, including social interactions, activities, work, and daily schedule because they take up much of the person's time (in excess of one hour daily) (APA, 2000).

The onset of postpartum OCD is different from the disorder experienced at other times in a woman's life. With the postpartum version of this disorder, the symptoms are primarily focused on the infant and on mother–infant interaction. For example, women with postpartum OCD report intrusive thoughts and fears of accidentally harming the baby (Abramowitz, Khandker, Nelson, Deacon, & Rygall, 2006; Abramowitz, Schwartz, & Moore, 2003; Arnold, 1999; Buttolph & Holland, 1990; Sichel, Cohen, Dimmock, & Rosenbaum, 1993; Wisner, Peindl, Gigliotti, & Hanusa, 1999). Unlike postpartum psychosis, women with postpartum OCD are aware that their intrusive thoughts are obsessive or troublesome and do not act on them (Ross & McLean, 2006). Frequent obsessions for these women are a fear that the fetus or newborn is contaminated (81 percent), preoccupation with symmetry or precision (50 percent), aggressive thoughts (43 percent), and religious preoccupations (38 percent)—as cited by Uguz et al. (2007). Two very common compulsive symptoms are repeatedly washing one's hands or disinfecting the environment in fear that the child will get sick (Wenzel, Gorman, O'Hara, & Stuart, 2001). In Uguz et al.'s (2007) research, 81 percent of women compulsively cleaned, 56 percent repeatedly checked things, and 44 percent were preoccupied by ordering and arranging items. Others have found that women with postpartum OCD will avoid specific activities (giving the baby a bath) or items (knives), may resort to praying quite often to prevent a feared tragedy, and fear that they may inadvertently harm the baby (Fairbrother & Abramowitz, 2007; Sichel, Cohen, Dimmock, & Rosenbaum, 1993). Some women experience recurrent disturbing thoughts such as stabbing the baby, unintentionally sexually abusing the baby, or accidentally drowning the child while giving the child a bath (Fairbrother & Abramowitz, 2007; Sichel, Cohen, Dimmock, & Rosenbaum, 1993). Over time, the woman negatively internalizes the intrusive thoughts, resulting in negative thoughts about herself such as, "I thought about hurting my child with a knife. This means I am a treacherous person and an unfit mother." Taken one step further, the woman may then think, "in order to protect the baby from myself, I had better be extra conscientious and careful to make sure that I do not harm my child" (Fairbrother & Abramowitz, 2007).

It may be that the type of obsessions and compulsions during pregnancy relate to the increase or decrease in symptoms postpartum. For example, Uguz et al. (2007) found that women who had aggressive or contamination obsessions with a primary focus on the fetus experienced a decline in or absence of obsessive–compulsive symptoms postpartum.

Fairbrother and Abramowitz (2007) and Abramowitz et al., (2003) proposed a cognitive behavioral-based model to understand the development of OCD in new mothers. They theorized that during pregnancy and following delivery, there are remarkable changes in responsibility and perceived threats to possible harmful outcomes to the fetus or baby. The combination of an exaggerated sense of responsibilities and an overestimated possibility of harm become the foundation for the development of obsessive and intrusive thoughts. Abramowitz, Nelson, Rygwall, and Khandker (2007) discussed previous findings from their research and integrated these findings to further the aforementioned model. When parents have high levels of obsessive thoughts or beliefs during the pregnancy, they are more likely than other parents to develop severe obsessive–compulsive symptoms during the postpartum period. Virtually all parents in their study had intrusive thoughts about sudden infant death syndrome, accidental suffocation, and accidents. Approximately 50 percent of parents had intrusive thoughts about contamination or the baby dying or experienced intrusive thoughts about intentionally harming the baby. Interestingly, both mothers and fathers had these intrusive thoughts with similar frequency. Having intrusive thoughts prior to delivery predicted the development of more severe obsessive–compulsive symptoms three months after delivery for both mothers and fathers. Preexisting psychological and physiological conditions were also related to the severity of postpartum obsessive–compulsive symptoms.

References

Abramowitz, J., Khandker, M., Nelson, C. A., Deacon, B. J., & Rygwall, R. (2006). The role of cognitive factors in the pathogenesis of obsessive-compulsive symptoms: A prospective study. *Behavior Research and Therapy, 44,* 1361–1374.

Abramowitz, J. S., Nelson, C. A., Rygwall, R., & Khandker, M. (2007). The cognitive mediation of obsessive–compulsive symptoms: A longitudinal study. *Journal of Anxiety Disorders, 21,* 91–104.

Abramowitz, J., Schwartz, S., A., & Moore, K. M. (2003). Obsessional thoughts in postpartum females and their partners: Content severity and relationship with depression. *Journal of Clinical Psychology in Medical Settings, 10,* 157–164.

Abramowitz, J., Schwartz, S., Moore, K., & Luenzmann, K. (2003). Obsessive–compulsive symptoms in pregnancy and the puerperium: A review of the literature. *Journal of Anxiety Disorders, 17,* 461–478.

Affleck, G., Tennen, H., Rowe, J., & Higgins, P. (1990). Mothers' remembrances of newborn intensive care: A predictive study. *Journal of Pediatric Psychology, 15,* 67–81.

American Pregnancy Association. (2009). *Statistics.* Retrieved from http://www.americanpregnancy.org/main/statistics.html

American Psychiatric Association. (1994). *Diagnostic and statistical manual of mental disorders* (4th ed.). Washington, DC: Author.

American Psychiatric Association. (2000). *Diagnostic and statistical manual of mental disorders* (4th ed. text rev.). Washington, DC: Author.

Areskog, B., Kjessler, B., & Uddenberg, N. (1982). Fear of childbirth in late pregnancy. *Gynecologic and Obstetric Investigation, 12,* 262–266.

Arnold, L. M. (1999). A case series of women with postpartum-onset obsessive-compulsive disorder. *Journal of Clinical Psychiatry, 1,* 103–108.

Ayers, S., & Pickering, A. D. (2001). Do women get posttraumatic stress disorder as a result of childbirth? A prospective study of incidence. *Birth, 28,* 111–118.

Balluffi, A., Kassam-Adams, N., Kazak, A., Tucker, M., Dominguez, T., & Helfaer, M. (2004). Traumatic stress in parents of children admitted to the pediatric intensive care unit. *Pediatric Critical Care Medicine, 5,* 547–553.

Bandelow, B., Sojka, F., Broocks, A., Hajak, G., Bleich, S., & Ruther, E. (2006). Panic disorder during pregnancy and postpartum period. *European Psychiatry, 21,* 495–500.

Beck, C. T. (1996). A concept analysis of panic. *Archives of Psychiatric Nursing, 10,* 265–275.

Beck, C. T. (1998). Post-partum onset of panic disorder. *Journal of Nursing Scholarship, 30*(2), 131–135.

Beck, C. T. (2004). Post-traumatic stress disorder due to childbirth: The aftermath. *Nursing Research, 53,* 216–224.

Beck, N. C., Siegel, L. J., Davidson, N. P., Kormeier, S., Breitenstein, A., & Hall, D. G. (1980). The prediction of pregnancy outcome: Maternal preparation, anxiety and attitudinal sets. *Journal of Psychosomatic Research, 24,* 343–351.

Beech, A. B., & Robinson, J. (1985). Nightmares following childbirth. *British Journal of Psychiatry, 147,* 586.

Bhagwanani, S. G., Seagraves, K., Dierker, L. J., & Lax, M. (1997). Relationship between prenatal anxiety and perinatal outcome in nulliparous women: A prospective study. *Journal of the National Medical Association, 89,* 93–98.

Boyce, P., & Todd. A. (1992). Increased risk of postnatal depression after emergency cesarean section. *Medical Journal of Australia, 157,* 172–174.

Brandes, M., Soares, C. N., & Cohen, L. S. (2004). Postpartum onset obsessive–compulsive disorder: Diagnosis and management. *Archives of Women's Mental Health, 7,* 99–110.

Breitkopf, C. R., Primeau, L. A., Levine, R. E., Olson, G. L., Wu, Z. H., & Berenson, A. B. (2006). Anxiety symptoms during pregnancy and postpartum. *Journal of Psychosomatic Obstetrics & Gynecology, 27*(3), 157–162.

Bronner, M. B., Knoester, H., Bos, A. P., Last, B. F., & Grootenhuis, M. A. (2008). Follow-up after paediatric intensive care treatment: Parental posttraumatic stress. *Acta Paediatrica, 97,* 181–186.

Burstein, I., Kinch, R. A., & Stern, L. (1974). Anxiety, pregnancy, labor, and the neonate. *American Journal of Obstetrics and Gynecology, 118,* 195–199.

Buttolph, L., & Holland, A. (1990). Obsessive–compulsive disorder in pregnancy and childbirth. In M. Jenike, I. Baer, & W. F. Minichiello (Eds.), *Obsessive–compulsive disorder: Theory and management* (pp. 89–95). Chicago: Yearbook Medical Publishers.

Cohen, L. S., Sichel, D. A., Dimmock, J. A., & Rosenbaum, J. F. (1994). Impact of pregnancy on panic disorder: A case series. *Journal of Clinical Psychiatry, 55,* 284–288.

Cohen, L. S., Sichel, D. A., Faraone, S. V., Robertson, L. M., Dimmock, J. A., & Rosenbaum, J. F. (1996). Course of panic disorder during pregnancy and the puerperium: A preliminary study. *Biological Psychiatry, 39,* 950–954.

Cohen, M. M., Ansara, D., Schei, B., Stuckless, N., & Stewart, D. E. (2004). Posttraumatic stress disorder after pregnancy, labor, and delivery. *Journal of Women's Health, 13,* 315–324.

Colville, G. A., & Gracey, D. (2006). Mothers' recollections of the paediatric intensive care unit: Associations with psychopathology and views on follow up. *Intensive Critical Care Nursing, 22,* 49–55.

Cowley, D. S., & Roy-Byrne, P. P. (1989). Panic disorder during pregnancy. *Journal of Psychosomatic Obstetrics & Gynecology, 10,* 193–210.

Creedy, D. K., Shochet, I. N., & Horsfall, J. (2000). Childbirth and the development of acute trauma symptoms: Incidence and contributing factors. *Birth, 27,* 104–111.

Czarnocka, J., & Slade, P. (2000). Prevalence and predictors of post-traumatic stress symptoms following childbirth. *British Journal of Clinical Psychology, 39,* 35–51.

Declercq, E. R., Sakala, C., Corry, M. P., & Applebaum, S. (2008). *New mothers speak out: National survey results highlight women's postpartum experiences.* New York: Childbirth Connection.

DiMatteo, M. R., Kahn, K. L., & Berry, S. H. (1993). Narratives of birth and the postpartum: Analysis of the focus group responses of new mothers. *Birth, 20,* 204–211.

Dion, X. (2002). Anxiety: A terrifying facet of postnatal depression. *Community Practitioner, 75,* 376–380.

Elliott, S. A., Rugg, A. J., Watson, J. P., & Brough, D. I. (1983). Mood changes during pregnancy and after the birth of a child. *British Journal of Clinical Psychology, 22*(Pt. 4), 295–308.

Enkin, M., Keirse, M. J., Renfrew, M., & Neilson, J. (1995). *A guide to effective care in pregnancy and childbirth* (2nd ed.). New York: Oxford University Press.

Fairbrother, N., & Abramowitz, J. S. (2007). New parenthood as a risk factor for the development of obsessional problems. *Behaviour Research and Therapy, 45,* 2155–2163.

Fairbrother, N., & Woody, S. R. (2007). Fear of childbirth and obstetrical events as predictors of postnatal symptoms of depression and post-traumatic stress disorder. *Journal of Psychosomatic Obstetrics & Gynecology, 28,* 239–242.

Field, T., Diego, M., Hernandez-Reif, M., Schanberg, S., Kuhn, C., Yando, R., & Bendell, D. (2003). Pregnancy anxiety and comorbid depression and anger: Effects on the fetus and neonate. *Depression and Anxiety, 17,* 140–151.

Fireman, B., Koran, L. M., Leventhal, J. L., & Jacobson, A. (2001). The prevalence of clinically recognized obsessive–compulsive disorder in a large health maintenance organization. *American Journal of Psychiatry, 158,* 1904–1910.

Fisch, R. Z. (1989). Postpartum anxiety disorder. *Journal of Clinical Psychiatry, 50,* 286.

Fisch, R. Z., & Tadmor, O. (1989). Iatrogenic post-traumatic stress disorder. *Lancet, 2,* 1397.

Fisher, J. R., Astbury, J., & Smith, A. (1997). Adverse psychological impact of operative obstetric interventions: A prospective longitudinal study. *Australian and New Zealand Journal of Psychiatry, 31,* 728–738.

George, D. T., Ladenheim, J. A., & Nutt, D. J. (1987). Effect of pregnancy on panic attacks. *American Journal of Psychiatry, 144,* 1078–1079.

Griez, E. J., Hauzer, R., & Meijer, J. (1995). Pregnancy and estrogen-induced panic. *American Journal of Psychiatry, 152,* 1688.

Hendrick, V. C., & Altshuler, L. L. (1997). Management of breakthrough panic disorder symptoms during pregnancy. *Journal of Clinical Psychopharmacology, 17,* 228–229.

Hill, D. A. (2000). *Cesarean section.* Retrieved from www.childbirthsolutions.com/articles/birth/cesarean/index.php

Holditch-Davis, D., Bartlett, T. R., Blickman, A. L., & Miles, M. (2003). Post-traumatic stress symptoms in mothers of premature infants. *Journal of Obstetric, Gynecologic, and Neonatal Nursing, 32,* 161–171.

Holditch-Davis, D., & Miles, M. (2000). Mothers' stories about their experiences in the neonatal intensive unit. *Neonatal Network, 19*(3), 13–21.

Holmes, T. H., & Rahe, R. H. (1967). The Social Readjustment Rating Scale. *Journal of Psychosomatic Research, 11,* 213–218.

Huber, C., Holditch-Davis, D., & Brandon, D. (1993). High-risk preterms at three years of age: Parental response to the presence of developmental problems. *Children's Health Care, 22,* 107–122.

Huizink, A. C., Mulder, E. H., Robles De Medina, P. G., Visser, G. H., & Buitelaar, J. K. (2004). Is pregnancy anxiety a distinctive syndrome? *Early Human Development, 79,* 81–91.

Judge, D., Nadel, S., Vergnaud, S., & Garralda, M. E. (2002). Psychiatric adjustment following meningococcal disease treated on a PICU. *Intensive Care Medicine, 28,* 648–650.

Kendall-Tackett, K. A. (2007). Violence against women and the perinatal period: The impact of lifetime violence and abuse on pregnancy, postpartum, and breastfeeding. *Trauma, Violence, & Abuse, 8,* 344–353.

Keogh, E., Ayers, S., & Francis, H. (2002). Does anxiety sensitivity predict post-traumatic stress symptoms following childbirth? *Cognitive Behavioral Therapy, 31,* 145–155.

Kessler, R. C., Berglund, P., Demler, O., Jin, R., Merikangas, K. R., & Walters, E. E. (2005). Lifetime prevalence and age-of-onset distributions of DSM-IT disorders in the National Comorbidity Survey Replication. *Archives of General Psychiatry, 62,* 593–602.

Kessler, R. C., Chiu, W. T., Demler, O., & Walters, E. E. (2005). Prevalence, severity and comorbidity of 12- month DSM-IV disorders in the National Comorbidity Survey Replication. *Archives of General Psychiatry, 62,* 617–627.

Kessler, R. C., McGonagle, K. A., & Zhao, S. (1994). Lifetime and 12 month prevalence of DSM-III-R psychiatric disorders in the United States. *Archives of General Psychiatry, 51,* 8–19.

Klein, D. F., Skrobala, A. M., & Garfinkel, R. S. (1994). Preliminary look at the effects of pregnancy on the course of panic disorder. *Anxiety, 1,* 227–232.

Kraus, R. P. (1989). Postpartum anxiety disorder. *Journal of Clinical Psychiatry, 50,* 268–269.

Kurki, T., Hiilesmaa, V., Raitasalo, R., Mattila, H., & Ylikorkala, O. (2000). Depression and anxiety in early pregnancy and risk for preeclampsia. *Obstetrics & Gynecology, 95,* 487–490.

Labad, J., Menchón, J. M., Alonso, P., Segalàs, C. Jiménez, S., & Vallego, J. (2005). Female reproductive cycle and obsessive-compulsive disorder. *Journal Clinical Psychiatry, 66,* 428–435.

Leifer, M. (1977). Psychological changes accompanying pregnancy and motherhood. *Genetic Psychology Monographs, 95,* 55–96.

Lewinsohn, P. M., Gotlib, I. H., Lewinsohn, M., Seeley, J. R., & Allen, N. B. (1998). Gender differences in anxiety disorders and anxiety symptoms in adolescents. *Journal of Abnormal Psychology, 107,* 109–118.

Loveland-Cook, C. A., Flick, L., Homan, S. M., Campbell, C., McSweeney, M., & Gallagher, M. E. (2004). Posttraumatic stress disorder in pregnancy: Prevalence, risk factors, and treatment. *Obstetrics & Gynecology, 103,* 710–717.

Lydiard, R. B., & Brawman-Mintzer, O. (1998). Anxious depression. *Journal of Clinical Psychiatry, 59*(Suppl. 18), 10–17.

MacLean, L. I., McDermott, M. R., & May, C. P. (2000). Method of delivery and subjective distress: Women's emotional responses to childbirth practices. *Journal of Reproductive and Infant Psychology, 18,* 153–162.

Maina, G., Albert, U., Bogetto, F., Vaschetto, P., & Ravizza, L. (1999). Recent life events and obsessive-compulsive disorder (OCD): The role of pregnancy/delivery. *Psychiatry Research, 89,* 49–58.

Mayou, R. A., & Smith, K. A. (1997). Post traumatic symptoms following medical illness and treatment. *Journal of Psychosomatic Research, 43,* 121–123.

Menage, J. (1993). Post-traumatic stress disorder in women who have undergone obstetric and/or gynecological procedures. *Journal of Reproductive and Infant Psychology, 11,* 221–228.

Metz, A., Sichel, D. A., & Goff, D. C. (1988). Postpartum panic disorder. *Journal of Clinical Psychiatry, 49,* 278–279.

Miles, M. S., & Holditch-Davis, D. (1995). Compensatory parenting: How mothers describe parenting their 3-year- old prematurely born children. *Journal of Pediatric Nursing, 10,* 243–253.

Miles, M. S., Holditch-Davis, D., Burchinal, P., & Nelson, D. (1999). Distress and growth outcomes in mothers of medically fragile infants. *Nursing Research, 48,* 129–140.

Neziroglu, F., Anemone, R., & Yaryura-Tobias, J. A. (1992). Onset of obsessive–compulsive disorder in pregnancy. *American Journal of Psychiatry, 149,* 947–950.

Northcott, C. J., & Stein, M. B. (1994). Panic disorder in pregnancy. *Journal of Clinical Psychiatry, 55,* 539–542.

O'Mara, L., & Johnston, C. (1989). Mothers' attitudes and their children's behavior in three-year-olds born prematurely and at term. *Journal of Developmental and Behavioral Pediatrics, 10,* 192–197.

Perrin, E. C., West, P. D., & Culley, B. S. (1989). Is my child normal yet? Correlates of vulnerability. *Pediatrics, 83,* 355–363.

Raphael-Leff, J. (2005). *Psychological processes of childbearing.* London: The Anna Freud Centre.

Rees, G., Gledhill, J., Garralda, M. E., & Nadel, S. (2004). Psychiatric outcome following pediatric intensive care unit (PICU) admission: A cohort study. *Intensive Care Medicine, 30,* 1607–1614.

Regier, D. A., Rae, D. S., Narrow, W. E., Kaelber, C. T., & Schatzberg, A. F. (1998). Prevalence of anxiety disorders in their comorbidity with mood and addictive disorders. *British Journal of Psychiatry, 173*(Suppl. 34), 24–28.

Reichman, S.R.F., Miller, A. C., Gordon, R. M., & Hendricks-Munoz, K. D. (2000). Stress appraisal and coping in mothers of NICU infants. *Children's Health Care, 29,* 279–293.

Rizzardo, R., Magni, G., Andreoli, C., Merlin, G., Andreoli, F., & Fabbris, L. (1985). Psychological aspects during pregnancy and obstetrical complications. *Journal of Psychosomatic Obstetrics and Gynecology, 4,* 11–22.

Ross, L. E., & McLean, L. M. (2006). Anxiety disorders during pregnancy and the postpartum period: A systemic review. *Journal of Clinical Psychiatry, 67,* 1285–1298.

Ryding, E. L., Wijma, K., & Wijma, B. (1997). Posttraumatic stress disorder after childbirth: A cross sectional study. *Journal of Anxiety Disorders, 11,* 587–597.

Ryding, E. L., Wijma, K., & Wijma, B. (1998). Experiences of emergency cesarean section: A phenomenological study of 53 women. *Birth, 25,* 246–251.

Ryding, E. L., Wijma, K., & Wijma, B. (1998). Predisposing psychological factors for posttraumatic stress reactions after emergency cesarean section. *Acta Obstetricia et Gynecologica Scandinavica, 77,* 351–352.

Ryding, E. L., Wijma, B., & Wijma, B. (2000). Emergency cesarean section: 25 women's experiences. *Journal of Reproductive and Infant Psychology, 18,* 33–39.

Seng, J. S., Oakley, D. J., Sampselle, C. M., Killion, C., Graham-Bermann, S., & Liberzon, I. (2001). Posttraumatic stress disorder and pregnancy complications. *Obstetrics and Gynecology, 97,* 17–22.

Shalev, A.Y., Schreiber, S., Galai, T., & Melmed, R. N. (1993). Post-traumatic stress disorder following medical events. *British Journal of Clinical Psychology, 32,* 247–253.

Sharp, H., & Bramwell, R. (2004). An empirical evaluation of a psychoanalytic theory of mothering orientation: Implications for the antenatal prediction of postnatal depression. *Journal of Reproductive and Infant Psychology, 22,* 71–89.

Shears, D., Nadel, S., Gledhill, J., & Garralda, M. E. (2005). Short-term psychiatric adjustment of children and their parents following meningococcal disease. *Pediatric Critical Care Medicine, 6,* 39–43.

Sichel, D. A., Cohen, L. S., Dimmock, J. A., & Rosenbaum, J. F. (1993). Postpartum obsessive–compulsive disorder: A case series. *Journal of Clinical Psychiatry, 54,* 156–159.

Sichel, D. A., Cohen, L. S., Rosenbaum, J. F., & Driscoll, J. (1993). Postpartum onset of obsessive–compulsive disorder. *Psychosomatics: Journal of Consultation Liaison Psychiatry, 34,* 227–279.

Simonds, V. M., & Whiffen, V. E. (2003). Are gender differences in depression explained by gender differences in co-morbid anxiety? *Journal of Affective Disorders, 77,* 197–202.

Sjogren, B. (1997). Reasons for anxiety about childbirth in 100 pregnant women. *Journal of Psychosomatic Obstetrics and Gynecology, 18,* 266–272.

Söderquist, J., Wijma, B., Thorbert, G., & Wijma, K. (2009). Risk factors in pregnancy for post-traumatic stress and depression after childbirth. *British Journal of Obstetrics and Gynecology, 116,* 672–680.

Soet, J. E., Brack, G. A., & Dilorio, C. (2003). Prevalence and predictors of women's experience of psychological trauma during childbirth. *Birth, 30,* 36–46.

Standley, K., Soule, B., & Copans, S. A. (1979). Dimensions of prenatal anxiety and their influence on pregnancy outcome. *American Journal of Obstetrics & Gynecology, 135,* 22–26.

Stuart, S., Couser, G., Schilder, K., O'Hara, M. W., & Gorman, L. (1998). Postpartum anxiety and depression: Onset and comorbidity in a community sample. *Journal of Nervous and Mental Disorders, 186,* 420–424.

Teixeira, J. M. A., Fisk, N. M., & Glover, V. (1999). Association between maternal anxiety in pregnancy and increased uterine artery resistance index: Cohort based study. *British Medical Journal, 318,* 153–157.

Uguz, F., Akman, C., Kaya, N., Sahingoz, M., & Cilli, A. S. (2008). One year follow-up of postpartum-onset obsessive–compulsive disorder: A case series. *Progress in Neuro-Psychopharmacology & Biological Psychiatry, 32,* 1091–1092.

Uguz, F., Gezginc, K., Zeytinci, I. E., Karatayli, S., Askin, R., Guler, O., et al. (2007). Course of obsessive-compulsive disorder during early postpartum period: A prospective analysis of 16 cases. *Comprehensive Psychiatry, 48,* 558–561.

van Bussel, J. C., Spitz, B., & Demyttenaere, K. (2009). Anxiety in pregnant and postpartum women: An exploratory study of the role of maternal orientations. *Journal of Affective Disorders, 114,* 232–242.

Verburg, C., Griez, E., & Meijer, J. (1994). Increase of panic during the second half of pregnancy. *European Psychiatry, 9,* 260–261.

Villeponteaux, V. A., Lydiard, R. B., Laraia, M. T., Stuart, G. W., & Ballenger, J. C. (1992). The effects of pregnancy on preexisting panic disorder. *Journal of Clinical Psychiatry, 53,* 201–203.

Vulink, N. C., Denys, D., Bus, L., & Westenberg, H. G. (2006). Female hormones affect symptom severity in obsessive–compulsive disorder. *International Clinical Psychopharmacology, 21,* 171–175.

Weisberg, R. B., & Paquette, J. A. (2002). Screening and treatment of anxiety disorders in pregnant and lactating women. *Women's Health Issues, 12,* 32–36.

Wenzel, A., Gorman, L., O'Hara, M. W., & Stuart, S. (2001). The occurrence of panic and obsessive compulsive symptoms in women with postpartum dysphoria: A prospective study. *Archives of Women's Mental Health, 4,* 5–12.

Wenzel, A., Haugen, E. N., Jackson, L. C., & Brendle, J. R. (2005). Anxiety symptoms and disorders at eight weeks postpartum. *Anxiety Disorders, 19,* 295–311.

White, T., Matthey, S., Boyd, K., & Barnett, B. (2006). Postnatal depression and post-traumatic stress after childbirth: Prevalence, course and co-occurrence. *Journal of Reproductive and Infant Psychology, 24,* 107–120.

Wijma, K., Ryding, E. L., & Wijma, B. (2002). Predicting psychological well-being after emergency caesarean section: A preliminary study. *Journal of Reproductive and Infant Psychology, 20,* 25–36.

Williams, K. F., & Koran, L. M. (1997). Obsessive-compulsive disorder in pregnancy, the puerperium, and the premenstruum. *Journal of Clinical Psychiatry, 58,* 330–334.

Wisner, K. L., Peindl, K. S., & Hanusa, B. H. (1996). Effects of childbearing on the natural history of panic disorder with comorbid mood disorder. *Journal of Affect Disorders, 41,* 173–180.

Wisner, K. L., Peindl, K. S., Gigliotti, T., & Hanusa, B. H. (1999). Obsessions and compulsions in women with postpartum depression. *Journal of Clinical Psychiatry, 6,* 176–180.

Zaers, S., Waschke, M., & Ehlert, U. (2008). Depressive symptoms and symptoms of post-traumatic stress disorder in women after childbirth. *Journal of Psychosomatic Obstetrics & Gynecology, 29,* 61–71.

Chapter 5

Postpartum Psychosis

Nearly 1 percent of the United States population will be diagnosed with schizophrenia. Men receive the diagnosis most frequently in their late teens to early twenties, whereas women most frequently receive the diagnosis in their late twenties to early thirties—during the reproductive years (American Psychiatric Association, 1994). On average, women are about 26 years of age when first experiencing postpartum psychosis and had typically functioned well prior to having the psychotic episode (Katona, 1982; Rohde, & Marneros, 1993).

The prevalence rate of postpartum psychosis is approximately one to two women per thousand, based on information provided by hospitalized women around the world. Population-based research finds up to four women per thousand births will experience postpartum psychosis (Oates, 1996). These rates are significantly lower in frequency than all the other postpartum mood disorders (PMDs) (Dean & Kendell, 1981; Kendell, Chalmers, & Platz, 1987; Klompenhouwer & van Hulst, 1991; Kumar, 1994; Kumar, Marks, Platz, & Yoshia, 1995; Meltzer, & Kumar, 1985; Okano et al., 1998). Yet, due to the dramatic nature of this disorder, it is the most commonly discussed PMD in the media. The disadvantage to this is that women who experience less severe, yet more common, postpartum mood changes become fearful that they are indeed "going crazy" and do not want to be labeled as such. Consequently, many women choose not to say anything and suffer in silence.

Postpartum psychotic symptoms occur two to four weeks after delivery; however, it is common to see symptoms as soon as two to three days postpartum (Heron, McGuinness, Blackmore, Craddock, & Jones, 2008; Okano et al., 1998; Sit, Rothschild, & Wisner, 2006). The risk for women to develop psychotic symptoms during their lifetime increases 16 times within the first postpartum month (Kendell et al., 1987; Nager, Johansson, & Sundquist, 2006). Rohde &

Marneros (2000) found that approximately one in three women in their study met the criteria for acute and transient psychosis for the first time in their life following delivery. Common symptoms include strange delusions, severe mood swings, insomnia, confusion, depersonalization, cognitive distortions, disordered behavior, paranoia, thought disorder, being excessively active and talkative, having difficulty restraining one's self, and grandiosity (Brockington & Cox-Roper, 1988; Fahim, Stip, Mancini-Marie, & Malaspina, 2007; Pritchard & Harris, 1996; Sit, Rothschild, & Wisner, 2006). The sooner psychotic symptoms are treated (within the first month after delivery), the better the prognostic outcomes (Pfuhlmann, Stoeber, & Beckmann, 2002; Robling et al., 2000).

The course of the illness is dependent on etiology. Approximately eight in 10 women who experience postpartum psychosis do so stemming from an underlying bipolar condition and do not exhibit psychotic symptoms again (Jabs, Pfuhlmann, & Bartsch, 2002; Sit et al., 2006). However, half of women who have underlying schizophrenia will continue to experience symptoms after their first postpartum psychosis experience, and more than one third will have postpartum psychosis again (Protheroe, 1969; Sit et al., 2006).

The first known designation of postpartum psychosis as different from other postpartum mood changes was the result of Marcé's work in 1858. His findings, that psychiatric symptoms following childbirth were different from those experienced at other periods in a woman's life cycle, needed further attention. In the early 1900s, Kraeplin's (1919) perspectives on schizophrenia became more clearly defined and Marcé's contributions were minimized. At this point, postpartum psychosis was no different from schizophrenia. The *Diagnostic and Statistical Manual of Mental Disorders* (DSM) continues to uphold Kraeplin's work by not designating PMDs as separate and distinct conditions but rather, considers it a subcategory to an Axis I diagnosis (for example, acute psychotic episode, postpartum onset rather than postpartum psychosis) (Bosanac, Buist, & Burrows, 2003). Sit, Rothschild, and Wisner (2006) described the situation of a woman (a physician) who had a normal delivery, and whose recovery appeared to be going well and as planned. Within two days after delivery, this woman started to accuse her husband of poisoning her food and believed that their baby was looking at her in an odd way. Then she began to report smelling and hearing horses galloping in the hall outside of her room. In discussions with her husband, she stated that voices were telling her to jump in front of a subway train while holding her baby. Sit et al.'s (2006) case presentation is a classic example of the rapid onset of the postpartum psychotic symptoms of delusions and hallucinations. Commendably, her husband sought out medical attention immediately.

Hallucinations and delusions experienced by women with postpartum psychosis appear contradictory to her affect and are untypical. She has a tendency to perceive that people or situations around her are "out to get" her or her baby (delusions of reference); believe that she is being ill-treated or victimized; express suspicion and distrust; or become "showy" or ostentatious, or feel an exaggerated sense of self-importance (grandiosity) (Dean & Kendell, 1981, Klompenhouwer & van Hulst, 1991; Sit et al., 2006; Wisner et al., 1994). These delusions co-occur with hallucinations that are visual, physical, or related to smell (American Psychiatric Association, 1994; Sit et al., 2006).

Diagnosis

Brief psychotic disorder (also known as acute or transient psychosis) is the experience of delusions, hallucinations, or behavior that does not make sense or speech that does not make sense. These symptoms can last from one to 30 days and are usually triggered by an extremely traumatic event or extreme distress (AllPsych Online, 2004). In contrast, schizophrenia is an umbrella term that encompasses five different schizophrenias, characterized by predominant symptoms. Symptoms of schizophrenia are similar to brief psychosis; however, symptoms do not resolve within one month, and over time, the person starts to develop other symptoms such as flattened affect or inappropriate emotional responses (AllPsych Online, 2004).

The diagnostic criteria for brief psychotic episode and schizophrenia, does not entirely encompass the experiences of women who suffer postpartum psychosis (Brockington, 1996; McGörry & Connell, 1990). To begin with, postpartum psychosis typically occurs within the first days to few months after delivery. Unless these symptoms resolve within one month, the diagnosis of schizophrenia needs consideration. Postpartum psychosis resolves within the first year or two postpartum, so the diagnosis of schizophrenia does not truly apply. As with postpartum depression and other postpartum anxiety conditions, postpartum psychotic symptoms focus primarily on the child; therefore, this does not completely meet the criteria for schizophrenia. Furthermore, women who have a preexisting schizophrenia diagnosis tend not to see an increase in postpartum psychotic symptoms (Meltzer & Kumar, 1985). Due to the difficulty of categorizing postpartum psychosis as a brief psychotic episode, schizophrenia, and the differing underlying conditions, it is hypothesized that physical and mental health reactions to childbirth are internalized as a trauma or major stressor and thereby trigger a psychotic break (Marneros, 2006; Riecher-Rössler & Rohde, 2005).

Another diagnostic consideration has been to classify women with atypical psychotic symptoms as schizoaffective (although the current edition of the DSM no longer includes this diagnosis). In a project conducted in Japan, two out of three women with schizoaffective disorder met the criteria for atypical psychotic symptoms, closer to affective psychotic symptoms rather than schizophrenic psychotic symptoms (Okano et al., 1998). Another option is to describe postpartum psychosis as a variant of bipolar disorder, where the woman will experience hypomanic or mixed bipolar symptoms shortly after delivery (Brockington et al., 1981; Chaudron & Pies, 2003; Sharma, Smith, & Khan, 2004). The early reported hypomanic or manic symptoms include an increase in excitation, feeling euphoric or high-spirited; an inability to sleep or felt minimal need to sleep; increase in energy and activity; and an increase in talking. These early symptoms can be a precursor for the development of postpartum psychosis. In women with a history of bipolar disorder, these symptoms should *not* be overlooked as a "normal," overjoyed reaction to having a baby. These hypomanic symptoms following childbirth can be similar to the experiences of women without hypomania, such as lack of sleep and euphoria about the birth. Kendell, Chalmers, and Platz (1987) suggested that postpartum psychosis, therefore, appears more related to bipolar disorder than to schizophrenia.

Diagnoses to Rule Out

Following childbirth, women are at risk of developing thrombophlebitis in pelvic or leg veins. Physiologically, this results in increased pressure in the skull, blocked veins in the brain, and pressure in the back that results in deficient blood flow (Brockington, 2007a). Symptoms resulting from cerebral vascular disease include headaches, vomiting, seizures, partial paralysis, and difficulty understanding or communicating language. These symptoms begin to appear during pregnancy and up to one month following delivery. Brockington (2007a) examined the causal effect of three types of cerebral vascular disease on the expression of postpartum psychosis symptomotology: arterial occlusion, postpartum cerebral angiopathy, and subarachnoid hemorrhage. Brockington revealed that each of these conditions can resemble postpartum psychotic symptoms. Arterial occlusion is a sudden blockage of blood flow due to a blood clot, air bubble, or amnion (the membrane that encloses the amniotic fluid). Symptoms from an arterial occlusion that resemble postpartum psychosis include confusion, hallucinations, and widely fluctuating emotions.

Postpartum cerebral angiopathy is a momentary spasm of arteries in the brain that results in a stroke. Incidentally, stroke occurs 13 times more frequently in women who are pregnant than in nonpregnant women and is the cause of 10 percent of perinatal deaths. However, the increased stroke rate appears to be linked to the postpartum period rather than pregnancy (Kittner et al., 1996; Knepper & Giuliani, 1995; Ursell et al., 1998; Wieber, 1985). One possible cause for postpartum cerebral angiopathy is the use of bromocriptine, which imitates the activity of dopamine in selectively reducing the release of prolactin (the hormone that stimulates or sustains lactation). Women who experience postpartum cerebral angiopathy may present with confusion and focal neurological deficits (such as limited functioning of a body part or difficulty speaking) (Brockington, 2007b; Ursell et al., 1998). A subarachnoid hemorrhage is bleeding that occurs underneath a thin lining of the spinal cord and brain. At times, subarachnoidal hemorrhages occur postpartum, after a miscarriage, or resulting from epidural anesthesia (Brockington, 2007b). Resulting symptoms that mimic postpartum psychotic symptoms include refusing to eat or drink, muteness, catatonia, appearing dazed and confused, widely fluctuating emotions, chaotic actions toward the newborn or other children, and attempting to hurt oneself.

Women with a lifetime history of epilepsy, who have not experienced preeclampsia (high blood pressure) during pregnancy, appear to be slightly more susceptible to postpartum psychosis than are women without this history (Brockington, 2007b). However, the discussion of this predisposition is based on case studies, some dating back nearly 100 years.

Brockington (2007b) also examined the historical case studies of women who have Sheehan's syndrome that results in hypopituitarism (underactive pituitary gland) and typically manifests up to 10 days following delivery. This condition impairs the HPA- and HPG-axes' function and can result in psychotic symptoms, such as confusion, agitation, disorientation, and hallucinations.

The presence of Krebs-Henseleit disorder in women can cause hyperammonemia. This condition frequently results in encephalopathy or death of the newborn. Hyperammonemia causes enzyme deficits that influence the development of postpartum psychotic symptoms such as speech changes or incoherency, memory loss, agitation, violent behavior, and disorientation (Brockington, 2007b; Enns, O'Brien, Kobayashi, Shinzawa, & Pellegrino, 2005).

England, Richardson, and Brockington (1998) noted four incidents of women who developed postpartum psychotic symptoms following early term delivery. Postpartum psychotic symptoms included elevated affect, an increase in talking and activity, insomnia, bizarre speech, disorientation, delusions or hallucinations, and a decrease in eating and taking fluids. Although the authors admitted the presence of other external risk factors for postpartum psychosis in each of these women's lives; they suggested that, although preterm delivery served as the triggering stressor for the onset of psychotic symptoms, hormonal levels at the point of the preterm delivery could influence the development of symptoms.

Early Indicators and Risk Factors

Unlike other PMDs, the onset of postpartum psychosis is rapid and dangerous because of the hallucinations and delusions with respect to the interactions between the mother and the baby. Therefore, it is imperative that symptoms of postpartum psychosis be acknowledged and addressed professionally as soon as possible to protect the lives of the mother and her child (Wisner, Peindl, & Hanusa, 1994). This is particularly the case for women who have a preexisting bipolar diagnosis, as 22 percent of psychotic symptoms tend to appear the first day after delivery and 50 percent of psychotic symptoms by the third day postpartum (Heron, Blackmore, McGuinness, Craddock, & Jones, 2007). In a 27-year study of first-time mothers in Sweden, several medically related postpartum psychosis risk factors were identified (Nager et al., 2008). These risk factors rested primarily on the health of the baby, including respiration difficulties, severe birth asphyxia, prematurity, perinatal death, and low birthweight. Mothers having C-sections were also more likely to develop postpartum psychosis symptoms. However, analysis from this study concluded that although these medically related risks were indicated, the most predictive factor, with the exception of prematurity and emergency C-section, was the mother's mental health history (both personal and familial) (Blackmore et al., 2006; Nager et al., 2008). Women in this study with a psychiatric hospitalization before pregnancy were nearly 100 times more likely to develop postpartum psychosis than were mothers without this history.

As childbirth is the stress-triggering event for postpartum psychosis, the medical model suggests that hormonally based underpinnings have an enormous influence on the development of psychotic symptoms. To recap hormonal theories from chapter 2, levels of estrogen, progesterone, melatonin, corticotrophin-releasing hormones and endorphins radically plunge immediately after delivery (Grof et al., 2000; Wieck et al., 1991). Estrogen, in particular, decreases close to 1,000 times that of third-trimester peak levels, which significantly affects the central serotonergic structure and orbitofrontal cortex functioning (Chow, 2000; Dolan, 1999; Fahim et al., 2007; Jones, Middle, McCandless, et al., 2000). Orbitofrontal cortex lesions in the brain are linked to personality changes and to the expression and regulation of social and emotional behaviors. Specific socioemotional behaviors include insensitivity toward significant others, increase in reckless behavior, mood fluctuations, lack of inhibition, and improper behaviors—all symptoms that, on the surface, resemble postpartum psychosis symptoms (Adolphs, 2001; Berlin, Rolls, & Iversen, 2005; Fahim et al., 2007; Schore, 2000; Zald & Kim, 2001). To examine orbitofrontal cortex functioning in women with postpartum psychosis, Fahim et al. (2007) used functional magnetic resonance imaging on one pair of monozygotic twins; one twin exhibited postpartum psychosis symptoms following childbirth; the other twin did not. The researchers discovered that the orbitofrontal cortex of the twin with postpartum psychosis was not activated, and the orbitofrontal cortex of the nonsymptomatic twin showed significant activation. The authors concluded that there may be a genetic predisposition to the expression of postpartum psychosis, but neuro-developmental or environmental stimuli after delivery can play a role as well.

Genetics

Women with first-degree relatives who have a bipolar diagnosis or have had postpartum psychosis are more likely to have a psychotic episode following delivery than are women without this family mental health history (Jones & Craddock, 2001). Approximately 60 percent of women who have these family mental health histories will experience postpartum psychosis (Jones & Craddock, 2001, 2005; Robertson et al., 2005). Jones and Craddock's (2001) study on family mental health history connected to postpartum psychosis found that approximately three out of four women who had a first-degree relative who experienced postpartum psychosis also suffered with the diagnosis. However, only one in three women who had a prior bipolar diagnosis but did not have a first-degree relative who experienced postpartum psychosis wound up developing the disorder.

Mental Health History

Studies indicate that between 25 percent to 50 percent of women with a bipolar diagnosis experience postpartum psychosis (Brockington, 1996; Jones & Craddock 2001). Other research estimates that eight in 10 women who have either bipolar or schizoaffective disorder will develop postpartum psychosis (Blackmore et al., 2006). Women who have bipolar-induced postpartum psychosis express manic-type symptoms within three days of delivery, with 90 percent of women showing symptoms within the first four weeks (Harlow et al., 2007; Heron et al., 2008). An estimated 40 percent of women with a history of psychiatric hospitalization for bipolar disorder were rehospitalized for psychosis following delivery (Harlow et al., 2007).

Only about one in 10 women who have a schizophrenia diagnosis will endure psychotic symptoms following delivery (Brockington, 1996; Sit, Rothschild, & Wisner, 2006; Wisner, Peindl, & Hanusa, 1995). Women who have a schizophrenia diagnosis, although less likely to develop postpartum onset of psychotic symptoms, tend to engage in behaviors that place them at risk for developing postpartum psychosis. Women with schizophrenia have a propensity for multiple sex partners and some, therefore, have unplanned pregnancies. These women are also more likely to be single during the pregnancy and postpartum (Miller & Finnerty, 1996). Those who do have partners are more likely to experience domestic abuse during pregnancy (Miller & Finnerty, 1996).

Effect on the Family

In general, psychosis has more deleterious effects on mother–infant bonding as compared with depression or anxiety conditions (Abel, Webb, Salmon, Wan, & Appleby, 2005; Chandra, Bhargavaraman, Raghunandan, & Shaligram, 2006; Jennings, Ross, Popper, & Elmore, 1999; Snellen, Mack, & Trauer, 1999). However, one small study revealed that women with postpartum psychosis bonded better with the infant than did the women with postpartum depression (Noorlander, Bergink, & van den Berg, 2008). The women with postpartum psychosis scored lower on scales that measured impaired bonding, anger, rejection, and anxiety about care. However, through the use of certain measurement instruments, it was found that interactions between the mother and baby were relatively the same for both groups of women. One key difference was observed by hospital nursing staff: Mother–child interactions were worse for women with postpartum psychosis when admitted but significantly improved upon release; this was not the case for women with postpartum depression. In addition, women with postpartum psychosis did not need hospital-based treatment as long as women with postpartum depression did. The differences in mother–infant bonding experiences appears linked to the general course of the PMDs: the duration of postpartum psychosis tends to subside more rapidly than do symptoms of postpartum depression, which can last six months to two years (Beck, 2002; Noorlander et al., 2008).

Approximately one in two mothers with a schizophrenia diagnosis is released from the hospital without her child or is discharged with social services supervision (Chandra et al., 2006; Howard, Shah, Salmon, & Appleby, 2003; Kumar et al., 1995). Women with a prior diagnosis of schizophrenia tend to have limited eye contact with their infant and do little to stimulate the infant. Furthermore, these women often fail to interpret baby cues correctly and show a high propensity for abusive behaviors, which in turn have a negative effect on the cognitive and emotional development of the child (Bosanac, Buist, Milgrom, & Burrows, 2004; Department of Human Services, 1996; Falcov, 1996; Stein, Gath & Bucher, 1991; Taylor, Norman & Murphy, 1991).

Due to postpartum psychotic symptoms including a preoccupation with hallucinations, delusions, and disorganized thinking, the baby is subjected to neglect or dangerous care (Kumar et al., 1995; Sit et al., 2006). In interviews, women with postpartum psychosis report feeling a sense of loss about being a mother after delivery and subsequent feelings of guilt and inadequacy about her abilities as a mom (Robertson & Lyons, 2003). Once these mothers were no longer having postpartum psychotic symptoms and felt more like themselves again, many reported the desire to "make up for lost time" with the baby. Women also report feeling upset that their psychotic symptoms could have caused emotional or other developmental problems for the child (Robertson & Lyons, 2003).

Many women with postpartum psychosis experience marital strains or a lack of partner support. Robertson and Lyons (2003) described three major strains on the marital relationship and family support for these women:

1. Male partners have difficulty managing spouses' psychotic symptoms while adjusting to being the primary caregiver for an infant.

2. Mothers are hospitalized with the baby, leaving her male partner alone and disillusioned about the situation.

3. Mothers use all available energy in trying to love and nurture the baby and neglect the emotional and adjustment needs of her partner.

In addition to marital strains, these women suffer alienation from friends and other "supports" as their symptoms can be confusing and frightening and the "supports" do not know how to respond (Robertson & Lyons, 2003).

When the Land Closes in Around Us
~ Brangwynne Purcell

It is a new unequaled life which has sprung
Sprung into devils and headaches
Sprung into great chasms before me
And things go on
fall in
without warning

Did you great friend
once know me for my great stoicism?
Here it is entirely escaped me....
as I sit down in the ground
face to the dirt
preferring the grave.

It is my husband who has not forgotten.
He forgives my backbone daily
as if to say: You are weak.
I am strong.

I say:
Fifty years from now
I wonder about your hairline
and my mind.

Infanticide

Perhaps one of the most publicized and disturbing aspects of postpartum psychosis is the catastrophic event of infanticide. Reportedly, infanticide during the first postpartum year accounts for one in three fatalities due to injury; in other words, one to two babies are killed daily in the United States as a result of postpartum psychosis (Herman-Giddens et al., 1999; McClain, Sacks, Froehlke, & Ewigman, 1993; Overpeck, Brenner, Trumble, Trifilletti, & Berendes, 1998). Nearly one in 10 postpartum psychotic women will have thoughts of harming the baby (Kumar, Marks, Platz, & Yoshida, 1995). One project in India found that 43 percent of women with postpartum mental health conditions thought about killing her baby and that 36 percent attempted to harm the child (Chandra, Venkatasubramanian, & Thomas, 2002).

Women who wind up harming the baby (and sometimes their other children) are usually experiencing command hallucinations or bizarre delusions (Chandra et al., 2006; Spinelli, 2004, 2005). Chandra et al.'s (2006) study of 105 psychiatrically hospitalized postpartum women examined the types of delusions experienced by women and related the psychotic symptoms to a mother's ability to take care of her baby. Six delusional categories identified in this study were as follows:

1. 36 percent believed that someone would kill or harm the baby.
2. 36 percent believed that the baby was predestined for evil or was the devil.
3. 29 percent had peculiar delusions (will discuss further).
4. 22 percent believed that the baby was actually someone else's.
5. 13 percent believed that the baby would be taken away by someone.
6. 13 percent believed that the baby was God.

Chandra et al. (2006) described specific examples of peculiar delusions that they were unable to categorize. These examples are worth quoting directly from their article:

- "I have still not delivered the baby"
- "The baby will be harmed if I breast feed as fumes are coming out of my breast"
- "The baby is dead"
- "A relative who died before marriage is born again as my daughter"
- "I will not be able to bear further children as this baby is female and my husband will remarry"
- "Someone has already killed my children"
- "My unmarried sister is bearing my child and my sister's child is inserted into my womb"
- "The nurse will poison my baby"
- "I have twins (actually had a single male child)" (p. 286).

Chandra et al. analyzed safety concerns for the baby by the types of delusions the women presented. They found the following:

1. Women who feared for the infant's safety were more likely to be loving and nurturing toward the baby but became upset when the baby was separated from them.
2. Women who believed the baby was predestined for evil or was the devil were more likely to yell, strike, or suffocate the baby.
3. Women who had peculiar delusions about the baby were reported by others to be at risk for harming the infant when left alone with him or her.

Suicide

Some women have postpartum psychosis with depressed symptoms. In one study from India, these women had the greatest risk of suicidal thoughts or actions (Babu, Subbakrishna, & Chandra, 2008). An estimated two out of every 1,000 women with postpartum psychosis commit suicide, but many more attempt it (CEMD, 2001). In 2001, the recent delivery of a child was responsible for one in three suicides in the United Kingdom, indicating suicide as the leading cause of maternal death (Oates, 2003a). The majority of women in this study who die by suicide had suffered severe postpartum psychosis within days following delivery (Jones & Craddock, 2005; Oates, 2003a).

Suicide attempts by women with postpartum psychosis are often severe and violent in nature, such as setting oneself on fire (Sit et al., 2006). Slightly less than 50 percent of women with postpartum psychosis who committed suicide in the United Kingdom had received prior psychiatric assistance (Jones & Craddock, 2005; Oates, 2003b). These women's lives could have been saved had appropriate assessment and preventive measures been taken.

Societal Impact: Legal, Ethical, and Cultural Issues

Recalling the sociopolitical theories about PMDs from chapter 2, the legislation that governs infanticide is largely dependent on the norms and values of a culture regarding motherhood (Oberman, 2002). Historically and currently in some countries, infanticide is used as a form of "birth control" or viewed as "survival of the fittest," as is the case for a community in Brazil (who leave some sick newborns to die to preserve life-giving resources for the remaining community) (Scheper-Hughes, 1992). In other countries where families may have one child by law (China) or where families are unable to afford marital dowries (India), male children are preferred. When a female baby is born, she may be abandoned—left to die by the side of a road or in a trash can. In other cultures, woman may have the baby (at times due to rape) and then kill it to avoid social stigmas or being outcast by her community (Indonesia, Vietnam) (Deutsche Presse Agentur, 2003; Spinelli, 2005).

It is interesting that infanticide became an illegal action only when the Christian church categorized it as a "mortal sin," due to an increase in mothers asphyxiating their babies by lying on top of them (Brockington, 1996; Oberman, 1996; Spinelli, 2005). Laws attempting to prevent infanticide became punitive in several countries around the world, including the United States. Punitive laws were particularly focused on unmarried women who had a baby and then killed it to avoid the stigma (Blaffer-Hardy, 1999; Spinelli, 2005).

By the late 1600s through the late 1800s, legal definitions differentiated infanticide and murder, with more severe penalties associated with murder than infanticide (Oberman, 1996; Spinelli, 2004, 2005). Women who committed infanticide were instead sentenced to probation and mandated to mental health treatment instead of imprisonment or torture under the Infanticide

Act (in the United Kingdom) (Spinelli, 2005). This attitude toward the mental health risks of postpartum women has been established in most westernized countries, particularly the countries that are the most up-to-date on caring for PMDs (such as Australia and New Zealand), with mandatory mental health intervention and shorter sentences compared with those of people convicted of manslaughter (Brockington, 1996; Linzer, 2001; Spinelli, 2005).

These laws and ethical values are different in the United States. Instead, women who commit infanticide typically receive long prison sentences, and even the death penalty, without much needed mental health treatment (Spinelli, 2005). A prominent example is Andrea Yates, who was convicted of capital murder and sentenced to life in prison after fewer than four hours of deliberation by the jury (Spinelli, 2005; Yardley, 2001). She received this sentence despite a clear history of postpartum mental health conditions, bipolarity in her family, and evidence of medical mismanagement (Denno, 2003).

One culturally based conflict is the notion of femininity and women as innate caretakers. Due to this perception, the media coverage of infanticide cases demonizes the mentally ill mother, thereby influencing the public, jury, and sentencing (Barnett, 2005). Advocates on behalf of these mothers point to the fact that both parents should be involved in child rearing, when one parent is not capable of safely attending to the infant's needs, the other parent has a responsibility to provide safe care for the infant and seek out medical or mental health treatment for the mother who is mentally sick (Barnett, 2005).

Another ethical and legal dilemma in the United States is that people are sympathetic to the abuse and murder of babies and children, yet the culture is not sympathetic to mental health conditions or providing preventive or proactive interventions that preclude a woman from making healthier and less violent choices (Spinelli, 2005). Unfortunately, in the case of infanticide due to postpartum psychosis, both mother and baby are wounded; the perpetrating woman who kills her infant is then revictimized by legal mandates, punishments, and a continued lack of mental health treatment (Spinelli, 2005). An additional legal concern is that individualized mandates are created separately by each state, making sentencing (such as life in prison, the death penalty, or probation) and a national response difficult to predict (Moss, 1988; Spinelli, 2005).

Of particular concern in creating these mandates is that there are no official mental health diagnoses in the DSM PMDs. Without a diagnosis, despite evidence to support the presentation of postpartum psychosis symptoms as distinct from current DSM diagnoses, some states are able to declare a woman legally sane at the time the infanticide occurred (Klompenhouwer et al., 1995; Spinelli, 2005). Add to this that many states base sentencing on laws that were created over 100 years ago. Most women in the United States who commit infanticide are not sentenced or treated appropriately by the legal system, mental health system, or the media (Meyer & Spinelli, 2002).

Sichel (2002) proposed that postpartum psychosis (and other mood disorders) results from indisputable neurophysiological changes (and other risk factors that result in physiological changes). The resulting mental health behaviors require outside intervention. When this outside intervention is not provided, the behavior that results (in this case, infanticide) ought to be addressed as outside of one's conscious control, necessitating updated U.S. laws that reflect this understanding. This would protect not only women who kill their babies due to an underlying condition they are unable to control but also the babies by increasing early intervention for these women (Spinelli, 2005). As a result, some experts are lobbying for the passage of the American Infanticide Act. This act would provide statutes, punitive measures, and mental health care similar to the systems currently in place in England and Canada (Stangle, 2008).

References

Abel, K. M., Webb, R. T., Salmon, M. P., Wan, M. W., & Appleby, L. (2005). Prevalence and predictors of parenting outcomes in a cohort of mothers with schizophrenia admitted for joint mother and baby psychiatric care in England. *Journal of Clinical Psychiatry, 66,* 781–789.

Adolphs, R. (2001). The neurobiology as social cognition. *Current Opinion in Neurobiology, 11,* 231–239.

Ahmad, A. J., Clark, E. H., & Jacobs, H. S. (1975). Water intoxication associated with oxytocin infusion. *Postgraduate Medical Journal, 51,* 249–252.

AllPsych Online. (2004). *The virtual psychology classroom: Brief psychotic disorder.* Retrieved from http://allpsych.com/disorders/psychotic/briefpsychotic.html

American Psychiatric Association. (1994). *Diagnostic and statistical manual for mental disorders* (4th ed.). Washington, DC: Author.

Babu, G. N., Subbakrishna, D. K., & Chandra, P. S. (2008). Prevalence and correlates of suicidality among Indian women with post-partum psychosis in an inpatient setting. *Australian & New Zealand Journal of Psychiatry, 42,* 976–980.

Barnett, B. (2005). Perfect mother or artist of obscenity? Narrative and myth in a qualitative analysis of press coverage of the Andrea Yates murders. *Journal of Communication Inquiry, 29*(1), 9–29.

Beck, C. T. (2002). Postpartum depression: A metasynthesis. *Quality Health Research, 12,* 453–472.

Berlin, H. A., Rolls, E. T., & Iversen, S. D. (2005). Borderline personality disorder, impulsivity, and the orbitofrontal cortex. *American Journal of Psychiatry, 162,* 2360–2373.

Blackmore, E. R., Jones, I., Doshi, M., Haque, S., Holder, R., Brockington, I., & Craddock, N. (2006). Obstetric variables associated with bipolar affective puerperal psychosis. *British Journal of Psychiatry, 188,* 32–36.

Blaffer-Hardy, S. (1999). *Mother nature: A history of mothers, infants and natural selection.* New York: Pantheon Books.

Bosanac, P., Buist, A., & Burrows, G. (2003). Motherhood and schizophrenic illnesses: A review of the literature. *Australian and New Zealand Journal of Psychiatry, 37,* 24–30.

Bosanac, P., Buist, A., Milgrom, J., & Burrows, G. (2004). General issues in research in motherhood and schizophrenic illness: A pilot study. *Stress and Health, 20,* 43–44.

Brockington, I. F. (1996). *Puerperal psychosis: Motherhood and mental health.* New York: Oxford University Press.

Brockington, I. F. (2007a). Cerebral vascular disease as a cause of postpartum psychosis. *Archives of Women's Mental Health, 10,* 177–178.

Brockington, I. F. (2007b). Postpartum psychoses due to other diseases with a specific link to childbirth. *Archives of Women's Mental Health, 10,* 241–242.

Brockington, I. F., Cernick, K. F., Schofield, E. M., Downing, A. R., Francis, A. F., & Keelan, C. (1981). Pueperal psychosis: Phenomena and diagnosis. *Archives of General Psychiatry, 38,* 829–833.

Brockington, I. F., & Cox-Roper, A. (1988). The nosology of puerperal mental illness. In R. Kumar & I. F. Brockington (Eds.), *Motherhood and mental illness* (pp. 1–17). London: Butterworths.

CEMD. (2001). *Confidential inquiries into maternal deaths: Why mothers die, 1997–99.* London: Royal College of Obstetricians and Gynaecologists.

Chandra, P. S., Bhargavaraman, R. P., Raghunandan, V.N.G., & Shaligram, D. (2006). Delusions related to infant and their association with mother–infant interactions in postpartum psychotic disorders. *Archives of Women's Mental Health, 9,* 285–288.

Chandra, P. S., Venkatasubramanian, G., & Thomas, T. (2002). Infanticideal ideas and infanticidal behavior in Indian women with severe postpartum psychiatric disorders. *Journal of Nervous and Mental Disease, 190,* 457–461.

Chaudron, L. H., & Pies, R. W. (2003). The relationship between postpartum psychosis and bipolar disorder: A review. *Journal of Clinical Psychiatry, 64,* 1284–1292.

Chow, T. W. (2000). Personality in frontal lobe disorders. *Current Psychiatry Report, 2,* 446–451.

Dean, C., & Kendell, R. E. (1981). The symptomatology of puerperal illnesses. *British Journal of Psychiatry, 139,* 128–133.

Denno, D. (2003). Who is Andrea Yates? A short story about insanity. *Duke Journal of Gender Law and Policy, 10,* 61–75.

Department of Human Services. (1996). *Understanding and responding to child abuse and neglect.* Melbourne, Australia: Protective Care/Prevention and Education Unit.

Deutsche Presse Agentur. (2003, May 18). *Mother who killed newborn given suspended sentence in Vietnam, Hanoi.*

Dolan, R. J. (1999). On the neurology of morals. *Nature Neuroscience, 2,* 927–929.

England, S., Richardson, B., & Brockington, I. F. (1998). Postpartum psychosis after short gestation. *Archives of Women's Mental Health, 1,* 143–146.

Enns, G. M., O'Brien, W. E., Kobayashi, K., Shinzawa, H., & Pellegrino, J. E. (2005). Postpartum 'psychosis' in mild arginosuccinate synthetase deficiency. *Obstetrics and Gynecology, 105,* 1244–1246.

Fahim, C., Stip, E., Mancini-Marie, A., & Malaspina, D. (2007). Orbitofrontal dysfunction in a monozygotic twin discordant for postpartum affective psychosis: A functional magnetic resonance imaging study. *Bipolar Disorders, 9,* 541–545.

Falcov, A. (1996). *Fatal child abuse and parental psychiatric disorder: Working together, part 8 reports* (Department of Health ACPC Series, No. 1). London: HMSO.

Gardner, D. (2003, February 9). Where have all the girls gone? Forty million women are missing in India. *Financial Times,* London.

Grof, P., Robbins, W., Alda, M., Berghoefer, A., Vojtechovsky, M., Nilsson, A., et al. (2000). Protective effect of pregnancy in women with lithium-responsive bipolar disorder. *Journal of Affective Disorders, 61,* 31–39.

Harlow, B. L., Vitonis, A. F., Sparen, P., Cnattingius, S., Joffe, H., & Hultman, C. M. (2007). Incidence of hospitalization for postpartum psychotic and bipolar episodes in women with and without prior prepregnancy or prenatal psychiatric hospitalizations. *Archives of General Psychiatry, 63,* 42–48.

Herman-Giddens, M. E., Brown, G., Verbiest, S., Carlson, P. J., Hooten, E. G., Howell, E., & Butts, J. D. (1999). Underascertainment of child abuse mortality in the United States. *JAMA, 282,* 463–467.

Heron, J., McGuinness, M., Blackmore, E. R., Craddock, N., & Jones, I. (2008). Early postpartum symptoms in puerperal psychosis. *BJOG: An International Journal of Obstetrics & Gynaecology, 115,* 348–353.

Heron, J., McGuinness, M., Blackmore, E. R., Craddock, N., & Jones, I. (2007). No 'latent period' in the onset of bipolar affective puerperal psychosis. *Archives of Women's Mental Health, 10,* 79–81.

Howard, L., Shah, N. Salmon, M., & Appleby, L. (2003). Predictors of social services supervision of babies of mothers with mental illness after admission to a psychiatric mother and baby unit. *Social Psychiatry and Psychiatric Epidemiology, 38,* 450–455.

Jabs, B. E., Pfuhlmann, B., & Bartsch, A. J. (2002). Cycloid psychoses: From clinical concepts to biological foundations. *Journal of Neural Transmission, 109,* 907–919.

Jennings, K. D., Ross, S., Popper, S., & Elmore, M. (1999). Thoughts of harming infants in depressed and nondepressed mothers. *Journal of Affective Disorders, 54,* 21–28.

Jones, I., & Craddock, N. (2001). Familiality of the puerperal trigger in bipolar disorder: Results of a family study. *American Journal of Psychiatry, 158,* 913–917.

Jones, I., & Craddock, N. (2005). Bipolar disorder and childbirth: The importance of recognising risk. *British Journal of Psychiatry, 186,* 453–454.

Jones, I., Middle, F., McCandless, F., Coyle, N., Robertson, E., Brockington, I., et al. (2000). Molecular genetic studies of bipolar disorder and puerperal psychosis at two polymorphisms in the estrogen receptor alpha gene (ESR 1). *American Journal of Medical Genetics, 96,* 850–853.

Katona, C. L. (1982). Puerperal mental illness: Comparisons with nonpuerperal controls. *British Journal of Psychiatry, 141,* 447–452.

Kendell, R., Chalmers, J., & Platz, C. (1987). Epidemiology of puerperal psychoses. *British Journal of Psychiatry, 150,* 662–673.

Kittner, S. J., Stern, B. J., Feeser, B. R., Hebel, J. R., Nagey, D. A., Buchholtz, D. W., et al. (1996). Pregnancy and the risk of stroke. *New England Journal of Medicine, 335,* 768–774.

Klompenhouwer, J., & van Hulst, A. M. (1991). Classification and postpartum psychosis: A study of 250 mother and baby admissions in the Netherlands. *Acta Psychiatrica Scandinavica, 84,* 255–261.

Klompenhouwer, J. L., van Hulst, A. M., Tulen, J.H.M., Jacobs, M. L., Jacobs, B. C., & Segers, F. (1995). The clinical features of postpartum psychosis. *European Psychiatry, 10,* 355–367.

Knepper, L. E., & Giuliani, M. J. (1995). Cerebrovascular disease in women. *Cardiology, 86,* 339–348.

Kraeplin, E. (1919). *Dementia praecox and paraphrenia.* Edinburgh, England: Livingstone.

Kumar, R. (1994). Postnatal mental illness: A transcultural perspective. *Social Psychiatric and Psychiatric Epidemiology, 29,* 250–264.

Kumar, R., Marks, M., Platz, C., & Yoshida, K. (1995). Clinical survey of a psychiatric mother and baby unit: Characteristics of 100 consecutive admission. *Journal of Affective Disorders, 33,* 11–22.

Linzer, L. (2001, August 13). When the blues turn deadly, where is the help? *Press Association.*

Marcé, L.V. (1858). *Traite de la folie des femmes encientes: Des nouvelles accouchees et des nourrices.* Paris: Baillerie.

Marneros, A. (2006). Beyond the Kraepelinian dichotomy: Acute and transient psychotic disorders and the necessity for clinical differentiation. *British Journal of Psychiatry, 189,* 1–2.

McClain, P.W., Sacks, J.J., Froehlke, R. G., & Ewigman, B. G. (1993). Estimates of fatal child abuse and neglect, US, 1979–88. *Pediatrics, 91,* 338–343.

McGörry, P., & Connell, S. (1990). The nosology and prognosis of puerperal psychosis: A review. *Comprehensive Psychiatry, 31,* 519–534.

Meltzer, E. S., & Kumar, R. (1985). Puerperal mental illness, clinical features and classification: A study of 142 mother-and-baby admissions. *British Journal of Psychiatry, 147,* 647–654.

Meyer, C., & Spinelli, M. G. (2002). Medical and legal dilemmas of postpartum psychiatric disorders. In M. Spinelli (Ed.), *Infanticide: Psychosocial and legal perspectives on mothers who kill* (pp. 167–184). Washington, DC: American Psychiatric Press.

Miller, L. J., & Finnerty, M. (1996). Sexuality, pregnancy, and childrearing among women with schizophrenia-spectrum disorders. *Psychiatric Services, 47,* 502–506.

Moss, D. C. (1988, August 1). Postpartum psychosis defense: New defensive measures for mothers who kill infants. *ABA Journal,* p. 22.

Nager, A., Johansson, L. M., & Sundquist, K. (2005). Are sociodemographic factors and year of delivery associated with hospital admission for postpartum psychosis? A study of 500,000 first-time mothers. *Acta Psychiatrica Scandinavica, 112,* 47–53.

Nager, A., Sundquist, K., Ramirez-Leon, V., & Johansson, L. M. (2008). Obstetric complications and postpartum psychosis: A follow-up study of 1.1 million first-time mothers between 1975 and 2003 in Sweden. *Acta Psychiatrica Scandinavica, 117,* 12–19.

Noorlander, Y., Bergink, V., & van den Berg, M. P. (2008). Perceived and observed mother-child interaction at time of hospitalization and release in postpartum depression and psychosis. *Archives of Women's Mental Health, 11,* 49–56.

Oates, M. (1996). Psychiatric services for women following childbirth. *International Review of Psychiatry, 8,* 87–98.

Oates, M. (2003a). Perinatal psychiatric disorders: A leading cause of maternal morbidity and mortality. *British Medical Bulletin, 67,* 219–229.

Oates, M. (2003b). Suicide: The leading cause of maternal death. *British Journal of Psychiatry, 183,* 279–281.

Oberman, M. (1996). Mothers who kill: Coming to terms with modern American infanticide. *American Criminal Law Review, 34,* 1–110.

Oberman, M. (2002). A brief history of infanticide and the law. In M. Spinelli (Ed.), *Infanticide: Psychosocial and legal perspectives on mothers who kill* (pp. 3–18). Washington, DC: American Psychiatric Press.

Okano, T., Nomura, J., Kumar, R., Kaneko, E., Tamaki, R,. Hanafusa, I., et al. (1998). An epidemiological and clinical investigation of postpartum psychiatric illness in Japanese mothers. *Journal of Affective Disorders, 48,* 233–240.

Overpeck, M. D., Brenner, R. A., Trumble, A. C., Trifilletti, L. B., & Berendes, H. W. (1998). Risk factors for infant homicide in the United States. *New England Journal of Medicine, 339,* 1211–1216.

Pfuhlmann, B., Stoeber, G., & Beckmann, H. (2002). Postpartum psychoses: Prognosis, risk factors, and treatment. *Current Psychiatry Reports, 4*(3), 185–190.

Pritchard, D. B., & Harris, B. (1996). Aspects of perinatal psychiatric illness. *British Journal of Psychiatry, 169,* 555–562.

Protheroe, C. (1969). Puerperal psychosis: A long-term study 1927–1961. *British Journal of Psychiatry, 115,* 9–30.

Riecher-Rössler, A., & Rohde, A. (2005). Diagnostic classification of perinatal mood disorders. In A. Riecher-Rössler & M. Steiner (Eds.), *Perinatal stress, mood and anxiety disorders from bench to bedside: Bibliotheka Psychiatrica, Vol. 1* (pp. 6–27). Basel, Switzerland: Karger.

Robertson, E., Jones, I., Hague, S., Holder, R., & Craddock, N. (2005). Risk of puerperal and non-puerperal recurrence of illness following bipolar affective puerperal (post-partum) psychosis. *British Journal of Psychiatry, 186,* 258–259.

Robertson, E., & Lyons, A. (2003). Living with puerperal psychosis: A qualitative analysis. *Psychology and Psychotherapy: Theory, Research and Practice, 76,* 411–431.

Robling, S., Paykel, E., Dunn, V., Abbott, R., & Katona, C. L. (2000). Long-term outcome of severe puerperal psychiatric illness: A 23-year follow-up study. *Psychological Medicine, 30,* 1263–1271.

Rohde, A., & Marneros, A. (1993). Postpartum psychosis: Onset and long-term course. *Psychopathology, 26*(3–4), 203–209.

Rohde, A., & Marneros, A. (2000). Bipolar disorders during pregnancy. In A. Marneros, & J. Angst (Eds.), *Bipolar disorders 100 years after manic depressive insanity* (pp. 127–137). Dordrecht, the Netherlands: Kluwer Academic Publishers.

Scheper-Hughes, N. (1992). *Death without weeping: The violence of everyday life in Brazil.* Berkeley: University of California Press.

Schore, A. N. (2000). Attachment and the regulation of the right brain. *Attachment in Human Development, 2,* 23–47.

Sharma, V., Smith, A., & Khan, M. (2004). The relationship between duration of labour, time of delivery, and puerperal psychosis. *Journal of Affective Disorders, 83,* 215–220.

Shoeb, I. H., & Hassan, G. A. (1990). Post-partum psychosis in the Assir Region of Saudi Arabia. *British Journal of Psychiatry, 157,* 427–430.

Sichel, D. A. (2002). Neurohormonal aspects of postpartum depression and psychosis. In M. Spinelli (Ed.), *Infanticide: Psychosocial and legal perspectives on mothers who kill* (pp. 235–256). Washington, DC: American Psychiatric Press.

Sit, D., Rothschild, A. J., & Wisner, K. L. (2006). A review of postpartum psychosis. *Journal of Women's Health, 15,* 352–368.

Snellen, M., Mack, K., & Trauer, T. (1999). Schizophrenia, mental state, and mother–infant interaction: Examining the relationship. *Australian and New Zealand Journal of Psychiatry, 33,* 902–911.

Spinelli, M. G. (2004). Maternal infanticide associated with mental illness: Prevention and the promise of saved lives. *American Journal of Psychiatry, 161,* 1548–1557.

Spinelli, M. G. (2005). Infanticide: Contrasting views. *Archives of Women's Mental Health, 8,* 15–24.

Stangle, H. L. (2008). Murderous Madonna: Femininity, violence, and the myth of postpartum mental disorder in cases of maternal infanticide and filicide. *William and Mary Law Review, 50,* 699–734.

Stein, A., Gath, D. H., & Bucher, J. (1991). The relationship between postnatal depression and mother–child interaction. *British Journal of Psychiatry, 158,* 46-52.

Taylor, C. G., Norman, J., & Murphy, M. (1991). Diagnosed intellectual and emotional impairment among parents who seriously mistreat their children. *Child Abuse & Neglect, 15,* 389–440.

Ursell, M. R., Marras, C. L., Farb, R., Rowed, D. W., Black, S. E., & Perry, J. R. (1998). Recurrent intracranial hemorrhage due to postpartum cerebral angiopathy: Implications for management. *Stroke, 29,* 1995–1998.

Wieber, D. O. (1985). Ischemic cerebrovascular complications of pregnancy. *Archives of Neurology, 42,* 1106–1113.

Wieck, A. Kumar, R., Hirst, A. D., Marks, M. N., Campbell, I. C., & Checkley, S. A. (1991). Increased sensitivity of dopamine receptors and recurrence of affective psychosis after childbirth. *British Medical Journal, 303,* 613–616.

Wisner, K., Peindl, K., & Hanusa, B. (1994). Symptomatology of affective and psychotic illnesses related to childbearing. *Journal of Affective Disorders, 30,* 77–87.

Wisner, K., Peindl, K., & Hanusa, B. (1995). Psychiatric episodes in women with young children. *Journal of Affective Disorders, 34,* 1–11.

Yardley, J. (2001, September 8). Despair plagued mother held in children's deaths. *New York Times,* p. A-07.

Zald, D. H., & Kim, S. W. (2001). The orbitofrontal cortex. In S. Salloway, P. Malloy, & J. Duffy (Eds.), *The frontal lobes and neuropsychiatric illness* (pp. 33–69). Washington DC: American Psychiatric Press.

_____ Chapter 6 _____

Newborns, Infants, Children, and Adolescents of Mothers with Postpartum Mood Disorders

W omen who experience postpartum depression have difficulty parenting their infants, especially those who continue to experience depression for one year or longer (Cornish et al., 2006). These difficulties can create a reciprocal relationship between the mother and the infant. The infant learns to respond to the mother in ways that disrupt developmental maturation and the mother becomes more distressed due to the infant's reactions. Over time, as the infant ages into a toddler, child, and adolescent, these developmental disruptions can become more serious; resulting in mental health concerns, neurobehavioral and cognitive disturbances, and difficulties relating to peers (Talge, Neal, Glover, & the ESTRTSN, 2007).

Mother–Infant Bonding and Interactions

I Know You
~ *Brangwynne Purcell*

I know this womb
and its thick walled cell
and the beating heart
of one child
after another

after another
resting there
waiting

And drawing from me
Me
drawing from this heart
and soul
some kind of underworld life
A life kept for my self
until your little hands touched it
took it
breathed it

It wasn't meant for you
This soul
so rich
of mine
It was meant for me
is, mine

Somehow
those years ago
at your conceptions
it got lost in depths
of lining and flesh
it got lost among
your entrails and cords
until it couldn't find its way back
to me
Up and out

Until its only choice was you
Your grip
soft hands groping,
touching,
holding

It stopped its dance and sway
gave up its host
to go another route
Down and out

As with all interpersonal relationships, mothers and babies develop interactions and effectual bonding through a reciprocal process that feeds off one another (Field, 1985, 1989; Field et al., 2005; Tronick, 1989). In other words, the baby will respond to the mother's behavior and interaction, which then leads to the mother responding to the baby's behavior and interaction, and so on. As these interchanges repeat over time, behavioral expectations are learned, expected, and continue to replicate. When these exchanges are positive, a strong, nurturing attachment between the mother and the infant develops that eventually influences the biopsychosocial development of the baby. However, when these exchanges are impaired or negative due to the mother's mental health, attachment, behavior, cognition, affective, motor/speech, and other developmental concerns develop in the infant. As Field and colleagues (2005) put it:

> The mother's role is to be sensitive to her infant's behaviors and respond contingently, taking care not to be overstimulating or understimulating. The infant can respond to optimal levels of stimulation but will become disorganized if the mother is under or overstimulating. (2005, p. 2)

One mother–infant bonding activity that supports the development of healthy attachment is breastfeeding. However, many times the experience of untreated PMDs can impair the woman's ability to breastfeed. Cognitive misperceptions of her ability to adequately feed the newborn can impair the mother's ability to nurse (Dennis & McQueen, 2007). Diminished self-efficacy and cognitive misperceptions influence a mother's perceived ability and duration of breastfeeding (Dennis & McQueen, 2007). Current research indicates that women with postpartum depression stop nursing most often between one month and four months postpartum, significantly sooner than women who did not suffer from postpartum depression (Akman et al., 2008; Dennis & McQueen, 2007). This decreased nursing duration may be an additional contributing factor to impaired mother–infant bonding in women with PMDs.

Attachment Styles

Mothers with PMDs, postpartum depression in particular, experience two major interacting styles with newborns and infants: withdrawn or intrusive (Cohn, Campbell, Matias, & Hopkins, 1990; Cohn, Matias, Tronick, Connell, & Lyons-Ruth, 1986; Field et al., 1996; Field, Healy, Goldstein, & Gurthertz, 1990; Field, Hernandez-Reif, & Diego, 2006a; Tronick & Field, 1986). Women who are withdrawn understimulate the baby, disengage emotionally from the baby, fail to respond to distress signals, and, although feeling emotionally upset at hearing an infant's cry, react as though uninterested (Field et al., 1990, Field et al., 2006a; Jones, Field, Hart, Lundy, & Davalos,

2001). These women limit touching, eye-to-eye contact, and vocalization with the baby. When withdrawn women do touch their babies, however, this touch tends to be positive, nurturing, and loving in nature (Malphurs et al., 1996; Malphurs, Raag, Field, Pickens, & Pelaez-Nogueras, 1996). In addition, when withdrawn women interact with their infant, the interaction is also in a nurturing and loving manner (Field, Diego, Hernandez-Reif, Shanberg, & Kuhn, 2003a, 2003b). In response to limited touch, eye contact, and vocalization, the baby learns not to keep eye contact with the mother but rather looks around at other objects or people. These babies are inactive, have limited facial expressions, and have limited expressions of distress (Cohn et al., 1990; Field et al., 1990; Field et al., 2006a).

At three months postpartum, infants of withdrawn mothers have higher dopamine levels than infants of nondepressed mothers without these mother–baby interaction styles (Jones et al., 1997). Neurological changes in the baby based on the mother's interaction style are further supported with right frontal EEG activation studies at three months postpartum, indicating patterns similar to those found in individuals with depression and withdrawal mannerisms (Dawson, Klinger, Panagitotides, Hill, & Speiker, 1992; Field et al., 2006a; Field, Fox, Pickens, & Nawrocki, 1995; Tomarken, Davidson, Wheeler, & Kinney, 1992).

Women, who have intrusive characteristics, express anger and annoyance toward the baby, respond in an impatient or angry manner to the sound of a baby's cry, verbalize loudly or rapidly, and touch the baby in a forceful manner (Field et al., 1990; Field et al., 2005; Field et al., 2006a; Jones et al., 2001). These women tend to poke, forcefully tickle, and tug at the baby (Field et al., 2006a). Intrusive women touch their babies up to two times more frequently than withdrawn mothers do and are more heavy-handed than withdrawn mothers (Malphurs et al., 1996a; Malphurs, Raag, et al., 1996b). In reaction, the baby learns to avoid contact with the mother and may increase or limit expressions of distress (Cohn et al., 1990; Field et al., 1990).

At three months postpartum, infants of intrusive mothers have higher dopamine levels than infants of nondepressed mothers without these mother–baby interaction styles (Jones et al., 1997). However, when tested at six months postpartum, the babies of intrusive mothers showed increased levels of left frontal EEG activation similar to the left frontal activation found in their intrusive mothers (Diego, Field, Jones, & Hernandez-Reif, 2005; Jones et al., 1997). These infants also had higher dopamine levels than the infants of withdrawn mothers, implying that there may be a link between dopamine levels and changes in left frontal lobe activation (Field et al., 2006a). At one year of age, babies of intrusive mothers appear to accommodate better, with better mental health development and exploratory play observations and testing scores, than do babies of withdrawn mothers (Hart, Jones, Field, & Lundy, 1999; Jones et al., 1997). This difference may be due to dopamine levels. High dopamine levels in children are linked to extroversion, higher energy levels, and normalized behaviors (Field et al., 2006a; Rogeness, Javors, & Pliszka, 1992); children with low dopamine levels more often express anxiety, depression, and inhibited behaviors (Field et al., 2006a; Rogenness et al., 1992).

Women with co-occurring high postpartum anxiety and depression smile, touch, use exaggerated facial expressions, imitate the baby's behaviors, play games with the baby, and verbally respond to the baby less often than women with low postpartum anxiety and depression symptoms (Field et al., 2005). Women who expressed high postpartum anxiety symptoms without co-occurring depression smiled less, cried more, and showed more facial indications of distress than did women with low postpartum anxiety symptoms without co-occurring depression (Field et al., 2005). These women—regardless of high or low levels of postpartum anxiety—show similar verbalization withthe baby, engage in motor activities, imitate the infant's behaviors, and engage in eye-to eye contact with the baby (Field et al., 2005). In response to high or low anxiety mothers, infants expressed less smiling and vocalizing. Babies also increased motor activities, imitating the mother—including the mother's facial expressions of distress, and crying frequency (Field et al., 2005).

Women with high expressions of anger co-occurring with postpartum depression spend less time smiling, playing games, and imitating their babies than women with postpartum depression and low expressions of anger (Field et al., 2005). However, these women were able to physically bond with their infant by moving the infant's limbs more frequently than their more angry and depressed counterparts. In response, babies of mothers who have high levels of anger spend less time smiling, vocalizing, making eye-to-eye contact, and imitating others than babies of mothers with low levels of anger (Field et al., 2005). These infants also showed greater frequency of distressed facial expressions, motor activity, and crying. In summary, the babies of women with higher co-occurring anxiety or co-occurring anger with postpartum depression express fewer positive reactions and increased negative reactions.

Physical Development

Growth

During pregnancy, fetuses of depressed women are very active, reactive, and tend to have high heart rates, yet their in vitro growth becomes stunted or delayed (Allister, Lester, Carr, & Liu, 2001; Dieter et al., 2001; Monk et al.,

2004). Maternal cortisol levels are the most influential factor of these symptoms. Other complications due to mood disorders during pregnancy include malformed placenta and preeclampsia (Field, Diego, & Hernandez-Reif, 2006; Jablesky, Morgan, Zubrick, Bower, & Yellachiach, 2005; Kurki et al., 2000).

Babies of women who are depressed during pregnancy are more likely to be delivered prematurely, have low birthweight, and be smaller in gestational age compared with babies whose mothers are not depressed during pregnancy (Field et al., 2004b; Field et al., 2008; Hoffman & Hatch, 2000; Orr, James, & Blackmore Prince, 2002). Diego et al. (2009) found that women with depression during pregnancy were five times more likely to have a low-birthweight baby and nearly two and a half times more likely to deliver prematurely. Many low-birthweight babies maintain slower growth rates through the first postpartum year (Patel, Rodrigues, & DeSouza, 2002; Rahman, Iqbal, Bunn, Lovel, & Harrington, 2003).

Eating

In the womb, the fetus begins to practice sucking behaviors that translate, within hours after birth, into suckling and nursing (DeVries, Visser, & Prechtl, 1985; Hepper, Shahidullah, & White, 1991; Mizuno & Ueda, 2001; Van Woerden, van Geijn, Caron, van der Valk, & Swartjes, 1988). In just a short time, infants are able to distinguish between sucking to feed and sucking for comforting (such as sucking on a pacifier) (Field & Goldson, 1984; Hernandez-Reif, Field, & Diego, 2004; Van Woerden et al., 1988). Hernandez-Reif and colleagues found that newborns of mothers who were depressed sucked two times more than did newborns of nondepressed mothers. They proposed that this increase in sucking frequency points to a difficulty in regulating stimulation and activity levels. In addition, increased sucking frequency may satisfy sensory needs not met by the mother–infant bond—in other words, self-nurturance.

During breastfeeding, beta-endorphins pass through the colostrum and milk. Beta-endorphins contribute to several developmental and physiological processes in the baby, including restfulness, steroid synthesis, cardiovascular functions, endocrine functions, the regulation of neuroimmune functions, and initiating a regular sleep–wake cycle in newborns (Facchinetti, Bagnoli, Bracci, & Genazzani, 1982; Ferrando et al., 1990; Graf, Hunter, & Kastin, 1984; Klein, Nambordirii, & Auerbach, 1981; Wadhwa, Sandman, Porto, Dunkel-Schetter, & Garite, 1993; Zanardo et al., 2001). Beta-endorphin concentrations decrease in postpartum women who experience anxiety and who have delivered vaginally (Zanardo et al., 2001). The assumption is that the pain during labor and vaginal delivery enhances beta-endorphin levels available for the newborn. Therefore, the negative effect of postpartum anxiety on the availability of beta-endorphins for the baby may influence the developmental delays commonly found in children of women with PMDs (Zanardo et al., 2001).

Sleeping

Researchers have detected a two-way relationship between the mother and fetal sleeping patterns (Field et al., 2007). In general, depressed individuals may experience sleep disturbances. During pregnancy, these sleep disturbances may increase due to hormonal, breathing, and other physiological changes, such as chronic pain in the legs and back due to the pregnancy (Field et al., 2007; Santiago, Nolledo, Kinzler, & Santiago, 2001). One hypothesis is that sleep disturbances experienced by pregnant, depressed women influence the sleeping patterns and activity levels of the fetus. In utero, fetal sleeping patterns are inconsistent and their activities are significantly greater than activity levels in mothers without prenatal depression (Dieter et al., 2001). This increased activity diminishes the ability or quality of the mother's sleep during pregnancy including frequently waking at night, difficulty falling asleep, difficulty falling into deep sleep, snoring, sleep apnea, and frequently feeling tired (Lee, Zaffke, & McEnany, 2000; Mindell & Jacobson, 2002; Sahota, Jain, & Dhand, 2003).

These sleep disturbances in depressed pregnant woman predict delivery complications, such as long labor and C-section procedures (Lee & Gay, 2005). These labor complications are also significant risk factors for PMDs. Furthermore, once born, these babies continue to experience inconsistent sleep patterns and increased activity levels, making it more difficult for the mother to return to a more normalized sleep pattern as well (Diego et al., 2003; Dieter et al., 2001; Field et al., 2004b; Jones, Field, Fox, Davalos, Lundy, & Hart, 1998).

Neurobiological, Psychological, and Emotional Development of Infants

Perinatally depressed mothers and their babies have higher levels of cortisol and norepinephrine, and lower dopamine levels than their nondepressed counterparts (Field, 1995; Field et al., 2004b; Lundy et al., 1999). Neonates have cortisol, dopamine, and serotonin levels similar to their mothers' (Field et al., 2004a; Gitau, Cameron, Fisk, & Glover, 1998; Glover, Teixeira, Gitau, & Fisk, 1999). These levels can negatively affect the newborn's development.

During gestation, approximately 40 percent of the mother's cortisol passes through the placenta and into the developing fetus. Exposure to these high cortisol levels and higher corticotropic hormones predict premature birth (Field et al., 2004a, 2004b; Sandman et al., 1999; Wadhwa, Porto, Garite, Chicz-DeMet, & Sandman, 1998). Premature birth puts the baby at risk for physical developmental delays and the mother at risk for postpartum mood changes.

Norepinephrine levels can decrease blood circulation. Replication of norepinephrine-linked decreases in blood circulation in the fetus is implied through evidence of increased artery resistance in the uterus, believed to influence poor fetal development and low birthweight (Field et al., 2004a, 2004b; Giannakoulopoulos, Teixeira, Fisk, & Glover, 1999). Decreased blood circulation is implicated in the following conditions of newborns: hypoxia (slow heart rates in the fetus), high blood pressure, and limited blood oxygen levels in fetal arteries (based on research conducted on rhesus monkeys) (Field et al., 2004a; Myers, 1975, 1977). This subsequently increases the likelihood of miscarriage, poor placental growth, and low birthweight.

Norepinephrine may also negatively influence the synthesis of dopamine in humans as it does in rat studies (Field et al., 2004a; Weiss, Demetnikopoulos, West, & Bonsall, 1996). Rats exposed to high norepinephrine levels experience reduced dopamine levels, resulting in depressed symptoms such as decreased psychomotor functioning. The combination of prenatal norepinephrine and dopamine levels in mothers who express symptoms of depression during pregnancy predicts these neurotransmitter levels in the baby at birth (Lundy et al., 1999).

Cognitive, Motor Skills, and Socioemotional Development

Babies with bonding and attachment difficulties with their mother due to a maternal PMD suffer from cognitive and emotional development difficulties (Murray & Cooper, 1997). Within the first day of life, babies are able to differentiate the sound of their mother's voice and respond to their mother's voice over all others (Maiello, 1995). As the baby's eyesight develops, by six weeks after delivery, the baby is able to make eye-to-eye contact with the mother and smile in preferential response to the mother's face (Maiello, 1995). Infants are finely attuned to their mother's reactions to this eye-to-eye contact and facial responses (smiling) (Emanuel, 2006; Maiello, 1995). Therefore, when the mother is unable to respond due to mental health concerns, the mother–infant interaction and bond is impaired, resulting in undesirable infant responses such as withdrawal and an increase in crying (Emanuel,

2006; Murray, 1988). By 18 months of age, toddlers of mothers who suffered a PMD have difficulty with secure attachment and difficulty on object permanence tests, indicative of delayed or impaired cognitive development (Emanuel, 2006; Hay, 1997). Infants and toddlers may also develop cognitive delays in response to limited and "self-focused" versus "infant-focused" verbalization from depressed mothers (Hay, 1997). These reactions of the infants and toddlers are reciprocal in nature—the infant's responses reinforce the mother's responses which, in turn, reinforce the infant's responses, and so forth. The more cognitive, socioemotional, and motor development delays or difficulties that the child expresses, the more the mother feels depressed and her self-efficacy to be a "good" parent decreases (Murray & Cooper, 1997).

There is growing evidence that babies born to women who are anxious or who experience extremely stressful situations during pregnancy also experience developmental delays. In one project, maternal anxiety during pregnancy was responsible for the mental and motor development delays in eight-month-old infants with greater frequency than no maternal anxiety during pregnancy (Huizink, Robles de Medina, Mulder, Visser, & Buitelaar, 2003).

Babies and infants are unable to verbalize their needs. Instead, they rely on nonverbal cues, crying, and other signals to get their needs met. When these infants of mothers who suffered PMDs grow into toddlers and children, they may appear shy and may experience language delays or anxiety (Kagan, Reznick, & Snidman, 1987, LaPlante et al., 2004; O'Connor, Heron, & Glover, 2002; O'Connor, Heron, Golding, Beveridge, & Glover, 2002; Talge et al., 2007). Mothers with PMDs are unable to pick up on these cues and signals, thereby increasing the frequency of infants' fussiness and crying to get their needs met. Moreover, infants cannot differentiate between life or death needs and socioemotional needs that can wait and may react similarly to both stimuli. For instance, the baby might feel excitement, fear, discomfort, loneliness, boredom, hunger, sleepiness, joy, or need a diaper change. Mothers with a PMD, who are unable to recognize the baby's needs, might not respond until the baby cries loudly, screams, kicks, bangs, or scratches to have these needs met. These disruptive behaviors are reinforced as strategies to have needs met (Emanuel, 2006; Murray & Cooper, 1997; Wurmser et al., 2006). This is unlike the reactions of mothers who are able to identify the communication style of the infant and relieve the child's distress without an increase in their own anxiety levels, thereby reinforcing to the infant that his or her needs are met (Emanuel, 2006). Instead, babies with nonpostpartum-mood-disordered mothers have decreased crying episodes, increased trust in communication, and an increase in security. Over time, this interaction becomes the foundation for the baby to develop the ability to manage his or her own feelings as a toddler, child, adolescent, and, eventually, an adult.

However, there are those infants who find an inner resiliency and give the appearance of not needing adult assistance with developmental maturation. Although some infants experience delayed motor skills development in response to maternal postpartum moods (Cornish et al., 2005), motor skills develop quickly in resilient children. Resilient infants learn that others in their environment will not help provide for their needs and become "self-sufficient and controlling" (Emanuel, 2006). Therefore, these infants prefer not to be held too much by their mother, and reach developmental markers early (sitting up, walking) to compensate for unmet needs through typical mother–infant communication. In reaction, mothers of resilient babies feel unneeded, useless, and inadequate as providers; this further reinforces cognitive distortions in the depressed mother.

Behaviors of Children and Adolescents

Children of depressed mothers may view others as intrusive or appear to others as withdrawn (Field et al., 2006a). For example, three-year-old preschool children exposed to their postpartum depressed mothers' acting injured respond in one of two ways: impatient and angry or distressed and uninterested (Jones, Field, & Davalos, 2000). Children of mothers who had postpartum depression expressed more frequent temper tantrums and showed difficulty interacting with their peers (Civic & Holt, 2000). These children also have difficulty containing or managing sadness, disappointment, fear, and behavioral responsiveness (Civic & Holt, 2000).

Over time, when babies are unable to use different strategies to get their needs met from their mothers, rather than externalizing their behavior, they may internalize or resolve that their needs will not be met, and appear depressed, similar to their mothers (Emanuel, 2006). These toddlers or children may appear difficult to reach and unreceptive to interactive communication with peers, teachers, or other adults. One study found that five-year-old twins of mothers with postpartum depression developed antisocial personality disorder (Kim-Cohen, Moffitt, Taylor, Pawlby, & Caspi, 2005). Furthermore, the mothers' experience of postpartum depression predicted the five-year-olds' antisocial personality disorder more so than a family history of antisocial personality disorder did.

The altered development of cognitive, social, and behavioral skills resulting from impaired mother–infant bonding sometimes results in long-term brain function changes. These delays and skills have been noted in children up to age four (Als et al., 2004; Milgrom et al., 2006). These toddlers and children are sometimes mislabeled as having low IQs due to their interactive styles (Emanuel, 2006; Williams, 1997).

Toddlers of women exposed to highly stressful events during pregnancy are at risk of developing language delays (LaPlante et al., 2004). Children between the ages of four and seven whose mothers showed signs of extreme anxiety levels during pregnancy are two times more at risk for developing behavioral problems (O'Connor et al., 2002b; O'Connor, Heron, Golding, & Glover, 2003; Talge et al., 2007).

PMDs may also influence the development of attention deficit/hyperactivity disorder (ADHD) in childhood and adolescence (Emanuel, 2006; O'Connor et al., 2002b; Talge et al., 2007; Van den Bergh et al., 2005). Van den Bergh and Marcoen (2004) found prenatal anxiety a strong indicator for the development of ADHD symptoms in children between the ages of eight and nine. Other work corroborates this evidence, with the experience of stressful events during pregnancy increasing the likelihood of an ADHD diagnosis twofold (Obel et al., 2003). Male infants of women with postpartum depression or anxiety during pregnancy are more susceptible to cognitive, social, and behavioral development issues, particularly ADHD (Carter, Garrity-Rokous, Chazan-Cohen, Little, & Briggs-Gowan, 2001; Milgrom, Ericksen, McCarthy, & Gemmill, 2006; Murray, Kempton, Woolgar, & Hooper, 1992; O'Connor et al., 2002b; Van den Bergh & Marcoen, 2004). One of the hypotheses for this link is impaired mother–infant interactions. The infant perceives and internalizes the mother's difficulty in identifying and reacting to the infant's needs as hostility or persecution. When a baby retaliates in an attempt to get its needs met (through screaming, crying, kicking, and other means), the baby's perception of hostility and persecution from the mother is internally strengthened (Emanuel, 2006). Over time, a cycle develops where the child externalizes frustration back onto the mother through increasingly antagonistic behaviors in the hope of receiving a response to its needs. These attention-seeking behaviors from the now toddler, child, or adolescent are classified as symptoms of ADHD at times. The child is now labeled for the creative ways of trying to get its needs met, as well as nonverbally attempting to express hurt feelings of hostility and persecution toward the mother due to her mental health symptoms.

As resilient infants grow into toddlers, children, and adolescents, they tend to have difficulty accepting assistance from others. In school, they become "perfectionists," wanting to have all the answers or be "all knowledgeable" about a subject, to not need assistance from other children or adults. For girls, that perfectionist, all-knowledgeable reaction can become the foundation for them to develop perinatal mood disorders when they have their own children. When these children are placed in positions where they need to be taught new subjects or new assignments or need to rely on others to move forward in education, they express frustration and anxiety—often directed toward themselves but nevertheless disruptive in a classroom environment (Emanuel, 2006). To control the situation, they may start to daydream rather than pay attention to the external environment where an individual or teacher is relaying information to them (Emanuel, 2006).

In summary, mood changes during pregnancy and the postpartum period have deleterious effects on infant, childhood, and adolescent development. It is imperative that women receive help for mental health changes to decrease the negative effects on children. However, as will be discussed in more detail in chapters 12 and 13, interventions should also include the child and, at times, the entire family.

References

Akman, I., Kuschu, M. K., Yurdakul, Z., Özdemir, N., Solakoğlu, M., Orhon, L., et al. (2008). Breastfeeding duration and postpartum psychological adjustment: Role of maternal attachment styles. *Journal of Paediatrics & Child Health, 44,* 369–373.

Allister, L., Lester, B. M., Carr, S., & Liu, J. (2001). The effects of maternal depression on fetal heart rate response to vibroacoustic stimulation. *Developmental Neuropsychology, 20,* 639–651.

Als, H., Duffy, F. H., McAnulty, G. B., Rivkin, M. J., Vajapeyam, S., & Mulkern. (2004). Early experience alters brain function and structure. *Pediatrics, 113,* 846–857.

Carter, A. S., Garrity-Rokous, F. E., Chazan-Cohen, R., Little, C., & Briggs-Gowan, M. J. (2001). Maternal depression and comorbidity: Predicting early parenting, attachment security, and toddler social–emotional problems and competencies. *Journal of the American Academy of Child and Adolescent Psychiatry, 40*(1), 18–26.

Civic, D., & Holt, V. L. (2000). Maternal depressive symptoms and child behavior problems in a nationally representative normal birthweight sample. *Maternal and Child Health Journal, 4,* 215–221.

Cohn, J. F., Campbell, S. B., Matias, R., & Hopkins, J. (1990). Face-to-face interactions of postpartum depressed and nondepressed mother–infant pairs at two months. *Developmental Psychology, 26,* 185–193.

Cohn, J. F., Matias, R., Tronick, E. Z., Connell, D., & Lyons-Ruth, K. (1986). Face-to-face interactions of depressed mothers and their infants. In E. Z. Tronick & T. Field (Eds.), *Maternal depression and infant disturbance.* San Francisco: Jossey-Bass.

Cornish, A. M., McMahon, C. A., Ungerer, J. A., Barnett, B., Kowalenko, N., & Tennant, C. (2005). Postnatal depression and infant cognitive and motor development in the second postnatal year: The impact of depression chronicity and infant gender. *Infant Behavior & Development, 28,* 407–417.

Cornish, A. M., McMahon, C. A., Ungerer, J. A., Barnett, B., Kowalenko, N., & Tennant, C. (2006). Maternal depression and the experience of parenting in the second postnatal year. *Journal of Reproductive and Infant Psychology, 24,* 121–132.

Dawson, G., Klinger, L., Panagitotides, H., Hill, D., & Spieker, S. (1992). Frontal lobe activity and affective behavior of infants of mothers with depressive symtpoms. *Child Development, 63,* 725–737.

Dennis, C. L. E., & McQueen, K. (2007). Does maternal postpartum depressive symptomatology influence infant feeding outcomes? *Acta Paediatrica, 96,* 590–594.

DeVries, J., Visser, G., & Prechtl, H. (1985). The emergence of fetal behavior, II: Quantitative aspects. *Early Human Development, 12,* 99–120.

Diego, M. A., Field, T., Hernandez-Reif, M., Schanberg, S., Kuhn, C., & Gonzalez-Quintero, V. H. (2009). Prenatal depression restricts fetal growth. *Early Human Development, 85* (1), 65–70.

Diego, M., Field, T., Jones, N., & Hernandez-Reif, M. (2005). Withdrawn and intrusive maternal interaction style and infant frontal EEG asymmetry shifts in infants of depressed and non depressed mothers. *Infant Behavior & Development, 29,* 220–229.

Dieter, J.N.I., Field, T., Hernandez-Reif, M., Jones, N. A., LeCanuet, J. P., Salman, F. A., & Redzepi, M. (2001). Maternal depression and increased fetal activity. *Journal of Obstetrics and Gynaecology, 21,* 468–473.

Emanuel, L. (2006). Disruptive and distressed toddlers: The impact of undetected maternal depression on infants and young children. *Infant Observation, 9,* 249–259.

Facchinetti, F., Bagnoli, F., Bracci, R., & Genazzani, A. R. (1982). Plasma opioids in the first hours of life. *Pediatric Research, 16,* 95–98.

Ferrando, T., Rainero, I., DeGennaro, T., Oggero, R., Mostert, M., Dattola, P., & Pinessi, L. (1990). ß-endorphin-like and a–MSH-like immunoreactivities in human milk. *Life Sciences, 47,* 633–635.

Field, T. (1985). Attachment as psychobiological attunement: Being on the same wavelength. In M. Reite & T. Field (Eds.), *Psychobiology of attachment and separation.* New York: Academic Press.

Field, T. (1989). Individual and maturational differences in infant expressivity. *New Directions for Child Development, 44,* 9–23.

Field, T. (1995). Infants of depressed mothers. *Infant Behavior and Development, 18,* 1–13.

Field, T., Diego, M., Dieter, J., Hernandez-Reif, M., Schanberg, S., Kuhn, C., et al. (2004). Prenatal depression effects on the fetus and the newborn. *Infant Behavior & Development, 27,* 216–229.

Field, T., Diego, M., & Hernandez-Reif, M. (2006). Prenatal depression effects on the fetus and newborn: A review. *Infant Behavior & Development, 29,* 445–455.

Field, T., Diego, M., Hernandez-Rief, M., Figueiredo, B., Schanberg, S., & Kuhn, C. (2007). Sleep disturbances in depressed pregnant women and their newborns. *Infant Behavior & Development, 30,* 127–133.

Field, T., Diego, M., Hernandez-Reif, M., Figueiredo, B., Schanberg, S., Kuhn, C., et al. (2008). Chronic prenatal depression and neonatal outcome. *International Journal of Neuroscience, 118,* 95–103.

Field, T., Diego, M., Hernandez-Reif, M., Schanberg, S., & Kuhn, C. (2003a). Depressed mothers who are "good interaction" partners versus those who are withdrawn or intrusive. *Infant Behavior and Development, 26,* 238–252.

Field, T., Diego, M., Hernandez-Reif, M., Schanberg, S., & Kuhn, C. (2003b). Pregnancy anxiety and comorbid depression and anger: Effects on the fetus and neonate. *Depression and Anxiety, 17,* 140–151.

Field, T., Diego, M., Hernandez-Reif, M., Schanberg, S., & Kuhn, C. (2004a). Massage therapy effects on the fetus and neonate. *Infant Behavior & Development, 27,* 216–229.

Field, T., Diego, M., Hernandez-Reif, M., Vera, Y., Gil, K., Schanberg, S., et al. (2004b). Prenatal maternal biochemistry predicts neonatal biochemistry. *International Journal of Neuroscience, 114,* 933–945.

Field, T., Estroff, D., Yando, R., del Vale, C., Malphurs, J., & Hart, S. (1996). "Depressed" mothers' perceptions of infant vulnerability are related to later development. *Child Psychiatry and Human Development, 27,* 43–53.

Field, T., Fox, N., Pickens, J., & Nawrocki, T. (1995). Relative right frontal EEG activation in 3- to 6-month-old infants of "depressed" mothers. *Developmental Psychology, 31,* 358–363.

Field, T., & Goldson, E. (1984). *Pacifying effects of nonnutritive sucking on term and preterm neonates during heelstick procedures, Pediatrics, 74,* 1012–1015.

Field, T., Healy, B., Goldstein, S., & Guthertz, M. (1990). Behavior state matching and synchrony in mother–infant interactions of nondepressed versus depressed dads. *Developmental Psychology, 26,* 7–14.

Field, T., Hernandez-Reif, M., & Diego, M. (2006a). Intrusive and withdrawn depressed mothers and their infants. *Developmental Review, 26,* 15–30.

Field, T., Hernandez-Reif, M., & Diego, M. (2006b). Newborns of depressed mothers who received moderate versus light pressure massage during pregnancy. *Infant Behavior & Development, 29,* 54–58.

Field, T., Hernandez-Reif, M., Vera, Y., Gil, K., Diego, M., Bendell, D., & Yando, R. (2005). Anxiety and anger effects on depressed mother-infant spontaneous and imitative interactions. *Infant Behavior & Development, 28,* 1–9.

Giannakoulopoulos, X., Teixeira, J., Fisk, N., & Glover, V. (1999). Human fetal and maternal noradrenaline responses to invasive procedures. *Pediatric Research, 45,* 494–499.

Gitau, R., Cameron, A., Fisk, N. M., & Glover, V. (1998). Fetal exposure to maternal cortisol. *Lancet, 352,* 707.

Glover, V., Teixeira, J., Gitau, R., & Fisk, N. M. (1999). Mechanisms by which maternal mood in pregnancy may affect the fetus. *Contemporary Reviews in Obstetrics and Gynecology,* September, 155–160.

Graf, M. V., Hunter, C. A., & Kastin, A. J. (1984). Presence of delta-sleep-inducing peptid-like material in human milk. *Journal of Clinical Endocrinology and Metabolism, 59,* 127–132.

Hart, S., Jones, N. A., Field, T., & Lundy, B. (1999). One-year-old infants of intrusive and withdrawn depressed mothers. *Child Psychiatry and Human Development, 30,* 111–120.

Hay, D. F. (1997). Postpartum depression and cognitive development. In L. Murray & P. J. Cooper (Eds.), *Postpartum depression and cognitive development in postpartum depression and child development.* New York: Guilford Press.

Hepper, P., Shahidullah, S., & White, R. (1991). Handedness in the human fetus. *Neuropsychologia, 29,* 1107–1111.

Hernandez-Reif, M., Field, T., & Diego, M. (2004). Differential sucking by neonates of depressed versus non- depressed mothers. *Infant Behavior & Development, 27,* 465–476.

Hoffman, S., & Hatch, M. C. (2000). Depressive symptomatology during pregnancy: Evidence for an association with decreased fetal growth in pregnancies of lower social class women. *Health Psychology, 19,* 535–543.

Huizink, A., Robles de Medina, P. G., Mulder, E.J.H., Visser, G.H.A., & Buitelaar, J. K. (2003). Stress during pregnancy is associated with developmental outcome in infancy. *Journal of Child Psychology and Psychiatry, 44,* 810–818.

Jablesky, A. V., Morgan, V., Zubrick, S. R., Bower, C., & Yellachiach, L. A. (2005). Pregnancy, delivery, and neonatal complications in a population cohort of women with schizophrenia and major affective disorder. *American Journal of Psychiatry, 162,* 79–91.

Jones, N. A., Field, T., & Davalos, M. (2000). Right frontal EEG asymmetry and lack of empathy in pre-school children of depressed mothers. *Child Psychiatry and Human Development, 30,* 189–204.

Jones, N. A., Field, T., Fox, N. A., Davalos, M., Lundy, B., & Hart, S. (1998). Newborns of mothers with depressive symptoms are physiologically less developed. *Infant Behavior & Development, 21,* 537–541.

Jones, N. A., Field, T., Fox, N. A., Davalos, M., Malphurs, J., Carraway, K., et al. (1997). Infants of intrusive and withdrawn mothers. *Infant Behavior & Development, 20,* 175–186.

Jones, N. A., Field, T., Hart, S., Lundy, B., & Davalos, M. (2001). Maternal self-perceptions and reactions to infant crying among intrusive and withdrawn depressed mothers. *Infant Mental Health Journal, 22,* 576–586.

Kagan, J., Reznick, J. S., & Snidman, N. (1987). The physiology and psychology of behavioral inhibition in children. *Child Development, 58,* 1459–1473.

Kim-Cohen, J., Moffitt, T., Taylor, A., Pawlby, S. J., & Caspi, A. (2005). Maternal depression and children's antisocial behavior: Nature and nurture effects. *Archives in General Psychiatry, 62,* 173–181.

Klein, D. C., Nambordirii, M.A.A., & Auerbach, D. A. (1981). The melatonin rhythm generating system, developmental aspects. *Life Sciences, 28,* 1975–1986.

Kurki, T., Hiilesmaa, V., Raitasalo, R., Mattila, H., & Ylikorkala, O. (2000). Depression and anxiety in early pregnancy and risk for preeclampsia. *Obstetrics and Gynecology, 95,* 487–490.

LaPlante, D. P., Barr, R. G., Brunet, A., DuFort, G. G., Meaney, M. J., Saucier, J. F., et al. (2004). Stress during pregnancy affects general intellectual and language functioning in human toddlers. *Pediatric Research, 56,* 400–410.

Lee, K. A., & Gay, C. L. (2005). Sleep in late pregnancy predicts length of labor and type of delivery. *American Journal of Obstetrics and Gynecology, 191,* 2041–2046.

Lee, K. A., Zaffke, M. E., & McEnany, G. (2000). Parity and sleep patterns during and after pregnancy. *Obstetrics and Gynecology, 95,* 14–18.

Lundy, B. L., Jones, N. A., Field, T., Nearing, G., Davalos, M., Peitro, P. A., et al. (1999). Prenatal depression effects on neonates. *Infant Behavior & Development, 22,* 119–129.

Maiello, S. (1995). The sound object: A hypothesis about prenatal auditory experience and memory. *Journal of Child Psychotherapy, 21,* 23–41.

Malphurs, J. E., Field, T., Larraine, C., Pickens, J., Pelaez–Nogueras, M., Yando, R., & Bendall, D. (1996a). Altering withdrawn and intrusive interaction behaviors of depressed mothers. *Infant Mental Health Journal, 17,* 152–160.

Malphurs, J. E., Raag, T., Field, T., Pickens, J., & Pelaez–Nogueras, M. (1996b). Touch by intrusive and withdrawn mothers with depressive symptoms. *Early Development and Parenting, 5,* 111–115.

Milgrom, J., Ericksen, J., McCarthy, R., & Gemmill, A. W. (2006). Stressful impact of depression on early mother–infant relations. *Stress and Health, 22,* 229–238.

Mindell, J. A., & Jacobson, B. (2002). Sleep disturbances during pregnancy. *Journal of Obstetrics and Gynecology of Neonatal Nursing, 29,* 590–597.

Mizuno, K., & Ueda, A. (2001). Development of sucking behavior in infants who have not been fed for 2 months after birth. *Pediatrics International, 43,* 251–255.

Monk, C., Sloan, R. P., Myers, M. M., Ellman, L., Werner, E., Jeon, J., Tager, F., & Fifer, W. P. (2004). Fetal heart rate reactivity differs by women's psychiatric status: An early marker for developmental risk? *Journal of the American Academy of Child and Adolescent Psychiatry, 43,* 283–290.

Murray, L. (1988). Effects of postnatal depression on infant development: Direct studies of early mother–infant interaction. In K. Kumar & I. Brockington (Eds.), *Motherhood and mental illness, Volume 2.* London: Wright.

Murray, L., & Cooper, P. J. (Eds.). (1997). *Postpartum depression and child development.* New York: Guilford Press.

Murray, L., Kempton, C., Woolgar, M., & Hooper, R. (1992). Depressed mothers' speech to their infants and its relation to infant gender and cognitive development. *Journal of Child Psychology and Psychiatry, 34,* 1083–1101.

Myers, R. E. (1975). Maternal psychological stress and fetal asphyxia: A study in the monkey. *American Journal of Obstetrics & Gynecology, 122,* 47–59.

Myers, R. E. (1977). Production of fetal asphyxia by maternal psychological stress. *Pavlovian Journal of Biological Science, 12,* 51–62.

Obel, C., Henriksen, T. B., Dalsgaard, S., Hedegaard, M., Linnet, K. M., Secher, N. J., et al. (2003). Does gestational anxiety result in children's attention disorders? *Ugeskr Laeger, 165,* 479.

O'Connor, T. G., Heron, J., & Glover, V. (2002a). Antenatal anxiety predicts child behavioral/emotional problems independently of postnatal depression. *Journal of the American Academy of Child and Adolescent Psychiatry, 41,* 1470–1477.

O'Connor, T. G., Heron, J., Golding, J., Beveridge, M., & Glover, V. (2002b). Maternal antenatal anxiety and children's behavioral/emotional problems at 4 years: Report from the Avon Longitudinal Study of Parents and Children. *British Journal of Psychiatry, 180,* 502–508.

O'Connor, T. G., Heron, J., Golding, J., & Glover, V. (2003). Maternal antenatal anxiety and behavioral/emotional problems in children: A test of a programming hypothesis. *Journal of Child Psychology and Psychiatry, 44,* 1025–1036.

Orr, S. T., James, S. A., & Blackmore Prince, C. (2002). Maternal prenatal depressive symptoms and spontaneous preterm births among African-American women in Baltimore, Maryland. *American Journal of Epidemiology, 156,* 797–802.

Patel, V., Rodrigues, M., & DeSouza, N. (2002). Gender, poverty, and postnatal depression: A study of mothers in Goa, India. *American Journal of Psychiatry, 159,* 1437–1438.

Rahman, A., Iqbal, Z., Bunn, J., Lovel, H., & Harrington, R. (2003). Impact of maternal depression on infant nutritional status and illness: A cohort study. *Archives of General Psychiatry, 61,* 946–952.

Rogeness, G., Javors, M., & Pliszka, S. (1992). Neurochemistry and child and adolescent psychology. *Journal of the American Academy of Child and Adolescent Psychiatry, 31,* 765–781.

Sahota, P. K., Jain, S. S., & Dhand, R. (2003). Sleep disorders in pregnancy. *Current Opinion Pulmonary Medicine, 9,* 477–483.

Sandman, C. A., Wadhwa, P., Glynn, L., Chicz-Demet, A., Porto, M., & Garite, T. J. (1999). Corticotropin-releasing hormone and fetal responses in human pregnancy. *Annals of New York Academic of Science, 897,* 66–75.

Santiago, J. R., Nolledo, M. S., Kinzler, W., & Santiago, T.V. (2001). Sleep and sleep disorders in pregnancy. *Annales International Medicine, 134,* 396–408.

Talge, N. M., Neal, C., Glover, V., & the Early Stress, Translational Research and Prevention Science Network: Fetal and Neonatal Experience on Adolescent Mental Health. (2007). Antenatal maternal stress and long-term effects on child neurodevelopment: How and why? *Journal of Child Psychology and Psychiatry, 48*(3/4), 245–261.

Tomarken, A., Davidson, R., Wheeler, R., & Kinney, L. (1992). Psychometric properties of resting anterior EEG asymmetry: Temporal stability and internal consistency. *Psychophysiology, 29,* 576–92.

Tronick, E. Z. (1989). Emotions and emotional communication in infants. *American Psychologist, 44,* 112–119.

Tronick, E. Z., & Field, T. (1986). *Maternal depression and infant disturbance.* San Francisco: Josey-Bass.

Van den Bergh, B.R.H., & Marcoen, A. (2004). High antenatal maternal anxiety is related to ADHD symptoms, externalizing problems, and anxiety in 8 and 9 year olds. *Child Development, 13,* 1085–1097.

Van den Bergh, B.R.H., Mennes, M., Oosterlaan, J., Stevens, V., Stiers, P., Marcoen, A., & Lagae, L. (2005). High antenatal maternal anxiety is related to impulsivity during performance on cognitive tasks in 14- and 15-year-olds. *Neuroscience and Biobehavioral Reviews, 29,* 259–269.

Van Woerden, E., van Geijn, H., Caron, F., van der Valk, A., & Swartjes, A. (1988). Fetal mouth movements during behavioral states 1F and 2F. *European Journal of Obstetrics Gynecology and Reproductive Biology, 29,* 97–105.

Wadhwa, P. D., Porto, M., Garite, T. J., Chicz-DeMet, A., & Sandman, C. A. (1998). Maternal corticotropin-releasing hormone levels in the early third trimester predict length of gestation in human pregnancy. *American Journal of Obstetrics and Gynecology, 179,* 1079–1085.

Wadhwa, P. D., Sandman, C. A., Porto, M., Dunkel-Schetter, C., & Garite, T. H. (1993). The association between prenatal stress and infant birth weight and gestational age at birth: A prospective investigation. *American Journal of Obstetrics and Gynecology, 169,* 858–865.

Weiss, J. M., Demetnikopoulos, M. K., West, C.H.K., & Bonsall, R. W. (1996). Hypothesis linking the noradrenergic and dopaminergic systems in depression. *Depression, 3,* 225–245.

Williams, G. (1997). Reflections on some dynamics of eating disorders: "No Entry" defenses and foreign bodies. *International Journal of Psycho-Analysis, 78,* 927–941.

Wurmser, H., Rieger, M., Domogalla, C., Kahnt, A., Buchwald, J., Kowatsch, M., et al. (2006). Association between life stress during pregnancy and infant crying in the first six months postpartum: A prospective longitudinal study. *Early Human Development, 82 ,* 341–349.

Zanardo, V., Nicolussi, S., Favaro, F., Faggian, D., Plebani, M., Marzari, F., & Freato, F. (2001). Effect of postpartum anxiety on the colostral milk ß-endorphin concentrations of breastfeeding mothers. *Journal of Obstetrics and Gynecology, 21,* 130–134.

_____ Chapter 7 _____

Fathers

Introduction

Several significant societal changes have strongly influenced the functions and roles of men in the family over the last 150 years. Until recently, the father's primary family role was financial provider in a two-parent family (Cabrera, Tamis-LeMonda, Bradley, Hofferth, & Lamb, 2000; LaRossa, 1997). Ten years ago, approximately 25 percent of children lived in two-parent families in which the father's primary role was described as being a monetary provider (Cabrera et al., 2000; Hofferth, 1998). Now, paralleling the concept of "super mom who does it all," fathers are starting to face role-demand conflicts: working, providing for the family, being actively involved in child and family life, co-parenting expectations and responsibilities, and for some fathers, the newly accepted stay-at-home dad and single-dad household (Barclay & Lupton, 1999). Many men who grew up in traditional households, without childhood modeling and encouragement are now expected to take on an active, highly involved, co-parenting roles in child rearing. This uncertainty can create anxiety about parenting and engagement abilities and skills, particularly when the father wants to be involved, affectionate, nurturing, receptive, but who himself had a father who was unengaged, passive and removed.

Several proposed models attempt to understand a father's involvement with his children. One suggests an exposure-based model implying that men who grew up in households where their father was nurturing and involved with their children tend to grow up and want to be involved with their own children (Cabrera et al., 2000; Hofferth, 1999). Another model indicates that men who have a genderless or equality-based view on parenting responsibilities and an emotional connection with his children are also more likely to develop strong father–child interactions and bonds (Cabrera et al., 2000; Gerson, 1993; Hofferth, 1998; Pleck, 1997).

A more comprehensive model elucidated by Lamb, Pleck, Chernov, and Levine (1987) implicates three factors that predict a father's interactions with his child: engagement, availability, and responsibility. Engagement refers to the direct contact that the father and child has. Availability is the child's ability to access his or her father and the presence of the father in the home. Finally, responsibility is the father's ability to provide resources (such as money) and involvement with day-to-day plans for the child (such as medical appointments and after-school activities). Palkovitz (2002) discussed a more recent version of this model. Cognitive, behavioral, and emotional involvement interact with the amount of time fathers spend with their children, the quality of these interactions, and accessibility (proximity) to the children. Characteristics of positive, healthy father–child involvement have been identified over the past 20 years. These include sharing in play, activities, and interests; availability; teaching and supporting education; engaging in discussions and nurturing the child's thinking and cognitive skills; being affectionate and giving emotional support; providing financial support and protection; and engaging in child care and related planning and errands (Amato, 1987; Cabrera, Fitzgerald, Bradely, & Roggman, 2007; Grossmann et al., 2002; Henderson & Berla, 1994; Lamb, 1997; MacDonald & Parke, 1986; McLanahan & Sandefur, 1994; Palkovitz, 2002; Paquette, 2004; Roggman, Boyce, & Cook, 2001).

Postpartum Mood Disorders in Fathers

Depression

Research on postpartum depression in fathers is rather limited. The available information estimates that 5 percent to 32 percent of fathers across the world experience moderate to severe postpartum depression symptoms (Areias, Kumar, Barros, & Figueiredo, 1996a, 1996b; Atkinson & Rickel, 1984; Ballard & Davies, 1986; Gao, Chan, & Mao, 2009; Pinheiro et al., 2005; Rees & Lutkins, 1971; Soliday, McCluskey-Fawcett, & O'Brien, 1999; Wang & Chen, 2006).

Despite much discussion about hormonal influences on the development of postpartum mood disorders (PMDs), these explanations are inadequate to explain the development of the condition in men. A stronger model to understand postpartum depression in fathers is the *diathesis theory*: having a biological predisposition to depression triggered by socioenvironmental stimuli.

A father's proclivity to experience postpartum depression increases when his partner also has postpartum depression (Marks & Lovestone, 1995; Roberts, Bushnell, Collings, & Purdie, 2006). Raskin, Richman, and Gaines (1990) found that nearly one in 10 couples experienced postpartum depression symptoms simultaneously; a more recent study found partner postpartum depression rates as high as 50 percent (Lovestone & Kumar, 1993). Characteristics of spouses that influence the onset of paternal postpartum depression include maternal personality or mental health, unresolved sexual abuse history, and perceiving the infant's temperament as difficult (Dudley, Roy, Kelk, & Bernard, 2001). Fathers with a spouse who has postpartum depression reported decreased marital satisfaction and sex life, and increased worry about parenting, family responsibilities, and household chore responsibilities (Goodman, 2008; Seimyr, Edhborg, Lundh, & Sjögren, 2004). Furthermore, some couples experience postpartum depression simultaneously when the father perceives his spouse as possessing more control, or the father has low levels of social support, and both partners received limited emotional support from each other (Buist, Morse, & Durkin, 2003; Goodman, 2008; Morse, Buist, & Durkin, 2000; Seimyr et al., 2004). Interestingly, men identify their support as that provided to the mother to help the baby (Bradley et al., 2004). One proposed reason for this comorbid experience of depression between partners is that men feel frustrated at not being able to "fix" their partner's depression and confused about what to do to help (Meighan, David, Thomas, & Droppleman, 1999). Preexisting marital discord and dissatisfaction are thought to play a role as well (Harvey & McGrath, 1988).

There Seem Many Apologies Awaiting Trial
~Brangwynne Purcell

I can make nothing up to you
for these first five months of
marriage and wailing
or the emotions
of an eleven year old girl I never knew
and you never knew and would like to forget
You married by default
a demon of fears
and walked into me before we knew better
But it is done

I can make nothing up to you
not by smiles or kisses or compliment
These you hate most from me
when you are thinking
and looking outside of me, beyond
into the nether land of redemption
I cannot reach you when you are there
or bring you home
I live by myself alone
in a book or with a poet
Until it is done

I can make nothing up to you
We will tell our children
stories of courtship
and how mother turned blue upon waking
from the romance
We ought to pretend
for the sake of our little souls
that I am not a mad woman
or one without controls
They will deserve better than
the one who bore them
and will believe what we say
So we will lie
And it will be done

I can make nothing up to you
and wish you not to think me hostile or pathetic
with the coming of age and poverty
I am young, a pre-mature woman
about to love you
Almost ready to be strong
more than beautiful: Heroic
but now
It is not yet done

Traditionally, men took on the role of the primary financial provider in the family. However, as previously discussed, this convention has changed significantly over the past 20 to 30 years. As a couple in today's society, parents both face competing demands for their time and attention. The influence of self, partner, other family member, and cultural norm expectations in conjunction with the pressures of maintaining optimal parenting, working, and interpersonal relationships make it difficult to fulfill any of these expectations adequately. Recall the discussion of Weaver and Ussher's (1997) "Myth of Motherhood" model in chapter 2, where the mother figure is expected to be caring, loving, patient, and ever suffering. I propose that men may suffer a similar plight: the "Myth of Fatherhood," in which the father figure provides financially for the family. In addition, it is expected for men to be the "anchor-stone" of the family and to now take on more of the traditionally feminine roles such as sharing household chores, changing diapers, feeding (formula or pumped breast milk from a bottle), playing, and preparing meals. Men may not mind sharing these responsibilities; however, many of today's men may not have been availed of the early childhood and adolescent rearing skills needed to be successful as a parent as many women have been over the centuries.

In addition, men tend to "want to do it right," want to provide, want to fix, and want to have clear direction on what to do and what not to do. Many men today had fathers who role-modeled how to provide financially, but not emotionally or psychologically. Therefore, despite the desire and increased expectation to share child care and family roles more equally, there is a gap in practical, "how-to" directives to follow, as well as difficulty relinquishing the role of primary financial provider. This is not due to a lack of interest but more to limited societally supported exposure, support, and education.

Given this situation, the father's partner may be the best person to provide guidance and share her expectations of the fatherhood role with him. However, a father's partner who is experiencing maternal postpartum depression is likely to have difficulty communicating these needs to her spouse to provide structured assistance.

Anxiety

In addition to postpartum depression, fathers may express heightened perinatal anxiety and anger (Buist et al., 2003). In 1994, Ferketich and Mercer's small study found that high anxiety levels in fathers predicted doubt in their ability to function in the paternal role. Another small study (half of whom were police officers) examined factors that influenced the development of high anxiety in fathers (Amanti Pollock, Amankwaa, & Amankwaa, 2005). This study found that financial responsibility for the family; work-related pressure, expectations, and stress; and difficulty identifying the infant's needs are the most significant indicators of postpartum stress in fathers. These are similar to findings from Zelkowitz and Milet's (1997) study of stress and support in paternal PMDs.

Other factors indicated in the experience of paternal anxiety are lack of sleep, time-management difficulties, desire to be a "good father," locating and obtaining a safe day care environment, cleaning, and decreased sexual activity. These anxiety-inducing factors are similar to those found by previous researchers, where first-time fathers reported difficulty managing multiple roles and difficulty understanding specific expectations in their roles as father and as husband (Barclay, Donovan, & Genovese, 1996; Bradley, MacKenzie, & Boath, 2004; Hall, 1992).

There is some indication that men experience higher rates of perinatal anxiety rather than depression (Matthey, Barnett, Kavanagh, & Howie, 2001). These high anxiety and depression levels occur in fathers with increased severity during pregnancy and usually decrease postpartum (Field et al., 2006). Heightened anxiety and depression levels during pregnancy may be due to anticipation of changes in lifestyle, roles, financial responsibilities, and the ability to meet these expectations. However, once the baby is born, fathers usually go into "action mode," able to perform caretaking and provider-related tasks.

In Matthey, Barnett, Howie, and Kavanagh's (2003) small study, one in two fathers experienced phobia for the first time in his lifetime after the birth of his child. In addition, pregnancy and childbirth may be the triggering event for the onset of obsessive-compulsive disorder (OCD) in some fathers. In a case study report, Abramowitz, Moore, Carmin, Wiegartz, and Purdon (2001), presented four cases in which fathers describe OCD symptoms developing shortly after the birth of their child. These fathers detailed ruminating thoughts of harming their child or their partner unintentionally; such as shaking the baby, accidentally stabbing the baby and other children in the family, having sexually obsessive thoughts about children, and repeating "rituals" in an attempt to keep the baby safe (checking electrical cords and the oven). Reactions to these thoughts were to avoid the baby and the partner, trying to self-distract from the thoughts, and feeling ashamed of these intrusive thoughts.

Father–Child Bonding

The increased societal acceptance of divorce has increased the number of female, single-parent homes and absentee fathers. This trend fueled father–child involvement research, as children in these households increasingly exhibited adjustment concerns, behavioral problems, peer relationship difficulties, and poor school performance (Amato & Keith, 1991; Biller, 1982; Blankenhorn, 1995; Hines, 1997; Vogel, Bradley, Raikes, Boller, & Shears, 2006). Results from these projects identified healthy and unhealthy father–child bonding characteristics.

A father who is positively involved and nurturing with his child helps the child learn how to regulate emotions, regulate behavioral control, and academically succeed (Cabrera et al., 2000; Furstenberg & Harris, 1993; Gottman, Katz, & Hooven, 1997; Levy-Shiff & Israelashvili, 1988; Nord, Brimhall, & West, 1997). The father's involvement with his child, regardless of whether or not he lives with the child, seems to specifically help the child self-regulate and manage aggressive behaviors (Vogel et al., 2006).

When parent-to-parent interactions are contentious, the benefit of individual parent-to-child interactions diminishes (Cabrera et al., 2000; Cummings & O'Reilly, 1997; Emery, 1994). In essence, family connectedness may be the more important influence on child development (Gable, Crnic, & Belsky, 1994; Lamb, 1986). This is particularly so in the case of two parents simultaneously experiencing postpartum depression. Goodman's (2008) study found that fathers had more difficulty interacting with their infant when their spouse was experiencing postpartum depression. In addition, the way that the mother felt about her interactions with her infant influenced how the father interacted with the infant.

Over the last 20 years, researchers have been paying more attention to the father–child relationship and how this relationship influences childhood development. This growing body of research has shown that the father–child interactions have similar effects on childhood development as do mother–child interactions (Cabrera et al., 2000; Lamb, 1997). For example, just as maternal postpartum depression increases the risk for social, behavioral, cognitive, and emotional difficulties for the child; paternal postpartum depression also increases these risks (Ramchandani, Stein, Evans, O'Connor, & the ALSPAC Study Team, 2005; Ramchandani et al., 2008). In Ramchandani et al.'s 2008 report, 12 percent of seven-year-old children with a father who had depression eight weeks after delivery were diagnosed with a psychiatric disorder; this was twice as frequent as seven-year-old children of non-postpartum depressed fathers. Similarly, children with fathers who have had postpartum depression were twice as likely to develop an oppositional or defiant conduct disorder as their counterparts—even when maternal postpartum depression is controlled (Ramchandani et al., 2008). This same study also found increased risks for seven-year-old children with a postpartum depressed father to develop hyperactivity, peer relationship difficulties, and conduct or behavioral difficulties. Current research on the influence of paternal postpartum depression yields a negative influence on the development of social and behavioral disorders in children, as compared with the influence of maternal postpartum depression, which yields a negative influence on the development of social, cognitive, behavioral, and emotional disorders in children (Murray & Cooper, 2003; Ramchandani et al., 2008; Ramchandani

& Psychogiou, 2009). In the future, more detailed, longitudinal research on the impact of paternal PMDs on childhood development independent of maternal influence is needed (Ramchandani et al., 2005, 2008).

References

Abramowitz, J., Moore, K., Carmin, C., Wiegartz, P., & Purdon, C. (2001). Acute onset of obsessive–compulsive disorder in males following childbirth. *Psychosomatics: Journal of Consultation Liaison Psychiatry, 42,* 429–431.

Amanti Pollock, M., Amankwaa, L. C., & Amankwaa, A. A. (2005). First-time fathers and stressors in the postpartum period. *Journal of Perinatal Education, 14*(2), 19–25.

Amato, P. R. (1987). Family processes in intact, one-parent, and stepparent families: The child's point of view. *Journal of Marriage and the Family, 49,* 327–337.

Amato, P. R., & Keith, B. (1991). Separation from a parent during childhood and adult socioeconomic attainment. *Social Forces, 70,* 187–206.

Areias, M. E., Kumar, R., Barros, H., & Figueiredo, E. (1996a). Comparative incidence of depression in women and men, during pregnancy and after childbirth: Validation of the Edinburgh Postnatal Depression Scale in Portuguese mothers. *British Journal of Psychiatry, 169,* 30–35.

Areias, M. E., Kumar, R., Barros, H., & Figueiredo, E. (1996b). Correlates of postnatal depression in mothers and fathers. *British Journal of Psychiatry, 169,* 36–41.

Atkinson, A. K., & Rickel, A. (1984). Postnatal depression in primiparous parents. *Journal of Abnormal Psychology, 99,* 115–119.

Ballard, C., & Davies, R. (1986). Postnatal depression in fathers. *International Review of Psychiatry, 8,* 65–71.

Barclay, L., Donovan, J., & Genovese, A. (1996). Men's experiences during their partners first pregnancy: A grounded theory analysis. *American Journal of Advanced Nursing, 13*(3), 12–23.

Barclay, L., & Lupton, D. (1999). The experience of new parenthood: A sociocultural analysis. *Journal of Advanced Nursing, 29,* 1013–1020.

Biller, H. B. (1982). Fatherhood: Implications for child and adult development. In B. B. Wolman & G. Stricker (Eds.), *Handbook of developmental psychology.* Englewood Cliffs, NJ: Prentice Hall.

Blankenhorn, D. G., Jr. (1995). *Fatherless America: Confronting our most urgent social problem.* New York: Basic Books.

Bradley, E., MacKenzie, M., & Boath, E. (2004). The experience of first-time fatherhood: A brief report. *Journal of Reproductive and Infant Psychology, 22*(1), 45–47.

Buist, A., Morse, C. A., & Durkin, S. (2003). Men's adjustment to fatherhood: Implications for obstetric health care. *Journal of Obstetric, Gynecologic, & Neonatal Nursing, 32,* 172–180.

Cabrera, N., Fitzgerald, H. E., Bradley, R. H., & Roggman, L. (2007). Modeling the dynamics of paternal influences on children over the life course. *Applied Development Science, 11*(4), 185–189.

Cabrera, N. J., Tamis-LeMonda, C. S., Bradley, R. H., Hofferth, S., & Lamb, M. E. (2000). Fatherhood in the twenty-first century. *Child Development, 71*(1), 127–137.

Cummings, E. M., & O'Reilly, A. W. (1997). Fathers in family context: Effects of marital quality on child adjustment. In M. E. Lamb (Ed.), *The role of the father in child development.* New York: Wiley.

Dudley, M., Roy, K., Kelk, N., & Bernard, D. (2001). Psychological correlates of depression in fathers and mothers in the first postnatal year. *Journal of Reproductive and Infant Psychology, 19*(3), 187–202.

Emery, R. E. (1994). *Renegotiating family relationships: Divorce, child custody and mediation.* New York: Guilford Press.

Ferketich, S. L., & Mercer, R. T. (1994). Predictors of paternal role competence by risk status. *Nursing Research, 43*(2), 80–85.

Field, T., Diego, M., Hernandez-Reif, M., Figueiredo, B., Deeds, O., Contogeorgos, J., & Ascencio, A. (2006). Prenatal paternal depression. *Infant Behavior & Development, 29,* 579–583.

Furstenberg, F. F., Jr., & Harris, K. M. (1993). When and why fathers matter: Impacts of father involvement on the children of adolescent mothers. In R. Lerman & T. Ooms (Eds.), *Young unwed fathers: Changing roles and emerging policies.* Philadelphia: Temple University Press.

Gable, S., Crnic, K., & Belsky, J. (1994). Coparenting within the family system: Influences on children's development. *Family Relations, 43,* 380–386.

Gao, L. L., Chang, S. W. C., & Mao, Q. (2009). Depression, perceived stress, and social support among first-time Chinese mothers and fathers in the postpartum period. *Research in Nursing & Health, 32,* 50–58.

Gerson, K. (1993). *No man's land: Men's changing commitments to family and work.* New York: Basic Books.

Goodman, J. H. (2008). Influences of maternal postpartum depression on fathers and on father–infant interaction. *Infant Mental Health Journal, 29,* 624–643.

Gottman, J. M., Katz, L. F., & Hooven, C. (1997). *Meta-emotion: How families communicate emotionally.* Hillsdale, NJ: Lawrence Erlbaum.

Grossmann, K., Grossmann, K. E., Fremmer-Bombik, E., Kindler, H., Scheuerer-Englisch, H., & Zimmerman, P. (2002). The uniqueness of the child-father attachment relationship: Fathers' sensitive and challenging play as the pivotal variable in a 16-year longitudinal study. *Social Development, 11,* 307–331.

Hall, W. A. (1992). Comparison of the experience of women and men in dual-earner families following the birth of their first infant. *Image: Journal of Nursing Scholarship, 24*(1), 33–38.

Harvey, I., & McGrath, G. (1988). Psychiatric morbidity in spouses of women admitted to a mother and baby unit. *British Journal of Psychiatry, 152,* 506–510.

Henderson, A. T., & Berla, N. (1994). *A new generation of evidence: The family is critical to student achievement.* Washington, DC: National Committee for Citizens in Education.

Hines, A. M. (1997). Divorce-related transitions, adolescent development, and the role of the parent–child relationship: A review of the literature. *Journal of Marriage and the Family, 59,* 75–88.

Hofferth, S. (1998). *Healthy environments, healthy children: Children in families.* Ann Arbor: Institute for Social Research, University of Michigan.

Hofferth, S. (1999). *Race/ethnic differences in father involvement with young children: A conceptual framework and empirical test in two-parent families.* Paper presented at the Urban Seminar on Fatherhood, Harvard University, Cambridge, MA.

Lamb, M. E. (Ed.). (1986). *The father's role: Applied perspectives.* New York: Wiley.

Lamb, M. E. (Ed.). (1997). *The role of the father in child development* (3rd ed.). New York: Wiley.

Lamb, M. E., Pleck, J. H., Charnov, E. L., & Levine, J. A. (1987). A biosocial perspective on paternal behavior and involvement. In J. B. Lancaster, J. Altmann, A. S. Rossi, & L. R. Sherrod (Eds.), *Parenting across the lifespan: Biosocial dimensions.* New York: Aldine de Gruyter.

LaRossa, R. (1997). *The modernization of fatherhood: A social and political history.* Chicago: University of Chicago Press.

Levy-Shiff, R., & Israelashvili, R. (1988). Antecedents of fathering: Some further exploration. *Developmental Psychology, 24,* 434–440.

Lovestone, S., & Kumar, K. (1993). Postnatal psychiatric illness: The impact on partners. *British Journal of Psychiatry, 163,* 210–216.

MacDonald, D., & Parke, R. D. (1986). Parent–child physical play: The effect of sex and age of children and parents. *Sex Roles, 15,* 367–378.

Marks, M., & Lovestone, S. (1995). The role of the father in parental postnatal mental health. *British Journal of Medical Psychology, 68,* 157–168.

Matthey, S., Barnett, B., Howie, P., & Kavanagh, D. J. (2003). Diagnosing postpartum depression in mothers and fathers: Whatever happened to anxiety? *Journal of Affective Disorders, 74,* 139–147.

Matthey, S., Barnett, B.E.W., Kavanagh, D. J., & Howie, P. (2001). Validation of the Edinburgh Postnatal Depression Scale for men, and comparison of item endorsement with their partners. *Journal of Affective Disorders, 64,* 175–183.

McLanahan, S., & Sandefur, G. (1994). *Growing up with a single parent: What hurts, what helps.* Cambridge, MA: Harvard University Press.

Meighan, M., David, M., Thomas, S., & Droppleman, P. (1999). Living with postpartum depression: The father's experience. *MCN: American Journal of Maternal/Child Nursing, 24*(4), 202–208.

Morse, C., Buist, A., & Durkin, S. (2000). First-time parenthood: Psychosocial influences on perinatal adjustment in fathers and mothers. *Journal of Psychosomatic Obstetrics and Gynaecology,* 21, 109–120.

Murray, L., & Cooper, P. (2003). Intergenerational transmission of affective and cognitive processes associated with depression: Infancy and the preschool years. In L. Goodyear, (Ed.), *Unipolar depression: A lifespan perspective* (pp. 17–46). New York: Oxford University Press.

Nord, C., Brimhall, D. A., & West, J. (1997). *Fathers' involvement in their children's schools.* Washington, DC: U.S. Department of Education, Office of Educational Research and Improvement.

Palkovitz, R. (2002). Involved fathering and child development: Advancing our understanding of good fathering. In C. S. Tamis-LeMonda & N. Cabrera (Eds.), *Handbook of father involvement.* Mahwah, NJ: Lawrence Erlbaum.

Paquette, D. (2004). Theorizing the father–child relationship: Mechanisms and developmental outcomes. *Human Development, 47,* 193–219.

Pinheiro, R. T., Magalhaes, P.V.S., Horta, B. L., Pinheiro, K.A.T., da Silva, R. A., & Pinto, R. H. (2005). Is paternal postpartum depression associated with maternal depression? Population-based study in Brazil. *Acta Psychiatrica Scandinavica, 113,* 230–232.

Pleck, E. H. (1997). Paternal involvement: Levels, sources, and consequences. In M. E. Lamb (Ed.), *The role of the father in child development* (3rd ed.). New York: Wiley.

Ramchandani, P., & Psychogiou, L. (2009). Paternal psychiatric disorders and children's psychosocial development. *Lancet, 374,* 646–653.

Ramchandani, P., Stein, A., Evans, J., O'Connor, T. G., & the ALSPAC Study Team. (2005). Paternal depression in the postnatal period and child development: A prospective population study. *Lancet, 365,* 3201–3205.

Ramchandani, P. G., Stein, A., O'Connor, T. G., Heron, K., Murray, L., & Evans, J. (2008). Depression in men in the postnatal period and later child psychopathology: A population cohort study. *Journal of the American Academy of Child and Adolescent Psychiatry, 47,* 390–398.

Raskin, V. D., Richman, J. A., & Gaines, C. (1990). Patterns of depressive symptoms in expectant and new parents. *American Journal of Psychiatry, 147,* 658–660.

Rees, W. D., & Lutkins, S. G. (1971). Parental depression before and after childbirth: An assessment with the Beck Depression Inventory. *Journal of the Royal College of General Practitioners, 21*(102), 26–31.

Roberts, S. L., Bushnell, J. A., Collings, S. C., & Purdie, G. L. (2006). Psychological health of men with partners who have post-partum depression. *Australian and New Zealand Journal of Psychiatry, 40,* 704–711.

Roggman, L. A., Boyce, L. K., & Cook, J. (2001). Widening the lens: Viewing fathers in infants' lives. In H. E. Fitzgerald, K. H. Karraker, & T. Luster (Eds.), *Infant development: Ecological perspectives.* New York: Routledge Falmer.

Seimyr, L., Edhborg, M., Lundh, W., & Sjögren, B. (2004). In the shadow of maternal depressed mood: Experiences of parenthood during the first year after childbirth. *Journal of Psychosomatic Obstetrics & Gynecology, 25,* 23–34.

Soliday, E., McClusky-Fawcett, K., & O'Brien, M. (1999). Postpartum affect and depressive symptoms in mothers and fathers. *American Journal of Orthopsychiatry, 69,* 30–39.

Vogel, C. A., Bradley, R. H., Raikes, H. H., Boller, K., & Shears, J. K. (2006). Relation between father connectedness and child outcomes. *Parenting: Science & Practice, 6*(2/3), 189–209.

Wang, S. Y., & Chen, C. H. (2006). Psychosocial health of Taiwanese postnatal husbands and wives. *Journal of Psychosomatic Research, 60,* 303–307.

Zelkowitz, P., & Milet, T. H. (1997). Stress and support as related to postpartum paternal mental health and perceptions of the infant. *Infant Mental Health Journal, 18,* 424–435.

_____ Chapter 8 _____

Spontaneous and Elective Abortion and Mood Concerns

Spontaneous Abortion

Every year, 600,000 women in the United States have a miscarriage (approximately one in six pregnancies) and 26,000 women will have a still-birth (American Pregnancy Association, 2009; Hemminki, 1998). During a spontaneous abortion (miscarriage), the woman experiences discomfort and bleeding, increasing the incidence of infections and embolisms, as the fetus is "birthed" (Saraiya et al., 1999). Hemorrhage-related complications are the second leading cause of death from miscarriages in the United States (Peloggia et al., 2006; Saraiya et al., 1999).

Despite the fairly common incidence of miscarriage, it was not until the early 1980s that bereavement was associated with the experience. Prior to this, miscarriage was viewed simply as a medical event, and accompanying grief and loss for the couple was neglected (Neugebauer & Ritsher, 2005). Since then, research on spontaneous abortion has shown that many women experience depressed symptoms for weeks to months afterward and sometimes develop major depressive disorder (Cordle & Prettyman, 1994; Neugebauer & Ritsher, 2005; Neugebauer et al., 1992a, 1992b; Neugebauer et al., 1997; Thaper & Thaper, 1992). Women from lower socioeconomic strata appear to be more likely to experience severe grief following miscarriage (Neugebauer & Ritsher, 2005).

Psychosocial Impacts

Prior to the 1990s, women's mental health following a miscarriage received minimal attention from researchers (Lok & Neugebauer, 2007) and was simply treated as a trivial, short-lived event. Even to this day, some families, friends, and professionals diminish the emotional and psychological impact of miscarriage on the mother and her partner, saying things such as, "I had five before I had your husband," or "your grandmother had two miscarriages … just continue to keep trying … it will happen." Evidence now shows that women who suffer a miscarriage are at increased risk of developing mental health symptoms, including depression, anxiety, grief, and guilt similar to the passing of any loved one (Refer to Table 8-1) (Griebel, Halvorsen, Golemon, & Day, 2005; Janssen, Cuisinier, Hoogduin, & de Graauw, 1996; Lok & Neugebauer, 2007; Neugebauer et al., 1997).

These symptoms typically appear shortly after the miscarriage and for up to two years later (Beutel, Deckardt, von Rad, & Weiner, 1995; Janssen et al., 1996; Janssen, Cuisinier, de Graauw, & Hoogduin, 1997; Leppert & Pahlka, 1984; Lin & Lasker, 1996; Neugebauer et al., 1992b; Neugebauer et al., 1997; Thaper & Thaper, 1992). A nationwide, seven-year, longitudinal, Finnish study found that 18 out of the 100,000 women who had a miscarriage that year had committed suicide, compared with six of 100,000 women who delivered a baby (Gissler, Hemminki, & Lonnqvist, 1996). This implies the possibility of a higher risk for the development of post-miscarriage depression, compared with women who have full-term deliveries.

Women most at risk for developing mental health symptoms following miscarriage do not currently have any children and wanted the pregnancy and the baby. Other risk factors include being single or being an older woman who previously miscarried (Friedman & Gath, 1989; Janssen et al., 1997; Lok & Neugebauer, 2007; Price, 2008). Both women and men are at risk for developing depressive symptoms following spontaneous abortions when the baby was seen during ultrasound examinations (Johnson & Puddifoot, 1996). Unlike postpartum depression, post-miscarriage depression does not appear to be linked to marital status, emotional adaptation, occupational status, social class, or infertility history (Forrest, Standish, & Baum, 1982; Klier, Geller, & Neugebauer, 2000; Neugebauer et al., 1992b; Neugebauer et al., 1997; Prettyman et al., 1993; Thaper & Thaper, 1992; Toedter, Lasker, & Alhadeff, 1988).

Research on racial and ethnic differences in cases of miscarriage is difficult to find. Price (2008) found that African American women experienced more miscarriages than women of other races and ethnicities in the study, yet there was no difference between the number of miscarriages and

Table 8-1 Surgical/Medical Procedure, Abortion Type, Procedure, Side Effects

Types	Procedure	Possible Side Effects
Dilation and Curettage (D&C)	• Occurs between 12 to 15 weeks into the pregnancy • Speculum is put into the vagina • Local anesthesia is used on the cervix • Dilation of the cervix is accomplished by cone-shaped rods • A curette is inserted into the uterus • The uterine lining, placenta, and fetus are scraped out using the curette • Cannula is introduced to ensure everything has been removed • Takes approximately 10 minutes • Recovery time in clinic is approximately five hours	• Cramps • Perspiration • Fainting • Nausea • Heavy protracted bleeding • Clotting • Perforated uterus • Injured cervix • Infection • Fever • Pain • Scar tissue
Dilation and Evacuation (D&E)	• Occurs between 15 and 21 weeks into the pregnancy • One day prior, a laminaria will be put into the cervix • 24 hours later, a tenaculum will be fastened to the cervix to uphold the uterus • Dilation of the cervix is accomplished by cone-shaped rods • Tissue is removed from the uterine lining by using a cannula • The uterine lining is further scraped by using a curette • Forceps are used to discard bigger fetal parts • The uterus is then suctioned to ensure all has been removed • Takes approximately half an hour • Recovery time varies and usually occurs in a hospital setting	Side effects two weeks after the procedure • Bleeding • Cramps • Nausea Other possible side effects • Clotting • Perforated uterus • Injured cervix • Infection • Uterine lining injury
Dilation and Extraction (D&X, Intrauterine Cranial Decompression, Intact D&X, Partial Birth Abortion)	• Occurs after 21 weeks into the pregnancy • Laminaria is put into the vagina to initiate dilation of the cervix two days prior to the procedure • Three days later, the woman's water will break • Forceps are used to draw the fetal appendages out of the birth canal • The doctor will cut into the fetal skull and suction the brain matter out through a catheter until the skull caves in • The remainder of the fetus is removed from the woman	Side effects two weeks after the procedure • Bleeding • Cramps • Nausea Other possible side effects • Clotting • Perforated uterus • Injured cervix • Infection • Uterine lining injury • Mental health and emotional adjustment difficulties

(continued)

Table 8-1 Surgical/Medical Procedure, Abortion Type, Procedure, Side Effects (*concluded*)

Types	Procedure	Possible Side Effects
Induced	• Used for pregnancies in which there are medical concerns or health problems in the woman or the fetus • Prostaglandins are put into the vagina while the woman receives intravenous pitocin • Dilation is initiated when laminaria is put into the cervix	Side effects two weeks after the procedure • Bleeding • Cramps • Nausea Other possible side effects • Clotting • Perforated uterus • Injured cervix • Infection • Uterine lining injury
Suction Aspiration (Suction Curetage or Vacuum Aspiration)	• Occurs between six to 12 weeks into the pregnancy • Speculum is put into the vagina • Local anesthesia is used on the cervix • Dilation of the cervix is accomplished by cone-shaped rods • A cannula hooked up to a suctioning machine is introduced into the uterus • The fetus and placenta are suctioned out of the uterus • Takes approximately 10 to 15 minutes • Recovery time in clinic is a couple of hours	• Cramps • Perspiration • Fainting • Nausea • Heavy protracted bleeding • Clotting • Perforated uterus • Injured cervix • Infection • Fever • Pain • Scar tissue

Source: Based on information from the American Pregnancy Association (2006).
Table 8.1: Corresponding Definitions (MedlinePlus Medical Dictionary, 2009)

Cannula: a small tube that is attached to a suction machine at one end and used in the uterus to suck out the placenta and fetus

Catheter: a small tube that is inserted into an incision in the fetal skull to suck out the brain matter

Curette: a device used in surgery to scrape or clean. It has a loop, ring, or scoop at the end.

Forceps: a device that is used to hold onto objects firmly

Laminaria: a type of kelp that is used during abortion procedures for cervical dilation

Pitocin: a medication that is used to induce labor

Prostaglandins: a type of unsaturated fatty acid that functions like hormones and assists in smooth muscle contraction

Speculum: a device that is inserted into the vagina to allow visualization of the cervix

Tenaculum: a device used to hold parts during surgery. It has a hook that is sharp and pointed at one end.

the symptoms of depression for African Americans. In this same research, white/Caucasian and Hispanic/Latina groups did show an interrelationship between the number of miscarriages and subsequent depression. These racial and ethnic differences were small, as was the sample size, so the ability to generalize these findings is difficult.

Depression and Grief

Between 20 percent and 55 percent of women experience depression symptoms following a spontaneous abortion (Janssen et al., 1996; Neugebauer et al., 1992a; Prettyman, Cordle, & Cook, 1993, Seibel & Graves, 1980). Approximately one in three women had depression symptoms immediately following the miscarriage and 40 percent were grappling with severe grief (brooding over the lost baby and pregnancy) two weeks following a miscarriage (Janssen et al., 2006; Neugebauer & Ritsher, 2005). One study found that over half of women who miscarried met the DSM criterion for major depression three months following the event (Garel, Blondel, Lelong, & Bonenfant, 1994). Of the women who were severely grieving, two in three were also symptomatic for depression. Women who had reached the stage of gestation when they could feel the baby moving are most likely to experience severe grief after the miscarriage. Twenty percent of women continued to experience severe grief six months after having the miscarriage. Nearly half (42 percent) of women who miscarry have a history of depression prior to becoming pregnant (Janssen et al., 1996).

In My Black Window
~ *Brangwynne Purcell*

I dreamt once of mansion and beadwork
and the sound of beauty coming through the screen
There was a moon, yellow
and she, my old friend
and too, there was a man
without figure or face
but coiled I think in poppies
picked by little girls

I am newer now than I was then
and washed
Ready for the cross probably
for what my god calls
Walking in Faith
to my demise, my dying

But the road he says is nicer
than I remember
It is clean
and ready also for me

Yesterday was when I wept in my husband's lap
and dreamt my world ending
I was covered
in the work of an old lady's hand
and felt no gratitude for her labour
I was thinking of the roads and the poppies
and the little girls I would bear

after solitude and sinking

Anxiety

Between 20 percent and 40 percent of women report anxiety symptoms following spontaneous abortion (Garel et al., 1992; Janssen et al., 1996; Prettyman et al., 1993). One in 10 women have acute stress disorder symptoms one month after a miscarriage (Bowles, James, Solursh, Yancey, et al., 2000). Over one year after the miscarriage, women continued to experience anxiety and experienced it more frequently than their male partners did (Cumming et al., 2007). Janssen et al. (1996) studied women who miscarried as compared with women who had a live birth. Those who had a miscarriage experienced higher levels of anxiety, somatization, and obsessive–compulsive behaviors up to six months following the event. Women at risk for post-miscarriage anxiety generally have prior mental health histories or other recent negative life events (Broen, Moum, Bödtker, & Ekeberg, 2006).

Between 3 percent and 25 percent of women suffer posttraumatic stress after miscarriage (Bowles et al., 2000; Engelhard, van den Hout, & Arntz, 2001; Lee et al., 1997; Salvesen, Oyen, Schmidt, Malt, & Eid-Nes, 1997; Wisner, Peindl, & Hanusa, 1996). These symptoms diminished over time, with 7 percent of women reporting posttraumatic stress at four months following the event (Engelhard et al., 2001). Common posttraumatic stress symptoms following miscarriage include reexperiencing the event (intrusive thoughts) and avoidance (Engelhard et al., 2001). As a result, these women may miss appointments, may choose not to get pregnant again, and may avoid having sex (Bowles et al., 2000; Engelhard, 2004). Women who have experienced several traumatic events in their lives and who have a propensity to feel lack of control over their emotions are more likely to have posttraumatic stress symptoms following a spontaneous abortion (Engelhard, 2004; Engelhard, van den Hout, Kindt, Arntz, & Schouten, 2003).

In Geller, Klier, and Neugebauer's (2001) study, miscarriage triggered an OCD reaction. Women who express feeling guilt over the miscarriage may ruminate about choices made during pregnancy that could have possibly prevented the miscarriage and fear about the possibility of having a miscarriage again in the future (Griebel et al., 2005; Nikcevic, Tunkel, & Nicolaides, 1998; Tunaley, Slade, & Duncan, 1993).

Effect on the Family

It is important to consider the emotional adjustment of the mother, partner, and couple as a unit (Carter, Misri, & Tomfohr, 2007). Although research is limited, available reports suggest that approximately 14 percent of men who lost a baby due to miscarriage, stillbirth, or sudden infant death express anxiety and depression two months following the death (Vance, Boyle, Najman, & Thearle, 1995). Men feel a sense of helplessness, sadness, and loss (Cummings, 1984; Murphy, 1998; Puddifoot & Johnson, 1997).

Each person in the couple is likely to grieve at varying intensities and durations and express their grief differently. Furthermore, one or both may deny the magnitude of the loss in his or her life personally and as a couple. The most frequent difficulties reported in the couple's relationship following multiple miscarriages are communication and the quality of their sex life (Serrano & Lima, 2006). Men believe it is their duty as the husband to "be strong" and to "be the protector" of the spouse who is grieving the loss of the baby. By doing this, however, these men do not address personal emotional grief and loss related to the miscarriage; rather, these men, repress emotional reactions (Kohn & Moffitt, 1992; Murphy, 1998). In addition, men who take on these roles express feelings of failure when the spouse cries or grieves over the loss (Hutti, 1989, 2005).

Friends and family supports may not address the loss or may try to minimize the effect of the miscarriage resulting in the couple feeling isolated in the grieving experience (Griebel et al., 2005). Women with minimal support from her partner or her social network experience intense grief responses to the miscarriage (Forrest et al., 1982; Friedman & Gath, 1989; LaRoche et al., 1982; Lok & Neugebauer, 2007; Toedter et al., 1988). In addition, women who have difficulty adjusting to marriage have more mental health difficulties following the miscarriage (Beutel et al., 1995; Lee et al.,1997; Lok & Neugebauer, 2007; Stirtzinger & Robinson, 1989).

Most often, women will become pregnant within two years following a miscarriage (Theut et al., 1989). Fantasies and thoughts race through parents' minds once discovering they are pregnant. These fantasies deepen as the fetus develops. As the pregnancy progresses, the fetus moves more and more. These dreams and thoughts solidify, coinciding with increased fetal movements. When dreams, fantasies, and attachment to the growing fetus are shattered by a spontaneous abortion, emotional attachment to future children becomes jeopardized. Children of women who are born AFTER miscarriages are sometimes referred to as the "replacement child" or the "vulnerable child" (Cain & Cain, 1964; Green & Solnit, 1964; Price, 2008). These children are at risk for a dichotomous reaction by the mother, partner, or both because of the following:

1. Attempts to re-create the emotional bonding that was lost when the prior pregnancy was spontaneously aborted, resulting in over-attachment (Perry, 2008); and

2. Emotional distancing from the infant as a form of self-preservation from the affective-pain experienced from the miscarriage (Armstrong, 2004; Côté-Arsenault & Marshall, 2000; Perry, 2008). This can result in insecure or disorganized attachment concerns (Heller & Zeanah, 1999; Perry, 2008).

Women who already have children face a difficult time attending to their needs as well as her personal psychosocial and grieving needs. This conflict has the potential to hinder mother-child attachments (Heller & Zeanah, 1999; Klier, Geller, & Ritsher, 2002).

Interventions

Medical Interventions

Going back to the late 18th century, dilation and sharp curettage (D&C) were the standard treatment for miscarriage to limit bleeding and other physical problems (Hemminki, 1998; Peloggia, Grimes, Lopez, & Nanda, 2006). Today, many doctors continue to prefer surgical evacuation (D&C or suction curettage [using a vacuum]) as the standard of care, particularly if there is evidence that the woman's condition is unstable (Griebel et al., 2005; Peloggia et al., 2006). Some women who do not have a D&C during the spontaneous abortion wind up having an incomplete miscarriage with tissue remaining in the uterus. Ultimately, these women need surgery to remove the tissue, resulting in increased bleeding (refer to List 8.1). Surgical evacuation increases women's health risks. Those women who opt for surgical evacuation are more likely to get an infection, experience physical trauma to the cervix or uterus, or develop scar tissue in the uterus.

The Peloggia et al. (2006) meta-analysis found no evidence to comprehensively support routine surgical evacuation but maintains that *expectant management*, waiting to see if medical intervention is truly needed, is in the best interest of the woman's health. During expectant management, the spontaneous abortion process is viewed as a naturally occurring process rather than a pathological event (Ankum, Wieringa-de Warrd, & Bindels, 2001). The woman receives support through the natural process. She is provided medical intervention as needed to prevent undue suffering or to save her life. Expectant management has successfully helped 82 percent to 96 percent of women avoid surgical evacuation (Ankum et al., 2001; Blohm, Friden, Platz, Christensen, Milsom, & Nielsen, 2003; Geyman, Oliver, & Sullivan, 1999; Griebel et al., 2005; Gronlund et al., 2002; Luise, Jermy, Collins, & Bourne, 2002; Nielsen & Hahlin, 1995; Sairam, Khare, Michailidis, & Thilaganathan, 2001). Women who receive managed miscarriage care experience less mental health complications afterward (Wieringa-De Waard et al., 2002).

In the late 1980s, the Dutch College of General Practitioners, and similar groups in the United Kingdom, Canada, and the United States supported the use of expectant management as the first strategy to use for miscarriage management and has since remained the protocol of choice (Ambulatory Sentinel Practice Network, 1998; Ankum et al., 2001; Dutch Society of General Practitioners, 1989; Everett, 1997; Wiebe & Janssen, 1998). In the aforementioned reports, expectant management occurred in a hospital setting or in the woman's home, monitored by general practitioners and family physicians. Yet, women most often call their gynecologist for symptoms of miscarriage (Engelhard, 2004). The majority of women seen by OB/GYN specialists receive surgical intervention for the miscarriage. Conclusions from Ankum et al.'s (2001) meta-analysis on expectant management compared to surgical procedures found:

1. Women who received surgical intervention after having a completed miscarriage were treated needlessly.

2. Women currently having a miscarriage should be observed through expectant management before other surgical options are considered.

3. Medication to assist the miscarriage did not provide additional assistance but increased gastrointestinal side effects and increased the cost of the event. Women who were provided medication assistance through the miscarriage experienced a decrease in their quality of life (Nansel, Doyle, Frederick, & Zhang, 2005).

Given these risks, each woman should make the choice to allow the spontaneous abortion to complete naturally or to undergo medical intervention (Peloggia et al., 2006). One way to make this decision easier is to conduct a pelvic ultrasound. This painless test detects any remaining tissue that may require surgical treatment (Haines, Chung, & Leung, 1994; Rulin, Bornstein, & Campbell, 1993).

Medication is another method used to aid in the spontaneous abortion process. The most researched medication is mifepristone (Mifeprex), administered during spontaneous or elective abortions up to the first seven weeks of pregnancy (Danco Laboratories, 2009). This medication blocks the hormone progesterone, thereby softening and breaking down the lining of the uterus. Once this occurs, another medication, misoprostol (Cytotec) is administered to cause contractions and complete the evacuation (Danco Laboratories, 2009; Pfizer, 2009). These medications appear to be helpful for some types of spontaneous abortions, but not in others (Griebel et al., 2005); therefore, women should discuss medication assistance with her physician for specific details.

Counseling and Support

Nine in 10 miscarrying women desire follow-up care for mental health symptoms. Yet, only one in three women receive this care from their medical care providers (Nikcevic et al., 1998), and many do not receive the support needed from friends or family (Hackett Renner, Verdekal, Brier, & Fallucca, 2000). Those who do receive care indicate an unpleasant experience and resentment toward the care provided (Brier, 1999; Cecil, 1994; Cuisinier, Kuijpers, Hoogduin, de Graauw, & Janssen, 1993; Friedman, 1989; Lee & Slade, 1996; Lok & Neugebauer, 2007; Speraw, 1994). In interviews with South African mothers who had miscarriages, many women reported experiencing difficulty after the event and wished that members of her support network would recognize her loss, be thoughtful, sensitive, listen to her talk about the experience, and provide affect support (Modiba & Nolte, 2007). These women were unable to find this assistance from health care providers.

Whereas medical professionals spend much of their time focusing on managing the physical risks involved in spontaneous abortion, the woman's and couple's psychological reactions and needs are often left unattended. In the UK National Women's Health Study, women who did not receive a medically related explanation for their miscarriage from a health professional in a supportive and caring manner resorted to intricate searches, attempting to attach meaning to the event (Simmons, Singh, Maconochie, Doyle, & Green, 2006). These women subsequently linked the miscarriage to themselves, their ability to be a mother, and "moral deservedness." Therefore, it is vitally important that medical professionals pay attention to these possible complications (Friedman, 1989; Stirtzinger & Robinson, 1989).

Today, support systems vary and we tend to rely more on external services and mental health providers for support. Several psychosocially based interventions are available to women and their partners who experience miscarriage such as support groups through hospice, hospitals, or other settings. Two national organizations may also assist women and their partners: Compassionate Friends and SHARE Pregnancy and Infant Loss Support, Inc. (Griebel et al., 2005).

Uprising
~ Brangwynne Purcell

What has come
to still these waters
and settle passions
into cave and canyon

A feather lifts, weightless
on the wing
of someone else
Maybe a child
Maybe my child

And so
down below
weighted with womb
and monthly debris
I long for flight

Lift me, child
on your wing
take me again
to my forgotten sky

Or to your sky
of blue and new
Lift me
carrying high this body
that has served you well
And then
let go

Drop your wing
and I will fall
without mass, up
And I will open
fingers, toes, lungs, legs
and breathe a breath
known to trees
and the wild

And falling up
I will see the bottomless-ness
of what lies below and above
and maybe
just maybe
the rose of my glasses
might return

Dead will rise
spirits
souls
mothers
All that has gone before
and not returned
will rise and call out a name
a name of a new born
or unborn
or not-yet-born

And the wind will speak in whispers
as if it too had voice
and I will remember
something bigger
and older
than I

Unfortunately, there is limited information about empirically researched psychosocial interventions for miscarriage (Griebel et al., 2005). One study of 14 women showed a 52 percent decrease in depression symptoms after receiving telephone-based interpersonal counseling for up to six weeks (Neugebauer et al., 2007). Grief counseling and support groups were available to women who had a stillbirth prior to being discharged from the hospital (Lake, Johnson, Murphy, & Knuppel, 1987). These women received follow-up support twice after discharge as well. Both the standard in-hospital support and follow-up support models were helpful in decreasing grief symptoms; however, those with follow-up support showed slightly more improvement than those who received in-hospital support only. A couple of documented projects analyze the effectiveness of nursing-based supportive counseling for women who had a miscarriage. Both showed improved mental health symptoms up to one-year post-miscarriage (Lok & Neugebauer, 2007; Swanson, 1999).

In 2000, the American Academy of Family Physicians recommended topics to discuss with a woman and her partner after experiencing spontaneous abortion (Deutchman, Eisinger, & Kelber, 2000), including the following:

- Assess, acknowledge, and normalize feelings of guilt and grief

- Provide information on how to bring up the topic of the miscarriage with friends, family, and others

- Offer support, comfort, and empathy with a focus on the future

- Provide information and preparation for the "anniversary phenomenon"—or the recollection of the event in the future.

Hutti (2005) has recommended three intervention steps. First, attempt to understand the meaning that the couple has ascribed to the pregnancy and to the loss of the baby. There are varying degrees to which the couple has attached to the baby. Attention may primarily go to the loss of the baby or to the health of the woman, often linked to the connectedness to and significance of the baby in the couple's life at the time of the miscarriage.

Second, assess the degree to which the miscarriage experience was what the couple expected it to be. That is, did the miscarriage proceed as the couple had imagined that it would, or were there complications that made the experience more traumatic for them? The extent of the difference between the actual experience and that which the couple had envisioned will determine the level of frustration, anger, and feelings of being traumatized. The final step Hutti (2005) recommends is to assess the couple's ability to lean on their family, friends, and each other for support through the grieving and healing process.

Elective Abortion

Approximately one in two pregnancies in the United States is unplanned with half of these pregnancies resulting in abortion (Alan Guttmacher Institute, 2002). An estimated 1.3 million abortions are performed annually in the United States (Alan Guttmacher Institute, 2002), with 43 percent of women having at least one abortion before age 45 (Alan Guttmacher Institute, 2002). Every year, twice as many women (1,200,000) experience pregnancy loss through medically assisted termination as compared to women (600,000) who experience spontaneous abortion in the United States (American Pregnancy Association, 2009). There are two types of elective abortion: surgical removal of the fetus and medication-induced evacuation of the fetus.

Unintentional pregnancy can be an extremely anxiety-provoking event, particularly if the woman is young, single, or career oriented. Even in the case of a planned pregnancy, circumstances such as divorce, death of a partner, maternal illness, or fetal health may influence a woman's choice to terminate the pregnancy, thereby increasing stress and mental health conditions (David, 1985; Rubin & Russo, 2004). When combined, the personal response to an unintended pregnancy, the political environment, and the presence of antiabortion activists can have severe repercussions on a woman's mental health (Rubin & Russo, 2004).

Surgical Removal

There are five accepted types of surgical abortion. The types, descriptions, and side effects can be found in List 8.1.

Medication-induced Abortion

Together with a prostaglandine, mifepristone is used to medicinally induce an abortion. Women who use this medicinal approach experienced longer duration and heavier bleeding than those who have the surgical abortion procedure (Hemmerling, Siedentopf, & Kentenich, 2005). Approximately one in three abortions performed in many European countries and China are medicinal in nature (Hemmerling et al., 2005). Several empirically based studies have shown mifepristone and prostaglandine administration to be successful and not dangerous (Ashok, Penney, Flett, & Templeton, 1998; Baird, Sukcharoen, & Thong, 1995; Schaff et al., 2000; Ulmann et al., 1992). The most common side effects of medicinal abortion are abdominal cramping, exhaustion, vomiting, and diarrhea. Interestingly, mifepristone appears to possess antidepressant properties, which may assist in reducing depression symptoms following the abortion

Since it was approved in 1995, the "morning after" pill (levonorgestrel) has seen a big increase in sales when it became available over-the-counter in Norway (Pedersen, 2008b). Although the "morning-after pill" is frequently used, it does not appear to aggregate into the abortion- rate statistics. One study in Norway found that women chose post-coital contraception two times more frequently than surgical abortion (Pedersen, 2007). Those who chose to use levonorgestrel versus surgical abortion differ in several ways. Women who chose the morning-after pill did not indicate any risk factors for use other than the fact that they came from families with high levels of education (Pedersen, 2008b). This is similar to the characteristics of women (higher levels of education and socioeconomic status) who opt for mifepriston-prostaglandine abortions (Bachelot, Cludy, & Spira, 1992; Hemmerling et al., 2005). Women who had surgical abortions, however, shared the following traits: They were found to have more complicated family environments; did not graduate from high school or had poor education;

showed early signs of depression, alcohol abuse, conduct disorder symptoms; and had a higher number of sexual partners (Pedersen, 2007, 2008a).

Psychosocial Impacts

The psychosocial effect of having an abortion due to ethical concerns, religious beliefs, fetal rights, and the mother's situation came to the forefront in the 1970s following the legalization of abortion in many countries around the world (Blanchard, 2002; Chen, 2004; Fergusson, Horwood, & Ridder, 2006; Hemmerling et al., 2005; Major, 2003). In fact, 90 percent of women showed no changes in mental health status following an elective abortion, especially when it occurred during the first trimester (Adler et al., 1992; Bracken, Klerman, & Bracken, 1978; Cohen & Roth, 1984; Faure & Loxton, 2003; A. Lazarus, 1985; Robbins & DeLamater, 1985; Rogers, Stoms, & Phifer, 1989; Stotland, 1992; Zolese & Blacker, 1992). However, a longitudinal, Norwegian-based study of 768 women found that younger adult women were at risk for developing depression following an induced abortion procedure (Pedersen, 2008a). When compared to women who delivered an unwanted first pregnancy, those who had an elective abortion reported fewer depression symptoms (Tanne, 2008).

In fact, research points to elevated depression levels prior to the abortion and a decrease in depression following the abortion. In one study, approximately two in three women felt depressed before having an abortion, which dropped to only one in ten women feeling depressed one month after the abortion (Urquhart & Templeton, 1991). This pattern appears to be similar for women who experience anxiety. In Hemmerling et al.'s (2005) study, approximately 30 percent of women had clinical levels of anxiety prior to the abortion while only about 4 percent showed symptoms of anxiety one month following the procedure. Women who chose medication-induced abortions reported lower anxiety levels compared to those who had surgical abortions (Hemmerling et al., 2005). Interestingly, the degree of support from friends, family, and partner did not predict anxiety or depression levels prior to or following the abortion.

Some research indicates that the mental health effects of having an elective abortion may not appear until a later time. These delayed mental health symptoms include unresolved loss, low self-esteem, and feelings of guilt related to terminating the pregnancy (Ney, Fung, Wickett, & Beaman-Dodd, 1994; Speckhard & Rue, 1992). There is also evidence that having an abortion can increase the risk of a woman developing low self-esteem, anxiety, depression, anger, irritability, substance abuse, and in some instances, bipolar disorder (Cougle, Reardon, & Coleman, 2003; Ferguson et al., 2006;

Reardon & Cougle, 2002; Reardon et al., 2003). Fergusson et al., (2006) examined 520 women from the New Zealand Longitudinal Christchurch Health and Development Study. The women participated in the project from birth through age 25 years. Results found that mental health symptoms were greatest for females who had had an abortion; conversely, mental health symptoms were lowest in those who did not become pregnant. Women (adolescents and young adults) who became pregnant before age 25 were characterized as having experienced socioeconomic disadvantages during childhood, dysfunctional family situations, adjustment difficulties, left child-hood home at an early age, and lived with her partner. Furthermore, women who became pregnant and had an abortion were most likely to experience depression, a greater number of mental health conditions, thoughts of sui-cide, and illegal drug dependency. Anxiety was not significant in women who had an abortion; however, anxiety was higher for women who became pregnant, but did not have an abortion.

Rubin and Russo (2004) hypothesized that women's mental health reac-tions to the abortion are predicated by the woman's intrapsychic factors including personality traits, cognitive patterns, coping mechanisms and resil-iency. These intrapsychic factors interact with situational or environmental factors such as the sociopolitical climate, financial status, and cultural values (R. Lazarus & Folkman, 1984; Russo & Green, 1993). The ways in which the woman manages the integration of intrapsychic factors and situational or environmental factors influences her mental health response to the abortion. These responses range from relief and empowerment to guilt and shame (Rubin & Russo, 2004).

Prior mental health and negative life experiences predict mental health symptoms following abortion (Sit, Rothschild, Creinin, Hanusa, & Wisner, 2007). Although not directly examined in most research, there are indica-tions that women who have prior mental health diagnoses and those who have experienced abuse (childhood physical or sexual abuse or domestic violence) are most likely to have postabortion mental health adjustment difficulties (Rubin & Russo, 2004). One project found that women who had at least one abortion were also more likely to have traumatic histories such as: physical or sexual abuse as a child, in a domestic violence situation, and rape (Russo & Denious, 2001).

There is evidence that some women have posttraumatic stress symptoms during the surgical termination procedure, particularly when

1. anesthesia is not administered correctly;
2. the woman experiences pain during the procedure;
3. the woman sees the fetus following the procedure;

4. the woman perceives the fetus dying; and

5. the woman is aware of blood loss during the procedure (Asmundson, Wright, & Stein, 2004; Osterman & van der Kolk, 1998; Slade, Heke, Fletcher, & Stewart, 1998; Urquart, & Templeton, 1991).

Postoperative PTSD symptoms include nightmares, flashbacks, and intrusive thoughts about the abortion. In one study, these symptoms occur most frequently in women who underwent general anesthesia (Slade et al., 1998), but Suliman et al.'s (2007) study did not find any long-term mental health differences in women who underwent general anesthesia.

Social Supports and Relationships

When abortions were illegal, many women did not discuss their pregnancy or "back alley" abortion decisions with anyone. However, since the legalization of abortion, nearly all women will consult with someone about her choices. Hemmerling et al. (2005) found that 97 percent of women shared the pregnancy and abortion plans with someone close to her.

The Hemmerling et al. (2005) study also found that one in 10 women did not discuss her decision to have an abortion with her partner. Of those women who did, two out of three partners supported her decision to abort the pregnancy and only one in sixteen partners disapproved of her decision. Nearly 50 percent of male partners accompany the woman to the abortion appointment. Approximately 66 percent of women feel reassured by the support of her male partner.

Family members tend to be less involved in the abortion process than the woman's partner. In one study, one in three women alerted family members about her decision to have an abortion and two in three alerted friends (Hemmerling et al., 2005). Generally, women report feeling encouraged and reassured by the family members and friends with whom she shared her decision (Hemmerling et al., 2005).

Sociopolitical Influences

For many women, the decision to either carry the baby to term and keep the child, carry the baby to term and allow the baby to be adopted, or terminate the pregnancy is a difficult one. By the time a woman presents herself to medical professionals, either to discuss abortion or to undergo the procedure, she has probably struggled internally about her decision. She may feel much anxiety and other emotional struggles with her decision yet intellectually is aware that this is the best decision for her, her future, and her relationships.

Unfortunately, individuals with extreme anti-abortion values and beliefs have used intimidation and harassment and have made this medical procedure even more stress provoking and stigmatizing (Rubin & Russo, 2004). These methods become more harmful than helpful. If the intention of these individuals is to protect life, this ought to occur in a loving manner, not in the form of vandalism; attacks on clinics, staff, doctors, and women seeking care; or through murderous attacks. Murdering a doctor contradicts the efforts to prevent the murder of another life—the fetus. Nonetheless, anxious women seeking an abortion need to be emotionally, psychologically, and physically prepared to walk through picket lines, through a barrage of negative slander, and see pictures of unborn fetuses. This, in itself, can be traumatic and result in feeling guilt, shame, or other mental health coping strategies later, and further undermine support-seeking from friends and family (Rubin & Russo, 2004).

Some anti-abortion activists refer to post-abortion syndrome, comparing the emotional aftermath of having an abortion to posttraumatic stress disorder symptoms (Barnard, 1990; Rue, Coleman, Rue, & Reardon, 2004; Speckhard & Rue, 1992). Yet research does not support this. Rather, the research on legal abortion indicates that

- women choose the abortion (which is different from being exposed to an traumatic event where one does not feel in control of the situation);

- abortion is experienced by close to half of the female population by age 45 (different from experiencing a traumatic event that most others in society do not experience); and

- women do not customarily fear for their lives during the abortion (different from experiencing a life-threatening traumatic situation typifying PTSD) (Rubin & Russo, 2004).

What to Do—What Not to Do

Social workers and other helping professionals need to assess a woman's coping strategies, particularly in regard to the abortion. Women who perceive the abortion as a temporary situation will most likely fare better following the procedure than will women who perceive the abortion as a traumatic event (Rubin & Russo, 2004). When viewed as a temporary situation, women are more likely to use their support network and have high self-efficacy in the ability to cope with the abortion. Using these "tools" to manage emotions and physical responses to the abortion will assist in the transition to life as it was prior to the abortion. Women who view the abortion as a trauma are more likely to alienate themselves from support networks, feel shame and guilt about the decision (Russo, 1992), and recall previous traumatic events or emotional reactions to these traumatic events, thereby having a more difficult time with mental health adjustment after the procedure (Rubin & Russo, 2004).

In response to the sociopolitical climate and for those who perceive the abortion as traumatic, social workers and other helping professionals need to take an empowering and strength-focused stance. Take time to acknowledge and speak to her internalization of societal labels and environmentally encouraged feelings of shame and guilt. Encourage her to express these feelings and make statements (positive reframe) to counteract these negative messages (Cozzarelli & Major, 1998; Major et al., 1998; Rubin & Russo, 2004).

Assessment of the woman's support system and her ability to use these supports is crucial to the adjustment process following an abortion. Sometimes women feel so much shame and guilt about becoming pregnant and having had the abortion that they will not speak to anyone or will speak to a limited few, who may or may not offer support. Other women may have been talked into or threatened to have the abortion by their partner, family members, or friends, which can influence their reliance on these individuals, all while adjusting to their emotional responses after the abortion (Alder et al., 1990, 1992; Lemkau, 1988; Rubin & Russo, 2004; Russo & Pope, 1993).

Although at face value, offering support groups to assist women through postabortion adjustment sounds promising, the evidence suggests just the opposite. One study regarding support groups that provide a venue to vent feelings and encourage event recall was found to be more damaging than helpful (Nolen-Hoeksema, 1987). However, the concept of a psychotherapeutic and cognitively based group treatment model may provide more positive results. This type of group, for women adjusting from having an abortion, has yet to be tested.

Social workers and mental health professionals need to be mindful of their own values, beliefs, and morals regarding the abortion issue. When working with postabortion women, it is imperative to avoid expressing personal prejudices through body language, tone, and statements. Personal prejudices may become internalized, coupled with sociopolitical stigmatization and statements made by others in her life, thereby increasing the likelihood of a more difficult mental health adjustment. Instead of focusing attention on the abortion event and personal values related to abortion itself, social work practitioners should focus on the biopsychosocial concerns that the woman had prior to making the decision to have the abortion. Topics such as finances, unsupportive partners, making a selfish decision, health concerns, going against cultural beliefs or values, and feelings of guilt because she felt relief after an abortion tend to be the most important mental health components to postabortion adjustment rather than judging the abortion procedure (Rubin & Russo, 2004). It was found that, to assist a woman in her mental health adjustment, it was best to offer strengths-based support. These include supporting her ability to make the decision, increased empowerment and control, and supporting a decision that was made in the best interest of the potential child.

References

Alan Guttmacher Institute. (2002). *Induced abortion: Facts in brief.* New York: Author.

Alder, N. E., David, H. P., Major, B. N., Roth, S. H., Russo, N. F., & Wyatt, G. E. (1990). Psychological responses after abortion. *Science, 248,* 41–44.

Alder, N. E., David, H. P., Major, B. N., Roth, S. H., Russo, N. F., & Wyatt, G. E. (1992). Psychological factors in abortion: A review. *American Psychologist, 47,* 1194–1204.

Ambulatory Sentinel Practice Network. (1998). Spontaneous abortion in primary care. *Journal of the American Board of Family Practice, 1,* 15–23.

American Pregnancy Association. (2006). *Surgical abortion procedures.* Retrieved from http://www.americanpregnancy.org/unplannedpregnancy/surgicalabortions.html

American Pregnancy Association. (2009). *Statistics.* Retrieved from http://www.americanpregnancy.org/main/statistics.html

Ankum, W. M., Wieringa-De Waard, M., & Bindels, P. J. (2001). Management of spontaneous miscarriage in the first trimester: An example of putting informed shared decision making into practice. *British Medical Journal, 322,* 1343–1346.

Armstrong, D. S. (2004). Impact of prior perinatal loss on subsequent pregnancies. *Journal of Gynecological and Neonatal Nursing, 33,* 765–773.

Ashok, P. W., Penney, G. C., Flett, G. M., & Templeton, A. (1998). An effective regimen for early medical abortion: A report of 2000 consecutive cases. *Human Reproduction, 13,* 2962–2965.

Asmundson, G.J.G., Wright, K. D., & Stein, M. B. (2004). Pain and PTSD symptoms in female veterans. *European Journal on Pain, 8,* 345–350.

Bachelot, A., Cludy, L., & Spira, A. (1992). Conditions for choosing between drug-induced and surgical abortions. *Contraception, 45,* 547–559.

Baird, D. T., Sukcharoen, N., & Thong, K. J. (1995). Randomized trial of misoprostol and cergem in combination with a reduced dose of mifepristone for induction of abortion. *Human Reproduction, 10,* 1521–1527.

Barnard, C. (1990). *The long-term psychological effects of abortion.* Portsmouth, NH: Institute for Pregnancy Loss.

Beutel, M., Deckardt, R., von Rad, M., & Weiner, H. (1995). Grief and depression after miscarriage: Their separation, antecedents, and course. *Journal of Psychosomatic Medicine, 57,* 517–526.

Blanchard, D. A. (2002). Depression and unintended pregnancy in young women. Readers should bear in mind potential conflict of interest. *British Medical Journal, 324,* 1097; author reply, 1097–1098.

Blohm, F., Friden, B., Platz, Christensen, J. J., Milsom, I., & Nielsen, S. (2003). Expectant management of first-trimester miscarriage in clinical practice. *Acta Obstetrica et Gynecologica Scandinavica, 82,* 654–658.

Bowles, S. V., James, L. C., Solursh, D. S., Yancey, M. K., Epperly, T. D., Folen, R. A., & Masone, M. (2000). Acute and post-traumatic stress disorder after spontaneous abortion. *American Family Physician, 61,* 1689–1697.

Bracken, M. B., Klerman, L. V., & Bracken, M. (1978). Abortion, adoption, or motherhood: An empirical study of decision-making during pregnancy. *American Journal of Obstetrics & Gynecology, 130,* 251–262.

Brier, N. (1999). Understanding and managing the emotional reactions to a miscarriage. *Obstetrics & Gynecology, 93,* 151–155.

Broen, A. N., Moum, T., Bödtker, A. S., & Ekeberg, O. (2006). Predictors of anxiety and depression following pregnancy termination: A longitudinal five-year follow-up study. *Acta Obstetricia et Gynecologica, 85,* 317–323.

Cain, A. C., & Cain, B. S. (1964). On replacing a child. *Journal of the American Academy of Child Psychiatry, 3,* 443–455.

Cannula. (2009). In *MedlinePlus medical dictionary.* Retrieved from Price, S. K. (2008). Stepping back to gain perspective: Pregnancy loss history, depression, and parenting capacity in the early childhood longitudinal study, birth cohort (ECLS-B). *Death Studies, 32,* 97–122.

Carter, D., Misri, S., & Tomfohr, L. (2007). Psychologic aspects of early pregnancy loss. *Clinical Obstetrics and Gynecology, 50,* 154–165.

Cecil, R. (1994). Miscarriage: Women's views of care. *Journal of Reproduction and Infant Psychology, 12,* 21–30.

Chen, J. (2004). *Campaign 2004: Huge abortion rights rally in DC.* CBSNEWS.com. Retrieved from www.cbsnews.com/stories/2004/02/09/politics/main598867.shtml

Cohen, L., & Roth, S. (1984). Coping with abortion. *Journal of Human Stress, 10*(3), 140–145.

Cordle, C. J., & Prettyman, R. J. (1994). A 2-year follow-up of women who have experienced early miscarriage. *Journal of Reproductive and Infant Psychology, 12,* 37–43.

Côté-Arsenault, D., & Marshall, R. (2000). One foot in-one foot-out: Weathering the storm of parenting after pregnancy loss. *Research in Nursing and Health, 23,* 473–485.

Cougle, J. R., Reardon, D. C., & Coleman, P. K. (2003). Depression associated with abortion and childbirth: A long-term analysis of the NLSY cohort. *Medical Science Monitor, 9,* CR105–CR112.

Cozzarelli, C., & Major, B. (1998). The impact of antiabortion activities on women seeking abortions. In L. J. Beckman & S. M. Harvey (Eds.), *The new civil war: The psychology, culture, and politics of abortion* (pp. 81–104). Washington, DC: American Psychological Association.

Cuisinier, M. C., Kuijpers, J. C., Hoogduin, C. A., de Graauw, C.P.H.M., & Janssen, H.J.E.M. (1993). Miscarriage and stillbirth: Time since the loss, grief intensity and satisfaction with care. *European Journal of Obstetrics & Gynecology and Reproductive Biology, 52*(3), 163–168.

Cumming, G. P., Klein, S., Bolsover, D., Lee, A. J., Alexander, D. A., Maclean, M., & Jurgens, J. D. (2007). The emotional burden of miscarriage for women and their partners: Trajectories of anxiety and depression over 13 months. *British Journal of Obstetrics and Gynecology, 114,* 1138–1145.

Cummings, D. D. (1984). The effects of miscarriage on a man. *Emotional First Aid, 1,* 47–50.

Danco Laboratories. (2009). *Mifeprex: The early option pill to end pregnancy.* Retrieved from http://www.earlyoptionpill.com/

David, H. P. (1985). Post-abortion and post-partum psychiatric hospitalization. *CIBA Foundation Symposium, 115,* 150–164.

Deutchman, M., Eisinger, S., & Kelber, M. (2000). First trimester pregnancy complications. In *ALSO: Advanced life support in obstetrics course syllabus* (4th ed., pp. 1–27). Leawood, KS: American Academy of Family Physicians.

Dutch Society of General Practitioners. (1989). Practice guideline (threatened) miscarriage [in Dutch]. *Huis Wetensch, 32,* 138–143.

Engelhard, I. M. (2004). Miscarriage as a traumatic event. *Clinical Obstetrics and Gynecology,* 547–551.

Engelhard, I., van den Hout, M., & Arntz, A. (2001). Posttraumatic stress disorder after pregnancy loss. *General Hospital Psychiatry, 61,* 1689–1697.

Engelhard, I. M., van den Hout, M. A., Kindt, M., Arntz, A., & Schouten, E. (2003). Peritraumatic dissociation and posttraumatic stress after pregnancy loss: A prospective study. *Behavioral Research and Therapy, 41,* 67–78.

Everett, C. (1997). Incidence and outcome of bleeding before the 20th week of pregnancy: Prospective study from general practice. *British Medical Journal, 315,* 32–34.

Faure, S., & Loxton, H. (2003). Anxiety, depression and self-efficacy levels of women undergoing first trimester abortion. *South African Journal of Psychology, 33*(1), 28–38.

Fergusson, D. M., Horwood, L. J., & Ridder, E. M. (2006). Abortion in young women and subsequent mental health. *Journal of Child Psychology and Psychiatry, 47,* 16–24.

Forrest, G. C., Standish, E., & Baum, J. D. (1982). Support after perinatal death: A study of support and counseling after perinatal bereavement. *British Medical Journal, 285,* 1475–1479.

Friedman, T. (1989). Women's experience of general practitioner management of miscarriage. *Journal of the Royal College of General Practice, 39,* 456–458.

Friedman, T., & Gath, D. (1989). The psychiatric consequences of spontaneous abortion. *British Journal of Psychiatry, 155,* 810–813.

Garel, M., Blondel, B., Lelong, N., & Bonenfant, S. (1994). Long-term consequences of miscarriage: The depressive disorders and the following pregnancy. *Journal of Reproductive and Infant Psychology, 124,* 233–240.

Geller, P. A., Klier, C. M., & Neugebauer, R. (2001). Anxiety disorders following miscarriage. *Journal of Clinical Psychiatry, 62,* 432–438.

Geyman, J. P., Oliver, L. M., & Sullivan, S. D. (1999). Expectant medical or surgical treatment of spontaneous abortion in first trimester of pregnancy? A pooled quantitative literature evaluation. *Journal of the American Board of Family Practice, 12,* 55–64.

Gissler, M., Hemminki, E., & Lonnqvist, J. (1996). Suicides after pregnancy in Finland, 1987–94: Register linkage study. *British Medical Journal, 313,* 1431–1434.

Green, M., & Solnit, A. (1964). Reactions to the threatened loss of a child: A vulnerable child syndrome. *Pediatrics, 34,* 58–66.

Griebel, C. P., Halvorsen, J., Golemon, T. B., & Day, A. A. (2005). Management of spontaneous abortion. *American Family Physician, 72,* 1243–1250.

Gronlund, L., Gronlund, A. L., Clevin, L., Andersen, B., Palmgren, N., & Lidegaard, O. (2002). Spontaneous abortion: Expectant management, medical treatment or surgical evacuation. *Acta Obstetricia et Gynecologica Scandinavica, 84,* 761–766.

Hackett Renner, C., Verdekal, S., Brier, S., & Gallucca, G. (2000). The meaning of miscarriage to others: Is it an unrecognized loss? *Journal of Personal & Interpersonal Loss, 5*(1), 65–76.

Haines, C. J., Chung, T., & Leung, D. Y. (1994). Transvaginal sonography and the conservative management of spontaneous abortion. *Gynecologic and Obstetric Investigation, 37,* 14–17.

Heller, S. S., & Zeanah, C. H. (1999). Attachment disturbances in infants born subsequent to perinatal loss: A pilot study. *Infant Mental Health Journal, 20,* 188–189.

Hemmerling, A., Siedentopf, F., & Kentenich, H. (2005). Emotional impact and acceptability of medical abortion with mifepristone: A German experience. *Journal of Psychosomatic Obstetrics & Gynecology, 26*(1), 23–31.

Hemminki, E. (1998). Treatment of miscarriage: Current practice and rationale. *Obstetrics & Gynecology, 91,* 247–253.

Hutti, M. H. (1989). *A study of parents' perceptions of the miscarriage experience.* (Unpublished doctoral dissertation). Indiana University at Indianapolis.

Hutti, M. H. (2005). Social and professional support needs of families after perinatal loss. *Journal of Obstetric, Gynecologic & Neonatal Nursing, 34,* 630–638.

Janssen, H.J.E.M., Cuisinier, M.C.J., de Graauw, K.P.H.M., & Hoogduin, K.A.L. (1997). A prospective study of risk factors predicting grief intensity following pregnancy loss. *Archives of General Psychiatry, 54,* 56–61.

Janssen, H.J.E.M., Cuisinier, M.C.J., Hoogduin, K.A.L., & de Graauw, K.P.H.M. (1996). Controlled prospective study on the mental health of women following pregnancy loss. *American Journal of Psychiatry, 153,* 226–230.

Johnson, M. P., & Puddifoot, J. E. (1996). The grief response in the partners of women who miscarry. *British Journal of Psychology, 69,* 313–327.

Klier, C. M., Geller, P. A., & Neugebauer, R. (2000). Minor depressive disorder in the context of miscarriage. *Journal of Affective Disorders, 59,* 13–21.

Klier, C. M., Geller, P. A., & Ritsher, J. B. (2002). Affective disorders in the aftermath of miscarriage: A comprehensive review. *Archives of Women's Mental Health, 5,* 129–149.

Kohn, I., & Moffitt, P. L. (1992). *Pregnancy loss: A silent sorrow.* London: Headway, Hodder, & Stoughton.

Lake, M. F., Johnson, T. M., Murphy, J., & Knuppel, R. A. (1987). Evaluation of a perinatal grief support team. *American Journal of Obstetrics and Gynecology, 157,* 1203–1206.

LaRoche, C., Lalinec-Michaud, M., Engelsmann, F., Fuller, N., Copp, M., & Vasilevsky, K. (1982). Grief reactions to perinatal death: An exploratory study. *Psychosomatics, 23,* 510–518.

Lazarus, A. (1985). Psychiatric sequelae of legalized elective first trimester abortion. *Journal of Psychosomatic Obstetrics & Gynecology, 4,* 141–150.

Lazarus, R., & Folkman, S. (1984). *Stress, appraisal, and coping.* New York: Springer.

Lee, C., & Slade, P. (1996). Miscarriage as a traumatic event: A review of the literature and new implications for intervention. *Journal of Psychosomatic Research, 40,* 235–244.

Lee, D.T.S., Wong, C. K., Cheung, L. P., Leung, H.C.M., Haines, C. J., & Chung, T.K.H. (1997). Psychiatric morbidity following miscarriage: A prevalence study of Chinese women in Hong Kong. *Journal of Affective Disorders, 43,* 63–68.

Lemkau, J. P. (1988). Emotional sequelae of abortion: Implications for clinical practice. *Psychology of Women Quarterly, 12,* 461–472.

Leppert, P. C., & Pahlka, B. S. (1984). Grieving characteristics after spontaneous abortion: A management approach. *Obstetrics & Gynecology, 64,* 119–122.

Lin, S. X., & Lasker, J. N. (1996). Patterns of grief after pregnancy loss. *American Journal of Orthopsychiatry, 66,* 262–271.

Lok, I. H., & Neugebauer, R. (2007). Psychological morbidity following miscarriage. *Best Practice & Research Clinical Obstetrics and Gynaecology, 21,* 229–247.

Luise, C., Jermy, K., Collins, W. P., & Bourne, T. H. (2002). Expectant management of incomplete, spontaneous first-trimester miscarriage: Outcome according to initial ultrasound criteria and value of follow-up visits. *Ultrasound Obstetrics and Gynecology, 19,* 580–582.

Major, B. (2003). Psychological implications of abortion: Highly charged and rife with misleading research. *Canadian Medical Association Journal, 168,* 1257–1258.

Major, B., Richards, C., Cooper, M. L., Cozzarelli, C., & Zubek, J. (1998). Personal resilience, cognitive appraisals, and coping: An integrative model of adjustment to abortion. *Journal of Personality and Social Psychology, 74,* 735–752.

Modiba, L., & Nolte, A. G. W. (2007). The experiences of mothers who lost a baby during pregnancy. *Health SA Gesondheid, 12*(2), 3–13.

Murphy, F. A. (1998). The experience of early miscarriage from a male perspective. *Journal of Clinical Nursing, 7,* 325–332.

Nansel, T. R., Doyle, F., Frederick, M. M., & Zhang, J. (2005). Quality of life in women undergoing medical treatment for early pregnancy failure. *Journal of Obstetric, Gynecologic & Neonatal Nursing, 34,* 473–481.

Neugebauer, R., Kline, J., Bleiberg, K., Baxi, L., Markowitz, J. C., Rosing, M., et al. (2007). Preliminary open trial of interpersonal counseling for subsyndromal depression following miscarriage. *Depression and Anxiety, 24,* 219–222.

Neugebauer, R., Kline, J., O'Connor, P., Shrout, P., Johnson, J., Skodol, A., et al. (1992a). Depressive symptoms in women in the six months after miscarriage. *American Journal of Obstetrics and Gynecology, 166,* 104–109.

Neugebauer, R., Kline, J., O'Connor, P., Shrout, P., Johnson, J., Skodol, A., et al. (1992b). Determinants of depressive symptoms in the early weeks after miscarriage. *American Journal of Public Health, 82,* 1332–1339.

Neugebauer, R., Kline, J., Shrout, P., Skodol, A., O'Connor, P., Geller, P. A., et al. (1997). Major depressive disorder in the six months after miscarriage. *JAMA, 277,* 383–388.

Neugebauer, R., & Ritsher, J. (2005). Depression and grief following early pregnancy loss. *International Journal for Childbirth Education, 20*(3), 21–24.

Ney, P. G., Fung, T., Wickett, A. R., & Beaman-Dodd, C. (1994). The effects of pregnancy loss on women's health. *Social Science and Medicine, 38,* 1193–1200.

Nielsen, S., & Hahlin, M. (1995). Expectant management of first-trimester spontaneous abortion. *Lancet, 345,* 84–86.

Nikcevic, A. V., Tunkel, S. A., & Nicolaides, K. H. (1998). Psychological outcomes following missed abortions and provision of follow-up care. *Ultrasound in Obstetrics and Gynecology, 11,* 123–128.

Nolen-Hoeksema, S. (1987). *Sex differences in depression.* Stanford, CA: Stanford University Press.

Osterman, J. E., & van der Kolk, B. A. (1998). Awareness during anesthesia and posttraumatic stress disorder. *General Hospital Psychiatry, 20,* 274–281.

Pedersen, W. (2007). Abortion or postcoital contraception? A longitudinal study of young women [in Norwegian]. *Tidsskr Nor Laegeforen, 127,* 3206–3209.

Pedersen, W. (2008a). Abortion and depression: A population-based longitudinal study of young women. *Scandinavian Journal of Public Health, 36,* 424–428.

Pedersen, W. (2008b). Emergency contraception: Why the absent effect on abortion rates? *Acta Obstetrica et Gynecologica, 87*(2), 132–133.

Peloggia, N. K., Grimes, D. A., Lopez, L. M., & Nanda, G. (2006). Expectant care versus surgical treatment for miscarriage. *Cochrane Database of Systematic Reviews, 2,* CD003518. DOI: 10.1002/14651858. CD003518.pub2.

Pfizer. (2009). *Pfizer products: Cytotec (misoprostol tablets).* Retrieved from http://www.pfizer.com/products/rx/rx_product_cytotec.jsp

Prettyman, R. J., Cordle, C. J., & Cook, G. D. (1993). A three-month follow-up of psychological morbidity after early miscarriage. *British Journal of Medical Psychology, 66,* 363–372.

Puddifoot, J. E., & Johnson, M. P. (1997). The legitimacy of grieving: The partner's experience at miscarriage. *Social Science Medicine, 45,* 837–845.

Reardon, D. C., & Cougle, J. R. (2002). Depression and unintended pregnancy in the National Longitudinal Survey of Youth: A cohort study. *British Medical Journal, 324,* 151–152.

Reardon, D. C., Cougle, J. R., Rue, V. M., Shuping, M. W., Coleman, P. K., & Ney, P. G. (2003). Psychiatric admissions of low-income women following abortion and childbirth. *Canadian Medical Association Journal, 168,* 1253–1256.

Robbins, J. M., & DeLamater, J. D. (1985). Support from significant others and loneliness following induced abortion. *Social Psychiatry, 20*(2), 92–99.

Rogers, J. L., Stoms, G. B., & Phifer, J. L. (1989). Psychological impact of abortion: Methodological and outcomes summary of empirical research between 1966 and 1988. *Health Care for Women International, 10,* 347–376.

Rubin, L., & Russo, N. F. (2004). Abortion and mental health: What therapists need to know. *Women & Therapy, 27*(3/4), 69–90.

Rue, V. M., Coleman, P. K., Rue, J. J., & Reardon, D. C. (2004). Induced abortion and traumatic stress: A preliminary comparison of American and Russian women. *Medical Science Monitor, 10*(10), SR5–SR16.

Rulin, M. C., Bornstein, S. G., & Campbell, J. D. (1993). The reliability of ultrasonography in the management of spontaneous abortion, clinically thought to be complete: A prospective study. *American Journal of Obstetrics and Gynecology, 168,* 12–15.

Russo, N. F. (1992). Psychological aspects of unwanted pregnancy and its resolution. In J. D. Butler & D. F. Walbert (Eds.), *Abortion, medicine and the law* (4th ed., pp. 593–626). New York: Facts on File.

Russo, N. F., & Denious, J. E. (2001). Violence in the lives of women having abortions: Implications for public policy and practice. *Professional Psychology: Research and Practice, 32,* 142–150.

Russo, N. F., & Green, B. L. (1993). Women and mental health. In F. L. Denmark & M. A. Paludi (Eds.), *Psychology of women: A handbook of issues and theories* (pp. 379–436). Westport, CT: Greenwood Press.

Russo, N. F., & Pope, L. (1993). *Implications of violence against women for reproductive health: Focus on abortion services.* Paper presented at the Conference on Psychology and Women's Health: Creating a Psychosocial Agenda for the 21st Century, Washington, DC.

Sairam, S., Khare, M., Michailidis, G., & Thilaganathan, B. (2001). The role of ultrasound in the expectant management of early pregnancy loss. *Ultrasound in Obstetrics and Gynecology, 17,* 506–509.

Salvesen, K., Oyen, L., Schmidt, N., Malt, U., & Eid-Nes, S. (1997). Comparison of long-term psychological responses of women after pregnancy termination due to fetal anomalies and after perinatal loss. *Ultrasound Obstetrics and Gynecology, 9,* 80–85.

Saraiya, M., Green, C. A., Berg, C. J., Hopkins, F. W., Koonin, L. M., & Atrash, H. K. (1999). Spontaneous abortion–related deaths among women in the United States—1981–1991. *Obstetrics & Gynecology, 94,* 172–176.

Schaff, E. A., Fielding, S. L., Westhoff, C., Ellerston, C., Eisinger, S. H., Stadalius, L. S., & Fuller, S. (2000). Vaginal misoprostol administered 1, 2, or 3 days after mifepristone for early medical abortion. *JAMA, 284,* 1948–1953.

Seibel, M., & Graves, W. L. (1980). The psychological implications of spontaneous abortions. *Journal of Reproductive Medicine, 25,* 161–165.

Serrano, F., & Lima, M. L. (2006). Recurrent miscarriage: Psychological and
relational consequences for couples. *Psychology and Psychotherapy: Theory,
Research and Practice, 79,* 585–594.

Simmons, R. K., Singh, G., Maconochie, N., Doyle, P., & Green, J. (2006).
Experience of miscarriage in the UK: Qualitative findings from the
National Women's Health Study. *Social Science & Medicine, 63,* 1934–1946.

Sit, D., Rothschild, A. J., Creinin, M. C., Hanusa, B. H., & Wisner, K. L.
(2007). Psychiatric outcomes following medical and surgical abortion.
Human Reproduction, 22, 878–884.

Slade, P., Heke, S., Fletcher, J., & Stewart, P. (1998). A comparison of medical
and surgical termination of pregnancy: Choice, psychological consequences and satisfaction with care. *British Journal of Obstetrics and Gynaecology, 105,* 1288–1295.

Speckhard, A. C., & Rue, V. M. (1992). Postabortion syndrome: An emerging
public health concern. *Journal of Social Issues, 48,* 95–119.

Speraw, S. R. (1994). The experience of miscarriage: How couples define
quality in health care delivery. *Journal of Perinatology, 14,* 208–215.

Stirtzinger, R. M., & Robinson, G. E. (1989). The psychological effects of
spontaneous abortion. *Canadian Medical Association Journal, 140,* 799–806.

Stotland, N. (1992). The myth of the abortion trauma syndrome. *JAMA,
268,* 2078–2079.

Suliman, S., Ericksen, T., Labuschgne, P., de Wit, R., Stein, D. J., & Seedat, S.
(2007). Comparison of pain, cortisol levels, and psychological distress in
women undergoing surgical termination of pregnancy under local anesthesia versus intravenous sedation. *BioMed Central Psychiatry, 7*(24), 1–9.

Swanson, K. M. (1999). Effects of caring, measurement, and time on miscarriage impact and women's well-being. *Nursing Research, 48,* 288–298.

Tanne, J. H. (2008). Abortion does not cause mental health problems, says
review. *British Medical Journal, 337,* 1374–1375.

Thaper, A. K., & Thaper, A. (1992). Psychological sequelae of miscarriage: A
controlled study using the General Health Questionnaire and the Hospital
Anxiety and Depression Scale. *British Journal of General Practice, 42,* 94–96.

Theut, S. K., Pedersen, F. A., Zaslow, M. J., Cain, R. L., Rabinovich, B. A., &
Morihisa, J. M. (1989). Perinatal loss and parental bereavement. *American
Journal of Psychiatry, 146,* 635–639.

Toedter, L. J., Lasker, J. N., & Alhadeff, J. M. (1988). The Perinatal Grief Scale:
Development and initial validation. *American Journal of Orthopsychiatry,
58,* 435–449.

Tunaley, J. R., Slade, P., & Duncan, S. B. (1993). Cognitive processes in psychological adaptation to miscarriage: A preliminary report. *Psychological Health, 8,* 369–381.

Ulmann, A., Silvestre, L., Chemama, L., Rezvani, &., Renault, M., Aguillaume, C. J., & Baulieu, E. E. (1992). Medical termination of early pregnancy with mifepristone (RU 486) followed by a prostaglandin analogue: Study in 16,369 women. *Acta Obstetricia et Gynecologica Scandinavica, 71*(4), 278–283.

Urquhart, D. R., & Templeton, A. A. (1991). Psychiatric morbidity and acceptability following medical and surgical methods of induced abortion. *British Journal of Obstetrics and Gynaecology, 98,* 396–399.

Vance, J. C., Boyle, F. M., Najman, J. M., & Thearle, M. J. (1995). Gender differences in parental psychological distress following perinatal death or sudden infant death syndrome. *British Journal of Psychiatry, 167,* 806–811.

Wiebe, E., & Janssen, P. (1998). Management of spontaneous abortion in family practices and hospitals. *Family Medicine, 30,* 293–296.

Wieringa-de Waard, M., Hartman, E. E., Ankum, W. M., Reitsma, J. B., Bindels, P.J.E., & Bonsel, G. J. (2002). Expectant management versus surgical evacuation in first trimester miscarriage: Health-related quality of life in randomized and non-randomized patients. *Human Reproduction, 17,* 1638–1642.

Wisner, K., Peindl, K., & Hanusa, B. (1996). Effects of childbearing on the natural history of panic disorder with comorbid mood disorder. *Journal of Affective Disorders, 41,* 173–180.

Zolese, G., & Blacker, C. V. (1992). The psychological complications of therapeutic abortion. *British Journal of Psychiatry, 160,* 742–749.

Chapter 9

Infertility and Mood Changes

Infertility

The World Health Organization (WHO) estimates that 8 percent to 12 percent, or one in seven, couples struggle with infertility in the world; and it appears, in the United States, to be more prevalent in African American women compared with Caucasian, or white, women (Human Fertilization and Embryology Authority, 2008; WHO, 2009). *Infertility* is the incapacity to become pregnant after consistently engaging in intercourse without contraception for a minimum of one year (some countries say up to two years). This period decreases by six months when the woman is over age 35 (Olshansky, 2003). Oddly, infertility rates have been increasing over time. This may be due to several factors:

- waiting to conceive
- decline in women's fertility with age
- primary infertility in men
- psychiatric history
- elevated number of those with a sexually transmitted disease
- birth control complications (for example, IUDs)
- botched or multiple abortions

◀ exposure to environmentally based contaminants (for example, lead, pesticide, radiation) (Downey & McKinney, 1992; Greenfeld, 1997; Morrow, Thoreson, & Penney, 1995).

In general, couples in which one or both partners are diagnosed as infertile experience more depression and anxiety symptoms than do fertile couples. At this point, it is unclear how psychological features interact with infertility. However, a growing base of knowledge indicates that high stress levels and symptoms of depression negatively affect conception rates (for example, hormonal levels, an environment unsuitable for conception, poor semen quality) (Barnea & Tal, 1991; Brkovich & Fisher, 1998; Lord & Robertson, 2005; Thiering, Beaurepaire, Jones, Saunders, & Tennant, 1993). Furthermore, heightened anxiety levels can also negatively influence insemination success and increase the likelihood of miscarriage (Demyttenaere, Nijs, Evers, & Koninckx, 1992).

Mental Health Reactions to Infertility

Discovering that one is infertile can be emotionally and psychologically devastating. Such symptoms include lowered self-image, confusion, identity concerns, frustration, sadness, resentment, guilt, blame, belief that one has a "defective body," depression, and anxiety (Beaurepaire, Jones, Thiering, Saunders, & Tennant, 1994; Belsky, Sapnier, & Rovine, 1983; Berg & Wilson, 1990; Covington, 2009; Möller & Fällström, 1991; Stanton & Golombok, 1993). Women with infertility experience more depression symptoms than women who are fertile (Domar, Broome, & Zuttermeister, 1992; Domar & Seibel, 1990). Nearly one in three infertile women experience depression (Garner, Arnold, & Gray, 1984).

In general, when the female partner is infertile, she reports distress, depression, anxiety, and somatic complaints more frequently when compared with men who are infertile (Abbey, Andrews, & Halman, 1994; Adashi et al., 2000; Demyttenaere et al., 1998; Henning & Strauss, 2002). These symptoms tend to be more severe in women when the etiological cause of her infertility cannot be determined (Oddens, den Tonkelaar, & Nieuwenhuyse, 1999; Wischmann, Stammer, Scherg, Gerhard, & Verres, 2001). In addition, remember that having a spontaneous abortion (miscarriage) can trigger mental health changes, including increases in depression and anxiety (Broen, Moum, Bødtker, & Ekeberg, 2005). The more miscarriages a woman has, it is logical to construe, the more susceptible she will be to mental health changes.

With regard to identity concerns, Olshansky has conducted extensive research on the development of an "infertility identity," which begins to replace the woman's other life roles (friend, wife, professional colleague).

This can lead a woman into social isolation and disconnection from others (Olshansky 1987a, 1987b, 1988a, 1988b, 1990, 1995, 1996, 2003). From the cultural–relational theory perspective, isolation and disconnection leads to depression and other mental health symptoms (Olshansky, 2003). When a woman who has identified herself through her infertility interacts with others, it is through the schema "I am innately flawed." This consumes her thoughts, behaviors, and discussions with others. She may alienate herself from friends who have children, from family members out of fear of being dismissed, and from her spouse for fear of being misinterpreted (Olshansky, 2003). When she actually becomes pregnant, this identity needs to change. This change is experienced by some as a kind of "death" or identity crisis, to reidentify as a pregnant woman and soon-to-be parent. When this re-identification does not naturally occur, the woman identifies herself as an "infertile pregnant woman" rather than a woman who is pregnant (Olshansky, 2003). This ego-dystonic or internally conflicting experience can cause confusion, anxiety, grief, a sense of loss, and depression, resulting in further self-isolation (Olshansky, 1990). After becoming a parent, women who had an "infertility identity" tend to feel guilty about normal adjustment feelings once the baby is born—indicating that they feel as if they do not have the "right" to express any negative feelings or exhaustion during the postpartum time period (Olshansky, 1995).

There are Stories
~ *Brangwynne Purcell*

Friend subject to childbirth
and pain and womanhood
I honor you now
And dream of holding Rosey
when he arrives.
Already my lullabies and lines
are waiting…

Books and music, your mother's face,
everything beautiful awaits you
in this cruel life.
I know that sweetness cannot cure
rogues and satan
I know now
that childhood is not innocence
but ignorance and maybe punishment.
I do not know anymore what
I once believed with passion

in my youth.
It is all past me, kept.
We who have gone before
make no promises
For all control has escaped us, fled.

And once before your birth
your parents dreamt you in the night
and named you.
You will not know that name
for they had forgotten it with waking
but I have not.
I will keep it for you.
Come to me when I am old
and have many children of my own.
We will teach you many things
about the walls and what they keep
for your children.

Couple's Reaction to Infertility

Infertility has the potential to negatively influence the couple's relationship and force them to re-evaluate life goals and social roles (Covington, 2009). Couples who have an infertility diagnosis also appear to experience higher anxiety levels than fertile couples (Thiering et al., 1993). Following the diagnosis, reports indicate that women feel less optimistic about their marriage and sexual relationship than the male partner (Bringhenti, Martinelli, Ardenti, & LaSala, 1997; Leiblum, Aviv, & Hamer, 1998; Monga, Alexandrescu, Katz, Stein, & Ganiats, 2004; Newton, Sherrard, & Glavac, 1999; Slade, Emery, & Lieberman, 1997). This feeling often persists throughout future infertility treatments.

In particular, sexual intimacy becomes difficult during infertility treatments as certain protocols need to be precisely followed, thereby increasing marital friction (Repokari et al., 2007). When infertility treatments last for a long time (up to years) and the couple experiences recurring treatment failure, marital distress, conflict, and unhappiness become amplified, resulting in decreased communication-based coping (Berg & Wilson, 1991; Gibson, Ungerer, Tennant, & Saunders; 2000; Guerra, Llobera, Veiga, & Barri, 1998; Hahn & DiPietro, 2001; Pasch, Dunkel-Schetter, & Christensen, 2002; Repokari et al., 2007; Schmidt, Holstein, Christensen, & Boivin, 2005). Specific events, such as a high number of failed assisted reproductive treatments (ART) procedures and miscarriages, are more likely to increase marital unhappiness in women.

Generally, the longer the couple is infertile, the greater the marital unhappiness and sexual dissatisfaction (Berg & Wilson, 1991; Connolly et al., 1992; Repokari et al., 2007). However, for some couples who undergo ART, the process strengthens their marriage, intimacy, quality of life, affection, trust, and companionship (Fisher, Hammarberg, & Baker, 2008). Successful ART has the potential to promote a stronger marital bond than the bond for couples who become pregnant without any assistance. The marital relationship strengthens when the couple mutually and equally supports each other through all ARTs and consoles one another's sorrow, bereavement, and disappointments as they occur (Pasch et al., 2002; Peterson, Newton, & Rosen, 2003; Repokari et al., 2007). However, couples who do not have a positive outcome, or who have multiple ART failures and do not support one another through the process, report an increase in marital discord (Benazon, Wright, & Sabourin, 1992; Berg & Wilson, 1991; Guerra et al., 1998; Slade et al., 1997; Sydsjö, Wadsby, Kjellberg, & Sydsjö, 2002).

Infertility Treatments

For approximately the last 25 years, infertility was understood as a physiological issue, influenced at times by psychosocial factors. Psychosocial factors may play a leading role in the 20 percent of infertility cases where etiology is undetermined (Oddens, den Tonkelaar, & Nieuwenhuyse, 1999; Wischmann et al., 2001). However, prior to these last 25 years, infertility was believed to stem from psychological issues in the woman. According to this perspective, an infertile woman was unsure if she wanted to be a mother, wanted to take on the mother role, or had unsettled differences with her own mother (Greenfeld, 1997). Today, as more evidence supports the physiological basis for infertility, the primary treatments involve medically assisted procedures or lifestyle changes.

Pharmaceutical Treatments for Infertility

Medicinal treatments aim at the specific cause of infertility. When infertility is due to ovulation malfunctions, drugs like clomiphene citrate (Clomid, Miophene, Serophene) may be prescribed to boost ovary production. When used for six months without any results, it is assumed that clomiphene citrate treatment is unsuccessful and other options are discussed (WebMd, 2008).

One side effect of this type of treatment is the generation of more than one viable egg, leaving open the possibility of a multiple-baby pregnancy (Speroff & Fritz, 2005). When infertility is due to sperm production, drugs can be prescribed to increase the quantity of the sperm (Health-Cares, 2005).

Assisted Reproductive Technologies

There are several types of ARTs available for couples based on the underlying cause of infertility. One of the more commonly discussed procedures, in vitro fertilization, was first successful in 1979. Therefore, most of the literature about ART and related mental health issues is still in the early investigative stages (Hammarberg, Fisher, & Wynter, 2008). Much of the following discussion in this chapter has the limited ability to be generalized but will provide insight into the findings over the past three decades.

Intrauterine Insemination

When sperm tallies are low, a large number of irregular sperm form, or the female has sperm antibodies in the cervix, intrauterine insemination (also known as artificial insemination or IUI) may be used (Health-Cares, 2005). This entails treating the sperm in a laboratory to improve fertilization odds. An excessive quantity of sperm is placed straight into the uterus for optimal entry into the fallopian tubes.

Gamete Intrafallopian Transfer

Women suffering from endometriosis or cervical disorders may have gamete intrafallopian transfer. Similar to in vitro fertilization, the female's eggs and male sperm are collected. However, rather than fertilizing the eggs in a test tube or laboratory dish, the eggs and the sperm are inserted into the woman's uterus to allow natural fertilization and implantation to take place (Health-Cares, 2005).

Zygote Intrafallopian Transfer

Zygote intrafallopian transfer (ZIFT) is similar to in vitro fertilization. The egg and sperm are fertilized in a test tube or laboratory dish. Then, rather than being inserted into the uterus, the fertilized egg is inserted into the fallopian tube. Typically, this procedure is recommended when the male produces abnormal sperm (Health-Cares, 2005).

Intracytoplasmic Sperm Injection

Intracytoplasmic sperm injection involves the insertion of one sperm into one egg, typically in a laboratory dish. To gather the egg, the preparation procedures for in vitro fertilization are followed. Once the egg is fertilized, it is either inserted into the fallopian tubes or allowed to mature in the laboratory dish for a few days and then inserted into the woman's uterus (Health-Cares, 2005).

Epididymal and Testicular Sperm Extraction

This procedure involves removing sperm, from either the testis or the epididymis, with a needle. One sperm is inserted directly into the egg as in intracytoplasmic sperm injection. Any leftover sperm is frozen for later use if needed (Health-Cares, 2005).

Men who experience certain types of infertility, such as azoospermia or spermatic cord abnormalities, may need to have an epididymal and testicular sperm extraction. The epididymis is a slender, tightly twisted tube that connects the efferent ducts from the back of the testicle to the vas deferens (Farlex, 2009). When sperm is formed in the testis, it enters the epididymis and is stored there, but these sperm lack the ability to swim until they reach a particular spot in the epididymis. The sperm fully matures in the woman's reproductive tract; this is called capacitation (Farlex, 2009).

There are three types of azoospermia. Obstructive azoospermia is when the sperm is created, but is unable to join ejaculatory fluids upon ejaculation. This is typically the result of a physically based obstacle (Farlex, 2009). When there is a problem with the formation and development of sperm, the male suffers from non–obstructive azoospermia (Farlex, 2009). Should a male infant be born with an abnormally developed vas deferens, then he suffers with congenital azoospermia (Farlex, 2009).

The vas deferens and the surrounding tissue that travels from the testicle up to the abdomen create the spermatic cord. A kink in the cord can cause significant and irreversible damage to the testicle by cutting off the blood supply (Farlex, 2009).

Surgical Intervention

A person might undergo surgical repair when the cause of infertility is blockage or damage in the female's fallopian tubes or the male sperm ducts (Health-Cares, 2005). Once surgically corrected, couples can try to conceive naturally.

In Vitro Fertilization Procedure

In vitro fertilization involves the removal of viable eggs from the woman's ovaries and the insertion of these eggs into a test tube or laboratory dish. To prepare the female body to produce viable eggs, she is injected (normally self-administered) with fertility drugs that stimulate several ova in the ovaries to "ripen" (Greenfeld, 1997). In step two of in vitro fertilization, the ripened eggs are gathered by laparoscopy or "needle guided aspiration" (Greenfeld, 1997). To induce fertilization, live sperm and the eggs are mixed. Once fertilized, one or more eggs are inserted into the woman's uterus in the hope that at least one will implant and pregnancy will result. Some couples are able to use the egg and sperm from one another. Other times, an egg or sperm donor is needed, which then includes contacting an agency and choosing the characteristics of the donor. In vitro fertilization is the treatment of choice when the cause of infertility is fallopian tube obstruction, irregular sperm, or endometriosis (Health-Cares, 2005).

Mental Health and Preparing for Interventions

In Vitro Fertilization

By the time a couple considers in vitro fertilization, they have often sought out other methods to become pregnant. These methods are often pursued for months to years before in vitro fertilization is even thought about. In these cases, the procedure is a last resort effort. Therefore, there is a lot of expectation, hope, and nervousness attached to the process (Covington, 2009).

In cases where donor sperm or egg is needed, couples need to integrate the concept of using another person's genetic material into the couple's dreams and aspirations of having a baby from their own genetic make-up. This can be difficult to come to terms with. The procedure is costly, involves timing intercourse, and is disruptive to normal, everyday activities. As a result, many couples compare the stress of preparing for in vitro fertilization to other major, life altering events such as the death of a loved one or divorce (Covington, 2009).

In the 1970s, Barbara Eck Menning, a nurse who experienced infertility, stated that the infertility interventions caused women anxiety instead of women's anxiety causing the state of infertility (Greenfeld, 1997; Menning, 1980). While the woman hormonally prepares her body for insemination, the couple locates a sperm or egg donor agency, decides on donor characteristics, financially secures the sperm or egg, and prepares for the possibility of multiple babies (Covington, 2009). All of these decisions are based on the couples' psychosocial background, religion, social impact or preferences, and financial means. It is obvious, as you recall the details for each of the ART procedures, that couples are under enormous stress. The characteristics of these stressors are similar to risk factors for perinatal mood disorders.

Following the medical insertion of the fertilized egg, the woman undergoes several sonograms in order to detect successful attachment. The time between insertion of the fertilized egg and determining embryo implantation is an extremely stressful time for the couple (Baram, Tourtelot, Muechler, & Huang, 1988; Boivin & Takeftnan, 1995; Daniluk, 1988; Ismail, Menezes, Martin, & Thong, 2004; Yong, Martin, & Thong, 2000). Women, more often than their male partners, experience anxiety and depression and express hostility (Ismail et al., 2004). In an effort to manage these emotions, women often seek out social support and the male partners tend to work longer hours (Ismail et al., 2004).

The preparation process can be difficult for the couple, but particularly for the woman who will be undergoing the procedure. Emotional responses while preparing can include extreme fluctuations in mood (from feeling hopeful to shame, disappointment, frustration, and embarrassment) and an increase in anxiety levels (Evert, 2007; Ismail et al., 2004). During preparation, women are subjected to numerous injections to alter hormone levels. This not only is disruptive to one's daily schedule, but also can result in several physiological symptoms including hot flashes, headaches, sore breasts, nausea, belated menses, and future health problems (Covington, 2009).

Obviously, some physiological symptoms are similar to the symptoms of pregnancy. Therefore, women who are initially undergoing ART to become pregnant may believe they are pregnant, when in actuality it is a side effect of the methods used to prepare the body to become pregnant. The realization that her physiological changes are not pregnancy related increases feelings of depression, anxiety, disappointment, and lack of hope for pregnancy (Sandelowski, Harris, & Holditch-Davis, 1990). Women who have been down this road before psychologically prepare themselves for another "failed attempt." When the woman finally becomes pregnant, she has a difficult time believing it, and feels shocked and confused (Olshansky, 1990; Sandelowski et al., 1990). Once pregnant, these women report an increase in anxiety symptoms rather than depressed symptoms (Klock & Greenfeld, 2000; McMahon, Tennant, Ungerer, & Saunders, 1999; Ulrich, Gagel, Hemmerling, Parstor, & Kentenich, 2004), particularly anxiety about possible miscarriage (Hammarberg et al., 2008). It is helpful to remember that these couples have typically gone through years of infertility and this is considered a "last shot deal." Two studies found that pregnancy in women who had ART can be more stressful and anxiety ridden than for women who did not use ART (Bernstein, Lewis, & Seibel, 1994; van Balen, Naaktgeboren, & Trimbos-Kemper, 1996). Anxious behaviors, such as repeatedly checking for "spotting" (vaginal bleeding), fear that the pregnancy will not last full term, irritability, and increased muscle tension are more prevalent in pregnant women who have had ART. Furthermore, these women tend to suffer recurrent, disturbing dreams (Bernstein, Lewis, & Seibel, 1994; Hjelmstedt, Widström, Wramsby, & Collins, 2003; McMahon, Ungerer, Beaurepaire, Tennant, & Saunders, 1997). Furthermore, these women are also more likely to express mother–baby separation anxiety prior to birth and are more likely to have a passionate, affective attachment to the unborn infant (Fisher et al., 2008). If the procedure fails, many couples suffer increased anxiety and depression (Baram et al., 1988; Ismail et al., 2005).

Postpartum Depression in Previously Infertile Mothers

Women with a history of infertility are still susceptible to postpartum mood disorder (PMD) symptoms, yet medical and mental health professionals often overlook these symptoms due to the misperception that these mothers struggled so hard to have her baby that they must feel overjoyed and elated (Olshansky, 2003). Consequently, these mothers may be more apt to hide negative (depressed or anxious) symptoms because she is socioculturally expected to be euphoric about the baby she worked so hard to have (Olshansky, 1995). Discussing postpartum depression symptoms was more difficult for women who had twins, triplets, or higher order multiples (often the result of ART), with only 27 percent of those with moderate to severe depression symptoms speaking to a health or mental health practitioner about their symptoms (Choi, Bishai, & Minovitz, 2009).

Studies in Australia have found that women who have undergone ART are approximately 25 percent more likely to need postpartum depression assistance (Fisher, Feekery, Amir, & Sneddon, 2002; Fisher, Hammarberg, & Baker, 2005). Another study conducted in Italy found high depression levels in women who had ART, particularly during the third trimester (Monti, Agostini, Fagandini, La Sala, & Blickstein, 2009).

Researchers are unclear whether depression influences a woman's infertility (with depression treatment improving the odds to become pregnant) or if the experience of infertility influences the development of depressed symptoms (Cousineau & Domar, 2007; Hunt & Monach, 1997; Olshansky, 2003; Thiering et al., 1993). In an older study, women who were infertile and had depression prior to becoming pregnant through medical assistance showed no decrease in their depressed symptoms after giving birth (Bernstein et al., 1988). These results imply that having a baby does not prevent previously infertile women from negative moods (Olshansky, 2003). What does seem to happen is a feeling of initial excitement about becoming pregnant, but these women find that the depression returns following delivery, which may point to postpartum depression (Herz, 1992).

As in the general population, previously infertile women who become pregnant may develop high-risk pregnancies. This experience can be nerve-racking for any woman. However, women with an infertility history have a tendency to blame her body for the high-risk pregnancy, as well as any other medically related problems that the newborn might have upon birth. Lind, Pruitt and Greenfeld (1989) found that previously infertile women's babies who needed intensive care psychologically blamed themselves for the baby's health. This way of thinking adds to the triggers for PMDs.

Multiple Births

Multiple births (twins, triplets, or greater) are a big risk factor when more than one fertilized egg is inserted into the uterus. One need only look at the "Octomom" to realize this potential. It is estimated that multiple births occur in one out of every four ART pregnancies (Human Fertilization and Embryology Authority, 1998; Lieblum, 1997). Between 1980 and 1997, the number of twin births increased by nearly 50 percent and the number of triplet or greater births increased by 404 percent, an increase linked to an increase in ARTs (Kalra, Milad, Klock, & Grobman, 2003; Martin & Park, 1999).

Multiple fetus pregnancies are typically high risk for the mother, and babies are sometimes born prematurely (Alexander, Kogan, Martin, & Papiernik, 1998a; ESHRE Capri Workshop Group, 2000; Pinborg et al., 2004). Based on estimates provided by Kalra et al. (2003), 20 percent to 30 percent of women pregnant with more than one fetus will experience postpartum depression and one in five will endure preeclampsia. Furthermore, these mothers are more likely to deliver via cesarean section (Lumley, 2004), which has been shown to increase anxiety about caring for the baby and about feeding problems in ART-multiple baby mothers' postpartum adjustment (Hammarberg, Fisher, & Rowe, 2008). Fifteen percent of multiple babies are born prematurely, one in 10 is of low birthweight, 7 percent are stillborn, and many need neonatal intensive care (Alexander, Kogan, Martin, & Papiernik, 1998b; Kovacs, Kirschbaum, & Paul, 1989; Long & Oats, 1987; Lumley, 2004; MacDorman, Minino, Strobing, & Guyer, 2002; Thorpe, Golding, MacGillivray, & Greenwood, 1991). Babies born prematurely are at increased risk for cognitive developmental delays or disabilities and behavioral problems (Bhutta et al., 2002; ESHRE Capri Workshop Group, 2000).

One option is multifetal pregnancy reduction, or aborting one or more of the implanted fetuses (Greenfeld, 1997). This can be difficult for the couple for three reasons:

1. Is there a doctor available near them who will do the procedure?

2. If so, how does one choose which fetuses to save? After trying so hard to have a baby, the concept of aborting one or more possible babies may be too hard to fathom.

3. The procedure contradicts the couple's religious beliefs or background.

Understandably, Garel, Stark, Blondel, Lefebre, et al. (1997), found that women can experience depression up to twelve months after undergoing multifetal pregnancy reduction.

Despite the increased biopsychosocial risks for the mother and baby, one study found that approximately two in three couples would have twins if ART was successful (Kalra et al., 2003). Another study found similar results with two out of three women indicating a desire for twins and one in two indicating a desire for triplets (Gleicher et al., 1995); this desire to have a multiple birth increased by the age of the woman.

Perinatal Mental Health

Many couples may not be cognitively prepared to understand the risks of a multiple-birth pregnancy and postpartum stressors after the long, arduous ART procedures (Fisher & Stocky, 2003). Couples who opt to proceed with the multiple-birth pregnancy are at an increased risk for marital tension or discord, financial demands, and postpartum mental health changes (Callahan et al., 1994; Thorpe et al., 1991; Glazebrook, Cox, Oates, & Ndukwe, 2001). Approximately one in four women who carry two or more babies to term will experience perinatal depression or anxiety (Garel, Salobir, & Blondel, 1997; Leonard, 1998; Parents of Multiple Births Association of Canada (PMBAC), 1993; Robin, Corroyer, & Casati, 1996; Thorpe, Greenwood, & Goodenough, 1995). The Glazebrook et al. (2001) study found that women who conceived twins or triplets from in vitro fertilization had high anxiety levels during pregnancy. An earlier study found that 40 percent of women who carried twins experienced moderate to high anxiety levels during pregnancy (Hay & O'Brien, 1984).

During the postpartum period, three out of four mothers of twins reported exhaustion and one in three reported depression symptoms (Hay et al., 1990). In this study, these mothers' anxiety was three times that of women who had one baby. At three months postpartum, mothers of twins had five times the rate of depression. This is similar to other accounts where 35 percent of mothers of twins and triplets had extreme emotional stress, and 29 percent to 40 percent of mothers of twins and triplets reported depression (Leonard, 1998; PMBAC, 1993; Robin, Bydlowski, Cahen, & Josse, 1991; Robin et al., 1996). Garel and Blondel's (1992) research with mothers of triplets found that one in four were receiving treatment for depression at 12 months postpartum.

Mothers of twins experience nine times the rate of exhaustion compared with mothers of one baby (Hay et al., 1990). Exhaustion is felt physically and emotionally. Nearly half of all mothers of twins or triplets experience loss of body strength, feel helpless, and have an increase in tension and irritability (Garel & Blondel, 1992). For mothers of triplets, fatigue, combined with mental health symptoms, continues for years after delivery. One in three women experience depression and anxiety at two years postpartum, with exhaustion and stress persisting four years after delivery (Garel et al., 1997; Leonard, 1998).

The father experiences additional stresses following ART-related multiple births with greater parent–child interaction difficulties as compared to the mother. This may be due to more father involvement than in single baby births, thereby increasing his experience of stress. The increased father involvement acts as a buffer for the mother, decreasing her levels of postpartum stress and depression (as postpartum depression levels were no different from prevalence rates in the general population) (Glazebrook et al., 2001).

Parenting Stress and Impact on the Family after ART

Parenting skills for the couple becomes a balancing act—meeting the needs for babies of the same age, adjusting to parenthood, addressing different parenting styles, meeting one another's individual needs, and simply enjoying the babies (Leonard, 1998). The parents of twins conceived via in vitro fertilization report higher parenting stress levels than do parents of twins conceived without assistance (Cook, Bradley, & Golombok, 1998; Glazebrook, Sheard, Cox, Oates, & Ndukwe, 2004). Olivennes et al. (2005) found that mothers of twins experienced less joy from the babies and more numerous reports of parenting-related stress, when compared to mothers of one baby. Parenting stresses, psychological symptoms, and other family or life obligations decreases the family's quality of life—fathers and mothers both report high stress, which increases with the number of children (Ellison et al., 2005; Sheard, Cox, Oates, Ndukwe, & Glazebrook, 2007). Sheard et al. (2007) found that mothers of multiples struggled to meet the needs of the babies collectively and individually. These results support the work of previous research (Beck, 2002; Garel & Blondel, 1992; Holditch-Davis, Roberts, & Sandelowski, 1999). Despite these struggles, added stressors seem to strengthen the couple's bonding with one another (Ellison & Hall, 2003).

ART and Impact on the Child

Although there is scant literature discussing the link between ART, mental health, and child development, the available research shows healthy parent-child bonding. One study of four- to eight-year-old children who were conceived through in vitro fertilization found better mother-baby interaction, emotional bonding, expression of warmth, and reported less parenting-related stress than did mothers of like-aged children who conceived without assistance (Glazebrook et al., 2001; Golombok, Cook, Bish, & Murray, 1995). Other studies, however, have found that women who conceived through in vitro fertilization have increased stress related to parenting skills (Glazebrook et al., 2001; McMahon, Ungerer, Tennant, & Saunders, 1997). Child protection record analysis, in one study, showed that being a twin predicted abuse and neglect—but this study had a small sample size (Glazebrook et al., 2001; Groothuis et al., 1982). Many mothers who conceived by in vitro fertilization give the children less freedom and independence, are overprotective, and perceive the children as unique compared to naturally conceived children (Colpin, Demyttenaere, & Vandemeulebroecke, 1995; Gibson et al., 2000; Hahn & DiPietro, 2001; Weaver, Clifford, Gordon, Hay, & Robinson, 1993).

Surrogacy

Purportedly, couples who seek out a surrogate are Caucasian or white, from a high socioeconomic status, have received high levels of education, and the female partner tends to be highly career focused (Braverman & Corson, 1992; Kleinpeter, 2002). The most frequently stated reasons for using a surrogate are as follows:

◖ to stop going through unsuccessful infertility treatments—particularly after a long period of time trying;

◖ to be genetically related to the child; and

◖ to avoid adoption complications (Kleinpeter, 2002; MacCallum, Lycett, Murray, Jadva, & Golombok, 2003).

There are two types of surrogacy. In cases where the woman is unable to produce viable eggs, a surrogate woman, willing to physically carry the couples' baby to term, is injected with the sperm of the male partner and follows artificial insemination procedures (Greenfeld, 1997). This is called partial or genetic surrogacy (Golombok, Murray, Jadva, MacCallum, & Lycett, 2004). The second type is full or nongenetic surrogacy, in which the woman follows in vitro fertilization procedures. The woman's eggs are harvested, fertilized by the male's sperm, and then inserted into the surrogate's womb (Golombok et al., 2004). This method is typically used if the female partner still has viable eggs but also has a congenital problem underlying her ability to carry the baby (Greenfeld, 1997).

There are two types of surrogates:

1. Altruistic surrogacy: A woman voluntarily carries the baby for the couple to allow the couple to have a baby of their own (commonly a relative or close friend)

2. Commercial surrogacy: A woman is monetarily compensated for carrying the couple's child (BioEdge, 2003; Federal Law Gazette, 1990; Tieu, 2009).

Statistically, surrogates are most likely to be white, have low education levels, have low to lower-middle socioeconomic status, are dissatisfied with traditional jobs, and are not under financial strain or motivated by monetary compensation (Aigen, 1996; Braverman & Corson, 1992). Psychologically, surrogates have a need to feel important to others, are extroverted, and seek excitement, but did not present with severe mental health conditions (Kleinpeter & Hohman, 2000).

Of primary importance when choosing a surrogate is assessing the surrogate's health, mental health, and reasons for becoming a surrogate. It is advised that counseling be undertaken by the contracting couple and the surrogate (and her partner if present) in order to address all current and potential health and mental health issues during the pregnancy and after delivery (Söderström–Antilla et al., 2002).

Mother's Emotional Reactions

As previously discussed, women who are infertile can feel anxious, depressed, frustrated, guilty, shameful, unable to fulfill her physiological role as a woman, and isolated. Sometimes, these feelings transfer to her perception of the surrogate who is able to fulfill the role she cannot. In addition, the woman (and the couple as a whole) may hide the fact that she is using a surrogate from family, friends, and others due to controversies about the practice, thereby further isolating herself from others (Golombok et al., 2004). However, this secrecy becomes a larger problem after the baby is born and the couple has to figure out a way to reveal their newborn to significant others (Golombok et al., 2004).

Surrogate Emotional Reactions

In efforts to promote healthy coping with the idea that another woman is carrying the couple's baby, there is a movement to encourage the objectification of the surrogate. Essentially, this means to view the surrogate as a means to have your baby and to separate from the surrogate as a person, but more as a vessel that holds and is providing a nourishing environment for your developing baby (Tieu, 2009). However, if the surrogate begins to view the baby in this way, she may emotionally have an easier time relinquishing the baby to the couple, but there is a risk for neonatal development problems. The majority of surrogate mothers enter the contract by cognitively distancing themselves from the baby, which does help to diminish maternal bonding with the baby throughout the pregnancy and improves her ability to hand the baby over to the couple (Ciccarelli & Beckman, 2005; Ragone, 1994; Tieu, 2009; van Zyl & van Niekerk, 2000). In the case of commercial surrogacy, emotional distancing through focus on payment also buffers the surrogate from emotional attachment to the baby (Baslington, 2002). When the surrogate does not use cognitive distancing strategies, the surrogate can experience postpartum depression (Baslington, 2002). To assist surrogate women with relinquishing the baby to the contracting couple, there are call-in support services (such as Childlessness Overcome Through Surrogacy), support through agencies that perform the fertilization procedures, and individual counseling (Blyth, 1994; Boseley, 1997; Smith, 1998). The majority of surrogates who seek out these support or counseling services are partial or genetic surrogates.

The majority of surrogates do not have difficulty emotionally letting go and giving the baby to the couple (Jadva, Murray, Lycett, MacCallum, & Golombok, 2003). Some women even appear to engage in commercial surrogacy as their "employment." In a 2003 United Kingdom report, one woman was on her ninth surrogate pregnancy (Anonymous)!

Parenting after Surrogacy

Currently, there does not appear to be any unusual parenting concerns due to genetic differences compared to couples who become pregnant naturally (Golombok et al., 1995, 2004; Golombok et al., 1996; Golombok, Brewaeys, et al., 2002; Golombok, MacCallum, Goodman, & Rutter, 2002; Golombok, Murray, Brinsden, & Abdalla, 1999; Raoul-Duval, Bertrand-Servais,

Letur-Konirsch, & Frydman, 1994; Söderström-Antilla, Sajaneimi, Tiitinen, & Hovatta, 1998). However, many parents who have a child through surrogacy do not divulge this information to the child, which can cause mental health and emotional dilemmas for the child later, should this information become known (Brewaeys, 1996, 2001; Turner & Coyle, 2000). For this reason, some surrogacy supporters also advocate for an open surrogacy arrangement (similar to an open adoption) where the surrogate has specified contact with the child, suggesting that this will ease developmental adjustments through understanding of their genetic background and history (Golombok et al., 2004). One study found that an estimated two in three surrogate mothers were in contact with the babies one year postpartum—although this study did not indicate how this contact influenced the babies or the contracting parents (Jadva, Murray, Lycett, MacCallum, & Golombok, 2003).

In the Golombok et al (2004) study of parent–child relationships in the first year of a baby's life, families who used a surrogate had better psychological health and had more easily adapted to parenting roles than did families who had a child naturally. Psychologically, both mothers and fathers who used a surrogate indicated less parenting-related stress, and the mothers indicated less depression symptoms than their non-surrogate-using counterparts did. In addition, surrogate-using parents were better able to express warmth, parent–child bonding, and joy about being a parent than the parents who conceived naturally.

Ethical and Legal Concerns

◀ When a couple chooses surrogacy, several ethical and legal issues need consideration.

◀ What will the surrogate's role be in the child's and couples' life after delivery?

◀ How will society, in general, view surrogacy?

Globally, each country has different legislation surrounding the practice, largely dependent on the religious, ethical, and moral traditions of the country. Some counties allow altruistic surrogacy; commercial surrogacy, a combination of the two; or outlaw the practice completely (Germany and Sweden, for example) (BioEdge, 2003; Federal Law Gazette, 1990; Reilly, 2007; Tieu, 2009). Places which currently allow surrogacy of some type include some states in the U.S., Canada, parts of Australia, France, the Netherlands, and Israel (Golombok et al., 2004; Honig, Nave, & Adam, 2000).

The United Kingdom passed the Surrogacy Arrangements Act in 1985 and the Human Fertilization and Embryology Act in 1990. The 1985 legislation made it illegal for commercial surrogacy agencies to accept money other than for sensible surrogate expenses, and the 1990 legislation, while allowing altruistic surrogacy, does not bind courts to signed surrogacy contracts (English & Sommerville, 1996; Roughley, 2007).

Israel's Surrogate Motherhood Law of 1996 permits surrogacy arrangements for women who were born without a uterus, had a hysterectomy, has complicating health conditions, or has had a minimum of eight to ten failed in vitro fertilization attempts. The sperm and egg are required to be provided by the contracting couple (Gagin, Cohen, Greenblatt, Solomon, & Itskovitz-Eldor, 2004). According to this act, the surrogate is allowed monetary compensation during the pregnancy through delivery and additional financial restitution for emotional suffering and lost wages; the surrogate is also legally allowed to change her mind, have an abortion, or legally pursue to keep the baby. The surrogate must be an Israeli resident, single, and match the contracting couple's religious background (Gagin et al., 2004; Honig et al., 2000; Oz, 1995; Zager, 1996).

To date, the United States has not enacted any federal laws about surrogacy; rather, policy institution is relegated to individual states. States that do allow surrogacy typically rely on multidisciplinary programs and lawyers to match couples with surrogates, provide health and mental health care, and formalize legal agreements (Kleinpeter & Hohman, 2000).

Informed Consent
Ethically and legally, the ability for a close friend or relative to provide uncoerced and objective informed consent to be a surrogate is questioned (Tieu, 2009). Family dynamic issues can interfere with the woman's decision, particularly if the potential surrogate does not want to see her close friend and family member suffer emotionally. Particularly salient for surrogates who are enmeshed in the couple's family or friend network is an underlying need to receive approval, love, self-worth, or self-esteem externally—from others in the family, other friends, or from the couple (Tieu, 2009). Furthermore, if the surrogate is a close friend or family member, how will she cope with the emotional separation from the baby after delivery, particularly if she is likely to be spending time with the baby after delivery at family functions and other activities? Will she be able to separate the role of physiologically carrying the baby and emotionally bonding with the baby while pregnant and being called aunt or friend after the baby is born (Tieu, 2009)?

Differing Personal Ethics and Values
Unforeseen events can negatively influence the surrogacy plan and wind up being resolved through the court system. For example, the couple may find

out through tests that the fetus has a disability and no longer want to continue with the surrogacy contract (Singer & Wells, 1983, 1985; Tieu, 2009). In this situation, should the surrogate continue with the pregnancy and keep the child? Should the surrogate be forced to have an abortion if the couple says that it is their preference? Alternatively, what if the couple wishes to have the baby despite the disability and the surrogate wishes to abort (Tieu, 2009)? This is similar to a case in California where the surrogate underwent in vitro fertilization and became pregnant with twins. The couple requested that the surrogate undergo multifetal pregnancy reduction to have only one baby. The surrogate refused, and the couple backed out from their contract (CNN, 2001; Tieu, 2009).

Motives for Surrogate

Another ethical concern is the underlying motives for becoming a surrogate. Some women simply enjoy the feeling of being pregnant, already have children, understand the emotional bonding concerns, and are happy to provide this service to a loved one. However, whenever altruism is involved, a myriad of underlying motives are often unrealized by others and even by the person acting in an altruistic manner. For instance, a surrogate may want to "make amends" for her own life choices that she now regrets, such as having given a baby up for adoption or having had abortions (Parker, 1983; Tieu, 2009). In one study, nearly one in four prospective surrogates had a past abortion and one in ten had adopted out her baby (Ragone, 1994).

Surrogate–Baby Bonding

A bioethical concern is raised due to the physiological attachment that naturally occurs between a mother and the fetus during pregnancy (Tieu, 2009). Van Zyl and van Niekerk (2000) found that a surrogate's commitment not only includes allowing medical procedures and restriction from specific behaviors, but also results in the conception and birth of a baby. This inextricably links the woman's biopsychoemotional response to the baby regardless of the surrogate's or contracting couple's social and moral interpretation of the act of surrogacy. Reportedly, estradiol levels increase and progesterone levels decrease approximately five weeks before delivery; these hormonal changes start a physiologically based attachment between the biological mother and the fetus (Klaus & Kennell, 1982; Smith, 1998).

Although surrogate mothers tend to use denial and cognitive strategies to manage the mother–fetal bond phenomenon (Fischer & Gillman, 1991), the fetus does not have this same coping ability. Neurohormonal and emotional bonds created in utero cannot simply be severed due to a legal contract (van Zyl & van Niekerk, 2000). As evidence of this biopsychoemotional bond, some surrogates have difficulty relinquishing the baby to the contracting parents and may seek out custody of the baby. In the United States, the surrogate mother of "Baby M" sued the contracting parents (unsuccessfully) in attempts to keep the child (Fischer & Gillman, 1991; Smith, 1998). Another case involved a surrogate in the United Kingdom who kept the baby and was subsequently sued by the commissioning parents for deceptively accepting money for her surrogacy-related expenses (Dyer, 1997).

Developmental models and theories point to the importance of uniting the mother and newborn as soon as possible after birth as touch stimulates and strengthens the growth of the mother–child bond. These bonds are so strong that some surrogate mothers find it difficult or are unable to surrender the baby to the couple. What happens if the couple sees the child and they do not feel that emotional parent–child connection, but the surrogate does? It is possible, should the baby have the genes of the father but not the mother, that the mother could resent the baby (and the surrogate) for not being genetically hers. What if the baby is born looking more like the surrogate than the mother? Not only do these reactions disrupt the potential mother–child bonding, but they induce an emotional and mental health crisis for the surrogate and the couple as well. Even though a contract is signed, legal and ethical problems ensue in this situation. With whom is the child better off—the surrogate who already has established physiologically and emotionally based bonds? Or the couple who has been relying and depending upon the surrogate to give them their baby (Tieu, 2009)? These situations have the potential to disrupt the family (as a whole), and friendships, and cost a lot of money in litigation—with the baby's developmental needs left unattended in a disharmonious environment.

To head off these potential outcomes, a balanced relationship between the surrogate and the couple must be attained so that there is enough emotional (objectification) distance to engage in the "business" aspect of the surrogacy role and enough emotional connectedness throughout the pregnancy for the couple to pseudo-bond with the baby and the surrogate to feel appreciated (Golombok et al., 2004). Others have suggested that the surrogate legally terminate her rights as a biological parent of the baby—even prior to becoming pregnant—in an attempt to avoid the aforementioned situations (Andrews, 1990; Tieu, 2009). Van Zyl and van Niekerk (2000) referred to this as the purchasing of "preconception termination of the mother's parental rights," because biologically, the surrogate is the actual biological mother. Following this line of thought, and borrowing from the concepts of adoption, the biological mother is rescinding her rights to a preconceived baby and legally binding the contracting mother as the intended "adoptive parent." In essence, the surrogate is not refuting that she is the mother of the baby, just refuting the right to raise the baby (van Zyl & van Niekerk, 2000). Another way of interpreting the surrogacy contract is that the unborn baby has been given permission to use the surrogate's body, thereby granting the contracting couple "control" of the surrogate's body by indicating what behaviors, perinatal care, lifestyle choices, nutritional choices, and medical procedures, are allowed during the designated time in which the fetus occupies the surrogate's body (van Zyl & van Niekerk, 2000). This perspective serves to objectify the surrogate, and the pregnancy and makes birth a business, an almost corporate venture rather than a biological, natural, species-related event. Supporting this, others argue that condensing and constricting motherhood to biology and genetics neglects the affective investment involved with actually being a parent—a mother (Snowdon, 1994).

References

Abbey, A., Andrews, F. M., & Halman, L. J. (1994). Infertility and parenthood: Does becoming a parent increase well-being? *Journal of Consulting and Clinical Psychology, 62,* 298–403.

Adashi, E. Y., Cohen, J., Hamberger, L., Jones, H. W. Jr., de Kretser, D. M., Lunenfeld, B., et al. (2000). Public perception on infertility and its treatment: An international survey. *Human Reproduction, 15,* 330–334.

Aigen, B. (1996). *Motivations of surrogate mothers: Parenthood, altruism, and self-actualization (a three-year study).* Retrieved from http://www.surrogacy.com/psychres/article/motivat.html

Alexander, G. R., Kogan, M., Martin, J., & Papiernik, E. (1998a). What are the fetal growth patterns of singletons, twins and triplets in the United States? *Clinical Obstetrics and Gynecology, 41,* 115–125.

Alexander, G. R., Kogan, M., Martin, J., & Papiernik, E. (1998b). When does intrauterine growth of multiples begin to differ from singletons? *Clinical Obstetrics and Gynecology, 41,* 116–126.

Andrews, L. B. (1990). Surrogate motherhood: The challenge for feminists. In L. Gostin (Ed.), *Surrogate motherhood: Politics and privacy.* Bloomington and Indianapolis: Indiana University Press.

Anonymous. (2003). A dedicated surrogate mother. *Reproductive BioMedicine Online,* 7(2), 144.

Baram, D., Tourtelot, E., Muechler, E., & Huang, K. (1988). Psychosocial adjustment following unsuccessful in vitro fertilization. *Journal of Psychosomatic Obstetrics and Gynecology, 9,* 181–190.

Barnea, E. R., & Tal, J. (1991). Stress-related reproductive failure. *Journal of In Vitro Fertilisation and Embryo Transfer, 8,* 15–23.

Baslington, H. (2002). The social organisation of surrogacy: Relinquishing a baby and the role of payment in the psychological detachment process. *Journal of Health Psychology, 7,* 57–71.

Beaurepaire, J., Jones, M., Thiering, P., Saunders, D., & Tennant, C. (1994). Psychological adjustment to infertility and its treatment: Male and female responses at different stages of IVF/ET treatment. *Journal of Psychosomatic Research, 38,* 299–240.

Beck, C.T. (2002). Mothering multiples: A meta-synthesis of qualitative research. *MCN: The American Journal of Maternal/Child Nursing, 27,* 214–221.

Belsky, J., Spanier, G. B., & Rovine, M. (1983). Stability and change in marriage across the transition to parenthood. *Journal of Marriage and Family, 45,* 567–577.

Benazon, N., Wright, J., & Sabourin, S. (1992). Stress, sexual satisfaction, and marital adjustment in infertile couples. *Journal of Sex & Marital Therapy, 18,* 273–284.

Berg, B. J., & Wilson, J. F. (1990). Psychiatric morbidity in the infertile population: A reconceptualization. *Fertility & Sterility, 53,* 654–661.

Bernstein, J., Lewis, J., & Seibel, M. (1994). Effect of previous infertility on maternal–fetal attachment, coping styles and self-concept during pregnancy. *Journal of Women's Health, 3,* 125–133.

Bhutta, A. T., Cleves, M. A., Casey, P. H., Cradock, M. M., & Anand, K.J.S. (2002). Cognitive and behavioral outcomes of school-aged children who were born preterm: A meta-analysis. *JAMA, 288,* 728–737.

BioEdge. (2003). Italy passes Europe's toughest IVF law. *BioEdge: Bioethics News for Health and Legal Professionals and the Media.* Retrieved from http://www.australasianbioethics.org/Newsletters/104-2003-12-12.html#italy

Blyth, E. (1994). "I wanted to be interesting. I wanted to be able to say I've done something with my life": Interview with surrogate mothers in Britain. *Journal of Reproductive and Infant Psychology, 12*(3), 189–198.

Boivin, J., & Takeftnan, J. E. (1995). Stress level across stages of in vitro fertilization in subsequently pregnant and non-pregnant women. *Fertility & Sterility, 64,* 802–810.

Boseley, S. (1997). Kiss and sell. *Guardian, 20*(Suppl. January), 2–3.

Braverman, A., & Corson, S. (1992). Characteristics of participants in a gestational carrier program. *Journal of Assisted Reproduction and Genetics, 9,* 353–357.

Brewaeys, A. (1996). Donor insemination: The impact on family and child development. *Journal of Psychosomatic Obstetrics and Gynecology, 17,* 1–13.

Brewaeys, A. (2001). Parent–child relationships and child development in donor insemination families. *Human Reproduction Update, 7,* 38–46.

Bringhenti, F., Martinelli, F., Ardenti, R., & LaSala, G. B. (1997). Psycho-logical adjustment of infertile women entering IVF treatment: Differ-entiating aspects and influencing factors. *Acta Obstetricia et Gynecologica Scandinavica, 76,* 431–437.

Brkovich, A. M., & Fisher, W. A. (1998). Psychological distress and infertility: Forty years of research. *Journal of Psychosomatic Obstetrics and Gyneacology, 19,* 218–228.

Broen, A., Moum, T., Bødtker, A., & Ekeberg, O. (2005). The course of mental health after miscarriage and induced abortion: A longitudinal, five-year follow-up study. *BMC Medicine, 3,* 14–18.

Callahan, T. L., Hall, J. E., Ettner, S. L., Christiansen, C. L., Greene, M. F., & Crowley, W. F. Jr. (1994). The economic impact of multiple gestation pregnancies and the contribution of assisted-reproduction techniques to their incidence. *New England Journal of Medicine, 331,* 244–249.

Choi, Y., Bishai, D., & Minkovitz, C. S. (2009). Multiple births are a risk factor for postpartum maternal depressive symptoms. *Pediatrics, 123,* 1147–1154.

Ciccarelli, J. C., & Beckman, L. J. (2005). Navigating rough waters: An over-view of psychological aspects of surrogacy. *Journal of Social Issues, 61,* 30–31.

CNN. (2001). *Surrogate mother sues California couple.* CNN.com/LawCenter. Retrieved from http://archives.cnn.com/2001/LAW/08/13/surrogate. dispute/

Colpin, H., Demyttenaere, K., & Vandemeulebroecke, L. (1995). New repro-ductive technology and the family: The parent–child relationship fol-lowing in vitro fertilization. *Journal of Child Psychology and Psychiatry and Allied Disciplines, 36,* 1429–1441.

Connolly, K. J., Edelmann, R. J., Cooke, I. D., & Robson, J. (1992). The impact of infertility on psychological functioning. *Journal Psychosomatic Research, 36,* 459–468.

Cook, R., Bradley, S., & Golombok, S. (1998). Preliminary study of parent-ing stress and child behavior in families with twins conceived by in vitro fertilization. *Human Reproduction, 13,* 3244–3246.

Cousineau, T. M., & Domar, A. D. (2007). Psychological impact of infertility. *Best Practice & Research: Clinical Obstetrics & Gynaecology, 21,* 293–308.

Covington, S. (2009). *Healthy parenting tip sheet—Preparing for in vitro fertiliza-tion: Emotional considerations.* Retrieved from http://www.helpstartshere. org/Default.aspx?PageID=1169

Daniluk, J. C. (1988). Infertility: Intrapersonal and interpersonal impact. *Fer-tility & Sterility, 49,* 982–990.

Demyttenaere, K., Bonte, L., Gheldof, M., Vervaeke, M., Meuleman, C., Vanderschuerem, D., & D'Hooghe, T. (1998). Coping style and depression level influence outcome in in vitro fertilization. *Fertility & Sterility, 69,* 1026–1033.

Demyttenaere, K., Nijs, S., Evers, K., & Koninckx, P. (1992). Coping and the ineffectiveness of coping influence the outcome of in vitro fertilization through stress response. *Psychoneuroendocrinology, 17,* 655–665.

Domar, A. D., Broome, B. A., & Zuttermeister, P. C. (1992). The prevalence and predictability of depression in infertile women. *Fertility & Sterility, 58,* 1158–1163.

Domar, A. D., & Seibel, M. M. (1990). Emotional aspects of infertility. In M. M. Seibel (Ed.), *Infertility: A comprehensive text* (pp. 30–43). Norwalk: Appleton and Lange.

Downey, J., & McKinney, M. (1992). The psychiatric stratus of women presenting for infertility evaluation. *Fertility & Sterility, 62,* 196–205.

Dyer, C. (1997). Surrogate mother refuses to give up baby. *British Medical Journal, 314* (7076), 250.

Ellison, M. A., & Hall, J. E. (2003). Social stigma and compounded losses: Quality-of-life issues for multiple-birth families. *Fertility & Sterility, 80,* 405–414.

Ellison, M. A., Hotamisligil, S., Lee, H., Rich-Edwards, J. W., Pang, S. C., & Hall, J. E. (2005). Psychosocial risks associated with multiple births resulting from assisted reproduction. *Fertility & Sterility, 83,* 1422–1428.

English, V., & Sommerville, A. (1996). Mothers in law. *Health Service Journal, 106*(5503), 6.

ESHRE Capri Workshop Group. (2000). Multiple gestation pregnancy. *Human Reproduction, 15,* 1856–1864.

Evert, J. (2007). In vitro fertilization: What to expect. *MentalHelp. net.* Retrieved from http://www.mentalhelp.net/poc/view_doc. php?type=doc&id=11289&cn=65

Farlex, Inc. (2009). *The free dictionary: Medical dictionary.* Retrieved from http://encyclopedia.thefreedictionary.com

Federal Law Gazette. (1990). Act for protection of embryos: The Embryo Protection Act. *Federal Law Gazette, Part I, 69,* 2746. Retrieved from http://78.35.36.94/files/-/1147/ESchG%20englisch.pdf

Fischer, S., & Gillman, I. (1991). Surrogate motherhood: Attachment, attitudes and social support. *Psychiatry, 54,* 13–20.

Fisher, J.R.W., Feekery, C. J., Amir, L. H., & Sneedon, M. (2002). Health and social circumstances of women admitted to a private mother baby unit. *Australian Family Physician, 31,* 966–971.

Fisher, J.R.W., Hammarberg, K., & Baker, G.H.W. (2005). Assisted conception is a risk factor for postnatal mood disturbance and early parenting difficulties. *Fertility & Sterility, 84,* 426–430.

Fisher, J.R.W., Hammarberg, K., & Baker, G.H.W. (2008). Antenatal mood and fetal attachment after assisted conception. *Fertility & Sterility, 89*, 1103–1112.

Fisher, J., & Stocky, A. (2003). Maternal perinatal mental health and multiple births: Implications for practice. *Twin Research, 6*, 506–512.

Gagin, R., Cohen, M., Greenblatt, L., Solomon, H., & Itskovitz-Eldor, J. (2004). Developing the role of the social worker as coordinator of services at the Surrogate Parenting Center. *Social Work in Health Care, 40*(1), 1–14.

Garel, M., & Blondel, B. (1992). Assessment at 1 year of the psychological consequences of having triplets. *Human Reproduction, 7*, 729–732.

Garel, M., Salobir, C., & Blondel, B. (1997). Psychological consequences of having triplets: A 4-year follow-up study. *Fertility & Sterility, 67*, 1162–1165.

Garel, M., Stark, C., Blondel, B., Lefebre, G., Vauthier-Brouzes, D., & Zorn, J. (1997). Psychological reactions after multifetal pregnancy reduction: A 2-year follow-up study. *Human Reproduction, 12*, 617–622.

Garner, C., Arnold, E., & Gray, H. (1984). The psychological impact of in vitro fertilization. *Fertility & Sterility, 41*, 28–31.

Gibson, F. L., Ungerer, J. A., Tennant, C. C., & Saunders, D. M. (2000). Parental adjustment and attitudes to parenting after in vitro fertilization. *Fertility & Sterility, 73*, 565–574.

Glazebrook, C., Cox, S., Oates, M., & Ndukwe, G. (2001). Psychological adjustment during pregnancy and the postpartum period in single and multiple in vitro fertilization births: A review and preliminary findings from an ongoing study. *Reproductive Technologies, 10*(2), 112–120.

Glazebrook, C., Sheard, C., Cox, S., Oates, M., & Ndukwe, G. (2004). Parenting stress in first-time mothers of twins and triplets conceived after in vitro fertilization. *Fertility & Sterility, 81*, 505–511.

Gleicher, N., Campbell, D., Chan, C. L., Karande, V., Rao, R., Balin, M., & Pratt, D. (1995). The desire for multiple births in couples with infertility problems contradicts present practice patterns. *Human Reproduction, 10*, 1079–1084.

Golombok, S., Brewaeys, A., Cook, R., Giavazzi, M. T., Crosignani, P. G., & Dexeus, S. (1996). The European Study of Assisted Reproduction Families: Family functioning and child development. *Human Reproduction, 11*, 2324–2331.

Golombok, S., Brewaeys, A., Giavazzi, M. T., Guerra, D., MacCallum, F., & Rust, J. (2002). The European Study of Assisted Reproduction Families: The transition to adolescence. *Human Reproduction, 17*, 830–840.

Golombok, S., Cook, R., Bish, A., & Murray, C. (1995). Families created by the new reproductive technology: The parent–child relationship following in vitro fertilization. *Journal of Child Psychology and Psychiatry, 36*, 1429–1441.

Golombok, S., MacCallum, F., Goodman, E., & Rutter, M. (2002). Families with children conceived by donor insemination: A follow-up at age 12. *Child Development, 73,* 952–968.

Golombok, S., Murray, C., Brinsden, P., & Abdalla, H. (1999). Social versus biological parenting: Family functioning and the socioemotional development of children conceived by egg or sperm donation. *Journal of Child Psychology and Psychiatry and Allied Disciplines, 40,* 519–527.

Golombok, S., Murray, C., Jadva, V., MacCallum, F., & Lycett, E. (2004). Families created through surrogacy arrangements: Parent–child relationships in the 1st year of life. *Developmental Psychology, 40,* 400–411.

Greenfeld, D. A. (1997). Infertility and assisted reproductive technology: The role of the perinatal social worker. *Social Work in Health Care, 24*(3/4), 39–46.

Groothuis, J. R., Altemeier, W. A., Robarge, J. P., O'Connor, S., Sandler, H., Vietze, P., & Lustig, J. V. (1982). Increased child abuse in families with twins. *Pediatrics, 70,* 769–773.

Guerra, D., Llobera, A., Veiga, A., & Barri, P. N. (1998). Psychiatric morbidity in couples attending a fertility service. *Human Reproduction, 13,* 1733–1736.

Hahn, C. S., & DiPietro, J. A. (2001). In vitro fertilization and the family: Quality of parenting, family functioning, and child psychosocial adjustment. *Developmental Psychology, 37,* 37–48.

Hammarberg, K., Fisher, J.R.W., & Rowe, H.J. (2008). Women's experiences of childbirth and post-natal healthcare after assisted conception. *Human Reproduction, 23,* 1567–1573.

Hammarberg, K., Fisher, J.R.W., & Wynter, K. H. (2008). Psychological and social aspects of pregnancy, childbirth and early parenting after assisted conception: A systematic review. *Human Reproduction Update, 14,* 395–414.

Hay, D., Gleeson, C., Davies, C., Lorden, B., Mitchell, D., & Patten, L. (1990). What information should the multiple birth family receive before, during and after the birth? *Acta Beneticae Medicae et Gemellolgiae, 39,* 259–269.

Hay, D., & O'Brien, P. (1984). The role of parental attitudes in the development of temperament in twins at home, school, and in test situations. *Acta Geneticae Medicae et Gemellologiae, 33,* 191–204.

Health-Cares. (2005). *What treatments are available to cure infertility? Health-Cares.net: Your fitness guides.* Retrieved from http://womens-health.health-cares.net/infertility-treatment.php

Henning, K., & Strauss, B. (2002). Psychological and psychosomatic aspects of involuntary childlessness: State of research at the end of the 1990's. In B. Strauss (Ed.), *Involuntary childlessness: Psychological assessment, counseling, psychotherapy.* Berlin: Hogrefe & Huber.

Herz, E. K. (1992). Prediction, recognition, and prevention. In J. A. Hamilton & P. N. Harberger (Eds.), Postpartum psychiatric illness: A picture puzzle. Philadelphia: University of Pennsylvania Press.

Hjelmstedt, A., Widström, A-M., Wramsby, H., & Collins, A. (2003). Patterns of emotional responses to pregnancy, experience of pregnancy and attitudes to parenthood among IVF couples: A longitudinal study. *Journal of Psychosomatic Obstetrics and Gynecology, 24,* 153–162.

Holditch-Davis, D., Roberts, D., & Sandelowski, M. (1999). Early parental interactions with and perceptions of multiple birth infants. *Journal of Advanced Nursing, 30,* 200–210.

Honig, D., Nave, O., & Adam, R. (2000). Israeli surrogacy law in practice. *Israel Journal of Psychiatry and Related Sciences, 37,* 115–123.

Human Fertilization and Embryology Authority. (1998). *Seventh annual report.* London: Human Fertilization and Embryology Authority.

Human Fertilization and Embryology Authority. (2008). *Facts and figures 2006: Fertility problems and treatment.* Retrieved from http://www.hfea.gov.uk/docs/Facts_and_Figures_2006_fertility_probs_and_treatment_2008-10-08.pdf

Hunt, J., & Monach, J. (1997). Beyond the bereavement model: The significance of depression for infertility counseling. *Human Reproduction, 12,* 188–194.

Ismail, W. A., Menezes, M. Q., Martin, C. W., & Thong, K. J. (2004). A comparison of psychological functioning in couples undergoing frozen-thawed embryo replacement in various stages of treatment using the Mean Affect Adjective Check List (MAACL). *Journal of Assisted Reproduction and Genetics, 21,* 323–327.

Jadva, V., Murray, C., Lycett, E., MacCallum, F., & Golombok, S. (2003). Surrogacy: The experiences of surrogate mothers. *Human Reproduction, 18,* 2196–2204.

Kalra, S. K., Milad, M. P., Klock, S. C., & Grobman, W. A. (2003). Infertility patients and their partners: Differences in desire for twin gestations. *Obstetrics & Gynecology, 102,* 152–155.

Klaus, M., & Kennell, J. (1982). *Parent-infant bonding* (2nd ed.). St. Louis: CV Mosby.

Kleinpeter, C. H. (2002). Surrogacy: The parents' story. *Psychological Reports, 91,* 201–219.

Kleinpeter, C. H., & Hohman, M. M. (2000). Surrogate motherhood: Personality traits and satisfaction with service providers. *Psychological Reports, 97,* 957–970.

Klock, S., & Greenfeld, D. A. (2000). Psychological status of in vitro fertilization patients during pregnancy: A longitudinal study. *Fertility & Sterility, 73,* 1159–1164.

Kovacs, B., Kirschbaum, T., & Paul, R. (1989). Twin gestations: Antenatal care and complications. *Obstetrics & Gynecology, 74,* 313–317.

Leiblum, S. (Ed.). (1997). *Infertility: Psychological issues and counseling strategies.* Chichester, England: John Wiley & Sons.

Leiblum, S. R., Aviv, A., & Hamer, R. (1998). Life after infertility treatment: A long-term investigation of marital and sexual function. *Human Reproduction, 13,* 3569–3574.

Leonard, L. G. (1998). Depression and anxiety disorders during multiple pregnancy and parenthood. *Journal of Obstetric, Gynecologic, and Neonatal Nursing, 27,* 329–337.

Lind, R. F., Pruitt, R. L., & Greenfeld, D. (1989). Previously infertile couples and the newborn intensive care unit. *Health & Social Work, 14,* 127–133.

Long, P., & Oats, J. (1987). Preeclampsia in twin pregnancy: Severity and pathogenesis. *Australian and New Zealand Journal of Obstetrics and Gynaecology, 27,* 1–5.

Lord, S., & Robertson, N. (2005). The role of patient appraisal and coping in predicting distress in IVT. *Journal of Reproductive and Infant Psychology, 23,* 319–332.

Lumley, J. (2004). O brave new world!: Commentary. *Birth, 31,* 315–316.

MacCallum, F., Lycett, E., Murray, C., Jadva, V., & Golombok, S. (2003). Surrogacy: The experience of commissioning couples. *Human Reproduction, 18,* 1334–1342.

MacDorman, M., Minino, A., Strobing, D., & Guyer, B. (2002). Annual summary of vital statistics –2001. *Pediatrics, 110,* 1037–1052.

Martin, J. A., & Park, M. M. (1999). Trends in twin and triplet births: 1980–1997. *National Vital Statistics Report, 47*(24), 1–16.

McMahon, C. A., Tennant, C., Ungerer, H. A., & Saunders, D. (1999). "Don't count your chickens": A comparative study of the experience of pregnancy after IVF conception. *Journal of Reproductive Infant Psychology, 17,* 345–356.

McMahon, C. A., Ungerer, J. A., Beaurepaire, J., Tennant, C., & Saunders, D. (1997). Anxiety during pregnancy and fetal attachment after in-vitro fertilization conception. *Human Reproduction, 12,* 176–182.

McMahon, C. A., Ungerer, J. A. Tennant, C., & Saunders, D. (1997). Psychological adjustment and the quality of the mother–child relationship at four months postpartum after conception by in vitro fertilization. *Fertility & Sterility, 68,* 492–500.

Menning, B. E. (1980). The emotional needs of infertile couples. *Fertility & Sterility, 34,* 313–319.

Möller, A., & Fällström, K. (1991). Psychological consequences of infertility: A longitudinal study. *Journal of Psychosomatic Obstetrics and Gynecology, 12,* 27–45.

Monga, M., Alexandrescu, B., Katz, S. E., Stein, M., & Ganiats, T. (2004). Impact of infertility on quality of life, marital adjustment, and sexual functioning. *Urology, 63,* 126–130.

Monti, F., Agostini, F. Fagandini, P., La Sala, G. B., & Blickstein, I. (2009). Depressive symptoms during late pregnancy and early parenthood following assisted reproductive technology. *Fertility & Sterility, 91,* 851–857.

Morrow, K., Thoreson, R., & Penney, L. (1995). Predictors of psychological distress among infertility clinic patients. *Journal of Consulting and Clinical Psychology, 63,* 163–167.

Newton, C. R., Sherrard, W., & Glavac, I. (1999). The fertility problem inventory: Measuring perceived infertility-related stress. *Fertility & Sterility, 72,* 54–62.

Oddens, B. J., den Tonkelaar, I., & Nieuwenhuyse, H. (1999). Psychosocial experiences in women facing fertility problems: Comparative survey. *Human Reproduction, 14,* 255–261.

Olivennes, F., Golombok, S., Ramogida, C., & Rust, J. (2005). Behavioral and cognitive development as well as family functioning of twins conceived by assisted reproduction: Findings from a large population study. *Fertility & Sterility, 84,* 725–733.

Olshansky, E. (1987a). Identity of self as infertile: An example of theory-generating research. *Advances in Nursing Science, 9,* 54–63.

Olshansky, E. (1987b). Infertility and its influence on women's career identities. *Health Care for Women International, 8*(2–3), 185–196.

Olshansky, E. (1988a). Married couples' experiences of infertility [Abstract]. *Communicating Nursing Research, 21,* 47.

Olshansky, E. (1988b). Responses to high technology infertility treatment. *Image: Journal of Nursing Scholarship, 20,* 128–131.

Olshansky, E. (1990). Psychosocial implications of pregnancy after infertility. *NAACOG's Clinical Issues in Women's Health and Perinatal Nursing, 1,* 342–347.

Olshansky, E. (1995). *Long-term psychological effects of infertility: Current state of knowledge.* Invited paper presentation for Workshop on the Psychobiology of Infertility. National Institute of Child Health and Human Development, National Institutes of Health, September 1995.

Olshansky, E. F. (1996). Theoretical issues in building a grounded theory: Application of an example of a program of research on infertility. *Qualitative Health Research, 6,* 394–405.

Olshansky, E. (2003). A theoretical explanation for previously infertile mothers' vulnerability to depression. *Journal of Nursing Scholarship, 35,* 263–268.

Oz, S. (1995). Genetic mother vs surrogate mother: Which mother does the law recognize? A comparison of Jewish Law, American Law, and English Law. *Touro International Law Review, 6*(1), 438–468.

Parents of Multiple Births Association of Canada. (1993). *Results of the national survey.* Stratford, Ontario, Canada: Author.

Parker, P. J. (1983). Motivation of surrogate mothers: Initial findings. *American Journal of Psychiatry, 140,* 117–118.

Pasch, L. A., Dunkel-Schetter, C., & Christensen, A. (2002). Differences between husbands' and wives' approach to infertility affect marital communication and adjustment. *Fertility & Sterility, 77,* 1241–1247.

Peterson, B. D., Newton, C. R., & Rosen, K. H. (2003). Examining congruence between partners' perceived infertility-related stress and its relationship with marital adjustment and depression among infertile couples. *Family Process, 42*(1), 59–70.

Pinborg, A., Loft, A., & Andersen, A. N. (2004). Neonatal outcome in a Danish national cohort of 8602 children born after in vitro fertilization or intracytoplasmic sperm injection: The role of twin pregnancy. *Acta Obstetrica et Gynecologica Scandinavica, 83,* 1071–1078.

Ragone, H. (1994). *Surrogate motherhood: Conception in the heart.* Boulder, CO: Westview Press.

Raoul-Duval, A., Bertrand-Servais, M., Letur-Konirsch, H., & Frydman, R. (1994). Psychological follow-up of children born after in-vitro fertilization. *Human Reproduction, 9,* 1097–1101.

Reilly, D. R. (2007). Surrogate pregnancy: A guide for Canadian prenatal health care providers. *Canadian Medical Association Journal, 176,* 483–485.

Repokari, L., Punamaki, R-L., Unkila-Kallio, L., Vilska, S., Poikkeus, P., Sinkkonen, J., et al. (2007). Infertility treatment and marital relationships: A 1-year prospective study among successfully treated ART couples and their controls. *Human Reproduction, 22,* 1481–1491.

Robin, M., Bydlowski, M., Cahen, F., & Josse, D. (1991). Maternal reactions to the birth of triplets. *Acta Beneticae Medicae et Gemellologiae, 40,* 41–52.

Robin, M., Corroyer, D., & Casati, I. (1996). Childcare patterns of mothers of twins during the first year. *Journal of Child Psychology and Psychiatry, 37,* 453–460.

Roughley, G. (2007). How would you feel about surrogacy? [Editorial]. *British Journal of Midwifery, 15,* 281.

Sandelowski, M., Harris, B. G., & Holditch-Davis, D. (1990). Pregnant moments: The process of conception in infertile couples. *Research in Nursing & Health, 13,* 273–282.

Schmidt, L., Holstein, B., Christensen, U., & Boivin, J. (2005). Does infertility cause marital benefit? An epidemiological study of 2250 women and men in fertility treatment. *Patient Education and Counseling, 59,* 224–251.

Sheard, C., Cox, S., Oates, M., Ndukwe, G., & Glazebrook, C. (2007). Impact of a multiple, IVF birth on post-partum mental health: A composite analysis. *Human Reproduction, 22,* 2058–2056.

Singer, P., & Wells, D. (1983, January). Spurned baby sparks action on surrogate births. *The Australian, 27,* 1.

Singer, P., & Wells, D. (1985). *The reproduction revolution: New ways of making babies.* Oxford: Oxford University Press.

Slade, P., Emery, J., & Lieberman, B. A. (1997). A prospective, longitudinal study of emotions and relationships in in-vitro fertilization treatment. *Human Reproduction, 12,* 183–190

Smith, M. (1998). Maternal-fetal attachment in surrogate mothers. *British Journal of Midwifery, 6*(3), 188–192.

Snowdon, C. (1994). What makes a mother? Interviews with women involved in egg donation and surrogacy. *Birth, 21,* 77–84.

Söderström-Antilla, V., Blomqvist, T., Foudila, T., Hippeläinen, M., Kurunmäki, H., Siegberg, R., et al. (2002). Experience of in vitro fertilization surrogacy in Finland. *Acta Obstetricia et Gynecologica Scandinavica, 81,* 747–752.

Söderström-Antilla, V., Sajaneimi, N., Tiitinen, A., & Hovatta, O. (1998). Health and development of children born after oocyte donation compared with that of those born after in-vitro fertilization, and parents' attitudes regarding secrecy. *Human Reproduction, 13,* 2009–2015.

Speroff, L., & Fritz, M. A. (2005). Induction of ovulation. In *Clinical gynecologic endocrinology and infertility* (7th ed.). Philadelphia: Lippincott, Williams & Wilkins.

Stanton, F., & Golombok, S. (1993). Maternal–fetal attachment during pregnancy following in vitro fertilization. *Journal of Psychosomatic Obstetrics and Gynecology, 14,* 153–158.

Sydsjö, G., Wadsby, M., Kjellberg, M., & Sydsjö, A. (2002). Relationships and parenthood in couples after assisted reproduction and in spontaneous primiparous couples: A prospective long-term follow-up study. *Human Reproduction, 17,* 3242–3250.

Thiering, P., Beaurepaire, J., Jones, M., Saunders, D., & Tennant, C. (1993). Mood state as a predictor of treatment outcome after in vitro fertilization/embryo transfer technology. *Journal of Psychosomatic Research, 37*(5), 481–491.

Thorpe, K., Golding, J., MacGillivray, I., & Greenwood, R. (1991). Comparison of prevalence of depression in mothers of twins and mothers of singletons. *British Medical Journal, 302,* 875–878.

Thorpe, K., Greenwood, R., & Goodenough, T. (1995). Does a twin pregnancy have a greater impact on physical and emotional well-being than a singleton pregnancy? *Birth, 22,* 148–152.

Tieu, M. M. (2009). Altruistic surrogacy: The necessary objectification of surrogate mothers. *Journal of Medical Ethics, 35*(3), 171–175.

Turner, A. J., & Coyle, A. (2000). What does it mean to be a donor offspring? The identity experiences of adults conceived by donor insemination and the implications for counseling and therapy. *Human Reproduction, 15,* 2041–2051.

Ulrich, D., Gagel, D. E., Hemmerling, A., Parstor, V-S., & Kentenich, H. (2004). Couples becoming parents: Something special after IVF? *Journal of Psychosomatic Obstetrics and Gynecology, 25,* 99–113.

van Balen, F., Naaktgeboren, N., & Trimbos-Kemper, T.C.M. (1996). In-vitro fertilization: The experience of treatment, pregnancy and delivery. *Human Reproduction, 11,* 95–98.

van Zyl, L., & van Niekerk, A. (2000). Interpretations, perspectives and intentions in surrogate motherhood. *Journal of Medical Ethics, 26,* 404–409.

Weaver, S. M., Clifford, E., Gordon, A. G., Hay, D. M., & Robinson, J. (1993). A follow-up study of "successful" IVF/GIFT couples: Social–emotional well-being and adjustment to parenthood. *Journal of Psychosomatic Obstetrics and Gynecology, 14,* 5–16.

WebMD. (2008). *Clomiphene citrate for infertility.* Retrieved from http://www.webmd.com/infertility-and-reproduction/clomiphene-citrate-for-infertility#zt1392

Wischmann, T., Stammer, H., Scherg, H., Gerhard, I., & Verres, R. (2001). Psychosocial characteristics of infertile couples: A study by the "Heidelberg fertility consultation service". *Human Reproduction, 16,* 1753–1761.

World Health Organization. (2009). *Assisted reproductive technologies (ARTs).* Retrieved from http://www.who.int/genomics/gender/en/index6.html

Yong, P., Martin, C., & Thong, J. (2000). A comparison of psychological functioning in women at different stages of in vitro fertilization treatment using the Mean Affect Adjective Check List. *Journal of Assisted Reproduction and Genetics, 17,* 553–556.

Zager, S. (1996). Legislative update. *Organization of Parents Through Surrogacy News, 15,* 8–12.

Chapter 10

Pre- and Postadoption
Depression

Approximately 3 percent of children ages 18 and under are adopted in the United States (Kreider, 2003). In general, there is the misconception that adoptive parents are excited, overjoyed, and looking forward to be parents. While this may be the case, the choice to adopt may include grief and loss over the inability to conceive as a couple (Silverstein & Kaplan, 1990). Stress levels increase due to agency evaluations, waiting for a baby to become available, social stigma, and thinking about possible health complications that the baby may have (Brodzinsky & Huffman, 1989; Senecky et al., 2009). Social stigma about adoption occurs when one or both members of a couple are infertile or unable to find a partner. When adopting a child of a different race or ethnicity or being a homosexual person trying to adopt a child, many people find they have to cope with racism and homophobia (Domar, Broome, Zuttermeister, Seibel, & Friedman, 1992). Furthermore, the dream of having a child may mask the radical life changes that occur once the baby has arrived (Lorant et al., 2003).

Adoption Process

The process of adoption is extremely stressful for some. This stress mimics that experienced by women during pregnancy, and can trigger post-adoption depression and anxiety. Approximately one in four women (in Israel) reported experiencing pre-adoption depression (Iancu, Horesh, Lepkifker, & Drory, 2003; Senecky et al., 2009). However, this depression appeared to decrease once the baby was in the home (Ceballo, Lansford, Abbey, & Stewart, 2004; Senecky et al., 2009). In Senecky et al.'s research conducted in Israel, pre- and post-adoption mothers had similar rates of depression. In addition, adoptive mothers may feel guilt or anxiety that she is not breastfeeding the baby, and this may cause health-related problems for the infant (Silverstein & Kaplan, 1990; Smith & Sherwen, 1988).

Most state laws mandate that adoptive parents pay for the prenatal care and some household expenses while the biological mother is pregnant—typically for two months prior to the birth. Other adoptive parents may go through advertisements and wind up paying for expenses longer or for extra items for the biological parent in an effort to ensure a healthy baby and to show their appreciation to the biological mother. Unfortunately, for the adopting parents, there is also legislation in place that gives the biological mother a specified period in which she can choose to keep the baby rather than continue with the adoption. This period can increase adoptive parents' depression and anxiety, and increase hesitancy to bond with the baby out of fear that the biological mother will change her mind. Women report feeling anxious, stressed, and depressed during this waiting period (Gair, 1999). This is further exacerbated when the parents are told that they will be called when a baby is ready to be adopted. When the call comes, some parents panic, have an increase in stress levels and sudden despair—wondering if they are actually ready.

Postadoption Mood Changes

As early as the 1950s, experts have described post-adoption depression after the baby arrives. However, even today, post-adoption depression receives limited attention (Melges, 1968; Van Putten & La Wall, 1981; Victoroff, 1952). Risk factors for the development of postadoption depression are similar to postpartum depression, such as increased workloads, decreased sleep, and increased responsibilities (Gair, 1999). Women can experience internal conflict due to adopting the child and coming to terms with her role as mother, particularly because she physically did not give birth or experience any physical postpartum changes (Melges, 1968).

There are similarities in adjusting to motherhood, regardless of whether the mother is biological or adoptive. Many new mothers face changes in independence, personal identity, career and employment, and in her relationship with her partner (Gair, 1999). Women who choose to delay motherhood to establish themselves professionally may have an increase in feelings of guilt, particularly if they waited too long, were not able to conceive a baby, and chose adoption instead.

A common trigger for postpartum depression is the disposition of the baby. Babies that cry often (particularly throughout the night), have colic, or have difficulty eating are often viewed negatively by the mother with post-partum depression, with the baby being blamed for her depressed feelings. Women who adopt may also experience this pattern, increasing susceptibility to post-adoption depression.

The concept of post-adoption depression has the potential to create etiological controversy, as mothers who adopt have obviously not experienced the hormonal fluctuations and obstetrical trauma risks associated with pregnancy or delivery. The only suggested biological influence on the development of post-adoption depression is the woman's history with premenstrual dysphoric disorder (Melges, 1968). Yet, other research into this potential hormonally based link between postpartum depression and premenstrual syndrome has been refuted by other research, making it unlikely that premenstrual syndrome is related to post-adoption depression at all (Davidson, 1972; O'Hara, Zekoski, Phillips, & Wright, 1990). Due to this, the development of post-adoption depression is primarily based on psychosocial and cultural factors. One proposal is that women who are mothers in contemporary Western societies express emotional responses related to the transition to motherhood and adapting to the expected mother roles (Gair, 1999).

Homosexual and Bisexual Couples Who Adopt

An estimated 1 million same-sex couples (gay, lesbian, and bisexual [GLB]) have children in the United States (Patterson & Friel, 2000). The majority of GLB individuals have stable mental health functioning. However, as I am discussing mental health changes, I am going to discuss some of the mental health statistics for this population here.

Mental health studies conducted with lesbians have shown that this population experiences higher rates of childhood abuse, low self-esteem, depression, and stress than their heterosexual counterparts (Hughes & Wilsnack, 1997; Ryan & Futterman, 1997; Trippet, 1994). Approximately one in five lesbian women have attempted suicide, slightly more than one in three had been physically abused, one in three had been sexually assaulted or raped, and one in five experienced incest as a child (Bradford & Ryan, 1994). By and large, lesbian and bisexual women will access mental health services more frequently in their lifetimes than will heterosexual women (Cochran & Mays, 2000; Cochran, Mays, & Sullivan, 2003). One project found that approximately three in four lesbian or bisexual women had received mental health care at some point in their lives and one in three had received mental health care within one year of the study (Steele, Ross, Epstein, Strike, &

Goldfinger, 2008). When seen for counseling, approximately one in two were suffering with depression symptoms (Bradford & Ryan, 1994, Rothblum & Factor, 2001). Common complaints are lack of family or friend support networks, feeling isolated from others, and feeling inferior in society (Oetjen & Rothblum, 2000; Safren & Heimberg, 1999; Savin-Williams, 1994). Those who openly live a homosexual lifestyle incur more violence and discrimination as a result, which negatively affects a person's health and mental health (Cochran & Mays, 2007). Yet others report more satisfaction with friends and in the workplace (D'Augelli, Hershberger, & Pilkington, 1998; Ellis & Riggle, 1996; Griffith & Hebl, 2002).

Parenthood Stressors

Several women who identify as lesbian or bisexual, whether in a same-sex partnership or single, seek to have children either through pregnancy, medically assisted methods, surrogacy, or adoption (Epstein, 2003; O'Hanlan et al., 2004). Unlike most heterosexual couples, homosexual couples see adoption as the first option to have children (Mallon, 2007; Turner, 1999). However, GLB couples may be denied the options due to homophobia and heterosexism (Baeten & Brewaeys, 2001; Strong & Schinfeld, 1984).

Some same-sex partners become pregnant and attend birthing classes and parenting classes. By and large, same-sex couples report having difficulty and feel anxious when attending these training courses—surrounded by heterosexual couples—finding it difficult to interact with other training course members due to homophobic reaction (Mallon, 2004, 2006; Mallon & Betts, 2005).

The Adoption Process

At times, homosexuals who apply to adopt a child are held to higher standards than are heterosexual counterparts. Therefore, some present themselves to the agency behaving in a conventional heterosexual, gender-stereotypical manner (Brodzinsky & the Staff of the Even B. Donaldson Adoption Institute, 2003; Brooks & Goldberg, 2001; Hicks, 2000). In Brodzinsky et al.'s (2003) study, adoption agencies that primarily placed domestically based children for adoption predominantly rejected same-sex couple's adoptions. Same-sex couples most likely receive adoption approval for children with special needs or international children. When adopting outside of the country, sexual orientation disclosure is not recommended (Ross et al., 2008). Not disclosing sexual orientation is exhausting. One person, who opted to keep her same-sex relationship private, reported feeling psycho-emotionally and physically exhausted by the constant questioning and threats by the agency to reject the adoption should a same-sex relationship be discovered (Ross et al., 2008).

Same-sex couples face heterosexism, oppression, stigma, and homophobic fears from those conducting the screening (Herek, 1988, 1990, 2000, 2004; Lobaugh, Clements, Averill, & Olguin, 2006). The intensity and fear involved during the agency screening process can cause a great emotional and mental health toll on same-sex couples. Approximately 70 percent of a small sample found that same-sex couples described the agency screening process as an "emotional rollercoaster" (Ross et al., 2008).

The screenings become more complex when taking into account the new political atmosphere about same-sex marriage, what constitutes a "family," and honoring state by state legislation about each—thereby adding an additional legislative level to the adoption assessment process for same-sex couples (Appell, 2001; Lobaugh et al., 2006). As of 2005, 13 states have approved same-sex-couple adoption, 14 states have approved these adoptions through lower court rulings, 21 states have yet to approve legislation for same-sex couples to adopt, and three states have disapproved adoption to same-sex couples (Lambda Legal, 2005; Lobaugh et al., 2006).

So, some same-sex couples need to evaluate their desire to adopt and go through the adoption assessment process but may also need to consider relocating to a state that approves of adoption to same-sex couples. These couples should also research adoption agencies that do not discriminate by sexual orientation (Brodzinsky, Patterson, & Vaziri, 2002; Lobaugh et al., 2006). If the couple chooses to relocate to adopt, this can decrease the parental and family support provided by family and friends due to location changes (Lobaugh et al., 2006). To recap, the agency screening process, the sociopolitical atmosphere surrounding heterosexism and the legalities of same-sex marriage, and the definition of family add to the stress, anxiety, and mental health concerns for homosexual couples seeking to adopt.

Contemporary Issues

One of the most predominant issues that surface when discussing homosexual couples who adopt is the welfare of the children in this family unit. Those that oppose same-sex-couple adoption argue that same-sex (particularly gay men) partners are less capable of healthy parenting skills as compared with heterosexual couples (Binger & Jacobsen, 1992; Maney & Cain, 1997; Mooney-Somers & Golombok, 2000). Over 30 years ago, when the acceptance of same-sex partnerships was less open than it is today, children from lesbian parents were no more likely to suffer from harassment, mental health conditions, or difficulty forming peer-to-peer relationships than were children from heterosexual, single-mother homes (Golombok, Spencer, & Rutter, 1983; Green, 1978; Green, Mandel, Hotvedt, Gray, & Smith, 1986; Kirkpatrick, Smith, & Roy, 1981; Mooney-Somers & Golombok, 2000). Children with same-sex parents have a similar sense of self-worth, future educational aspirations, and maturity level as do children with heterosexual parents (Stacey & Biblarz, 2001). There are no noted differences in development or well-being. Children adopted by lesbians have no different gender identity, sexual orientation, morals, social judgment, intellectual capabilities, and concept of self than other children (Anderssen, Amlie, & Ytteroy, 2002).

One issue commonly raised is the fear that children with same-sex parents will develop abnormal gender identity and roles. In the extreme, some hold the belief that gay male couples are seeking to adopt to encourage their children to lead a gay lifestyle later in life (Green et al., 1986). Those who hold this belief contend that children of same-sex couples wind up becoming homosexual later in life, show gender confusion, and express gender-inappropriate behaviors (Mooney-Somers & Golombok, 2000). However, some children from heterosexual parents grow up and identify as gay, lesbian, bisexual, or transgendered—obviously not a result of being influenced by homosexual parents. In addition, sociocultural environment influences and defines gender stereotypes, not necessarily the parents (Mooney-Somers & Golombok, 2000). Past research shows no difference in feminine or masculine behaviors in girls or boys, respectively, of homosexual or heterosexual mothers (Drexler, 2006; Golombok et al., 1983; Green et al., 1986; Kirkpatrick et al., 1981; Mitchell, 2008; Mooney-Somers & Golombok, 2000). In one study, nine out of 10 children who grew up with two female parents identified as heterosexual when assessed as young adults (Golombok & Tasker, 1996; Tasker & Golombok, 1997). Often, lesbian partners who adopt male children try to find supportive male role models (Brewaeys, Olbrechts, Devroey, & Van Steirteghem, 1989; Drexler, 2006; Hare & Richards, 1993; Kirkpatrick et al., 1981; Mooney-Somers & Golombok, 2000). Children of lesbian mothers who were divorced (from a heterosexual marriage) had more contact with their fathers than did heterosexual couple's children (Golombok et al., 1983).

Contrary to the aforementioned argument against same-sex couple adoption, many male adolescents have better social conduct, are less aggressive, and are more sexually controlled than their heterosexual-parented counterparts (Stacey & Biblarz, 2001). A study of children raised by lesbian couples found that the mothers were more likely to be committed to and engaged in the child's life, to cultivate a healthy emotional environment for development, and to have had better synchronization in parenting perspectives (Stacey & Biblarz, 2001). Research shows no attachment style differences between children raised by heterosexual and homosexual parents (Ridge & Feeney, 1998; Shaver & Hazan, 1993). Instead, it is argued, that maintaining a healthy and stable environment in which to grow up is the most important quality that children who are adopted need, just as it is with other children who are not adopted (Lobaugh et al., 2006; Silverman, 2002).

Another argument is that homophobia is rampant in United States society and it is unfair to subject children to potential societal disenfranchisement. The result of this exposure can lead to mockery and discrimination; conflicts with peers; becoming depressed, anxious, or suicidal; and disruption of the development of healthy peer-to-peer relationships (Cochran & Mays, 2000; Mooney-Somers & Golombok, 2000).

The National Association of Social Workers states that children reared with hetero- or homosexual parents are no different (Crisp & Padilla, 2004). Through an extensive literature search, Lobaugh et al. (2006) found no medical or mental health professional organization that condemned same-sex parents from adopting, stating that organizational support is based on empirical research—but public and societal opinion, heterosexism, homophobia, and stigma may have a stronger influence on legislative changes.

Postpartum and Postadoption Mood Changes

Unfortunately, there is little information about perinatal mental health effects on same-sex couples (Ross, 2005; Trettin, Moses-Kolko, & Wisner, 2006). When lesbian women become pregnant, either through medically assisted procedures or through prearranged sexual intercourse with a chosen male, perinatal mood changes may be greater due to stigmas by medical professionals and due to normal risks that all women face (Steele & Stratmann, 2006; Trettin et al., 2006). In general, lesbians are at increased risk to develop depression due to the constant stress of living in a homophobic and heterosexist society, as well as the detrimental events that often occur for lesbians who are open about their sexual orientation (Matthews, Hughes, Johnson, Razzano, & Cassidy, 2002). However, female same-sex partners may also possess protective factors that heterosexual couples tend not to have, such as a planned pregnancy, more balanced and equal sharing of child care, and better communication skills (Ross, 2005).

The neurochemical increases in stress hormones may result from living with constant stressors (Trettin et al., 2006). When a lesbian becomes pregnant, she experiences the normal hormonal changes while living in a homophobic environment—a constant stressor. Combine these constant stressors with the physical and emotional effect of pregnancy and you have a formula for high-risk perinatal mood disorder conditions. One study found that lesbian and bisexual mothers had higher levels of postpartum depression than their heterosexual counterparts (Ross, Steele, Goldfinger, & Strike, 2007).

Lesbian and bisexual mothers who adopt report high Edinburgh Perinatal Depression Scale scores, indicating high levels of post-adoption depression (Ross et al., 2007). This may indicate a greater risk for post-adoption depression due to discrimination, legal concerns, high prevalence rate for a pre-existing depression and anxiety diagnoses, and limited social supports, but further research needs to be conducted (Cochran, 2001; Gilman et al., 2001; Matthews et al., 2002; O'Hara & Swain, 1996; Robertson, Grace, Wallington, & Stewart, 2004; Ross, Sellers, Gilbert-Evans, & Romach, 2004; Ross et al., 2007; Sandfort, de Graaf, Bijl, & Schnabel, 2001).

One risk factor for mood changes during the first postadoption year is adapting to lifestyle changes related to having a baby in the family (Bennett, 2003; Shelley-Sireci & Ciano-Boyce, 2002). Lesbian couples who adopt reported decreased support from same-sex friends (Bennett, 2003) and may already have strained relationships or little support from family members due to their sexual orientation. In addition, many lesbian couples who adopt find limited support from other couples who have had medically assisted pregnancies or who are younger same-sex couples, further isolating the couple's support network (Bennett, 2003). In short, same-sex couples who adopt are at a substantial risk for social, communitywide, and familial isolation.

Another risk factor is that same-sex couples are likely to adopt children who have special needs (Brooks et al., 2001), thereby increasing the risk to develop mental health changes (McGlone, Santos, Kazama, Fong, & Mueller, 2002). These mental health risks are not researched sufficiently in the same-sex adopting community and, therefore, are expressed here as suppositions based on general research about adopting children with special needs (Ross et al., 2008).

Access to Care

Pregnant and postpartum lesbian women most often receive mental health care from psychologists, psychotherapists, or obstetricians. One in five lesbian women received mental health care from her obstetrician during pregnancy or while she tried to conceive (Steele et al., 2008). In Steele et al.'s study, lesbian or bisexual women who were the nonbiological parents of the child (assumed here to be adoptive parents) sought out mental health services less frequently than did those who were attempting to become pregnant. Women in this study who reported that their mental health needs were not being met were more likely to have become pregnant by engaging in prearranged intercourse with a man as compared with women who became pregnant by an anonymous sperm donor from a sperm bank. In addition, women who were pregnant but concealed their sexual orientation were more likely to have sought out mental health care close to the time of the study.

One barrier to perinatal health and mental health is heterosexism and homophobia from medical professionals, which negatively affects appropriate perinatal care. This barrier increases should a woman also be a member of two to three minority groups (for example, being a minority woman who is also homosexual) (Trettin, Moses-Kolko, & Wisner, 2006). Whereas one study estimated one in three women disclosed her sexual orientation to her medical provider (Lehmann, Lehmann, & Kelly, 1998), more recent research shows that nine in 10 only disclosed this information to the doctor with whom they visited most often (Steele et al., 2008). Of those who disclosed this personal information, approximately one in four indicated that the disclosure harmfully influenced her health care (van Dam, Koh, & Dibble, 2001).

References

Anderssen, N., Amile, C., & Ytteroy, E. A. (2002). Outcomes for children with lesbian or gay parents. A review of studies from 1978 to 2000. *Scandinavian Journal of Psychology, 43,* 335–351.

Appell, A. R. (2001). Lesbian and gay adoption. *Adoption Quarterly, 4,* 75–86.

Baeten, P., & Brewaeys, A. (2001). Lesbian couples requesting donor insemination: An update of the knowledge with regard to lesbian mother families. *Human Reproduction Update, 7,* 512–519.

Bennett, S. (2003). International adoptive lesbian families: Parental perceptions of the influence of diversity on family relationships in early childhood. *Smith College Studies in Social Work, 47*(1), 73–91.

Binger, J., & Jacobsen, R. (1992). Adult responses to child behavior and attitudes toward fathering: Gay and nongay fathers. *Journal of Homosexuality, 233*(3), 99–111.

Bradford, J., & Ryan, C. (1994). National Lesbian Health Care Survey: Implications for mental health care. *Journal of Consulting and Clinical Psychology, 62,* 228–243.

Brewaeys, A., Olbrechts, H., Devroey, P., & Van Steirteghem, A. V. (1989). Counselling and selection of homosexual couples in fertility treatment. *Human Reproduction, 4,* 850–853.

Brodzinsky, D. M., & Huffman, L. (1989). Transition to adoptive parenthood. *Marriage and Family Review,* 267–286.

Brodzinsky, D. M., Patterson, C. J., & Vaziri, M. (2002). Adoption agency perspectives on lesbian and gay prospective parents: A national study. *Adoption Quarterly, 5*(3), 5–23.

Brodzinsky, D. M., & the staff of the Even B. Donaldson Adoption Institute. (2003). Adoption by lesbians and gays: A national survey of adoption agency policies, practices, and attitudes. *Adoption Quarterly, 3*(5), 5–23.

Brooks, D., & Goldberg, S. (2001). Gay and lesbian adoptive and foster care placements: Can they meet the needs of waiting children? *Social Work, 46,* 147–157.

Ceballo, R., Lansford, J. E., Abbey, A., & Stewart, A. J. (2004). Gaining a child: Comparing the experiences of biological parents, adoptive parents and stepparents. *Family Relations, 53*(1), 38–48.

Cochran, S. D. (2001). Emerging issues in research on lesbians' and gay men's mental health: Does sexual orientation really matter? *American Psychologist, 56,* 931–947.

Cochran, S., & Mays, V. (2000). Lifetime prevalence of suicide symptoms and affective disorders among men reporting same sex-sexual partners: Results from the NHANES III. *American Journal of Public Health, 90,* 573–578.

Cochran, S. D., & Mays, V. M. (2007). Physical health complaints among lesbians, gay men and bisexual and homosexually experienced heterosexual individuals: Results from the California Quality of Life Survey. *American Journal of Public Health, 97,* 2048–2055.

Cochran, S. D., Mays, V. M., & Sullivan, J. G. (2003). Prevalence of mental disorders, psychological distress, and mental health services use among lesbian, gay, and bisexual adults in the United States. *Journal of Consulting and Clinical Psychology, 71,* 53–61.

Crisp, K., & Padilla, Y. (2004). *Gay, lesbian, and bisexual issues.* Retrieved from the National Association for Social Workers Web site: www.socialworkers.org/da/da2005/2005comments/documents/glb.pdf

D'Augelli, A. R., Hershberger, S. L., & Pilkington, N. W. (1998). Lesbian, gay, and bisexual youth and their families: Disclosure of sexual orientation and its consequences. *American Journal of Orthopsychiatry, 68,* 361–371.

Davidson, J. (1972). Postpartum mood changes in Jamaican women: A description and discussion of its significance. *British Journal of Psychiatry, 121,* 659–663.

Domar, A. D., Broome, A., Zuttermeister, P. C., Seibel, M., & Friedman, R. (1992). The prevalence and predictability of depression in infertile women. *Fertility & Sterility, 58,* 1158–1163.

Drexler, P. (2006). *Raising boys without men.* Emmaus, PA: Rodale.

Ellis, A. L., & Riggle, E. D. (1996). The relation of job satisfaction and degree of openness about one's sexual orientation for lesbians and gay men. *Journal of Homosexuality, 30* (2), 75–85.

Epstein, R. (2003). Lesbian families. In M. Lynn (Ed.), *Voices: Essays on Canadian families* (pp. 76–102). Toronto: Nelson Canada.

Gair, S. (1999). Distress and depression in new motherhood: Research with adoptive mothers highlight important contributing factors. *Child & Family Social Work, 4*(1), 55–66.

Gilman, S. E., Cochran, S. D., Mays, V. M., Hughes, M., Ostrow, D., & Kessler, R. C. (2001). Risk of psychiatric disorders among individuals reporting same-sex sexual partners in the National Comorbidity Survey. *American Journal of Public Health, 91,* 933–939.

Golombok, S., Spencer, A., & Rutter, M. (1983). Children in lesbian and single-parent households: Psychosexual and psychiatric appraisal. *Journal of Child Psychology and Psychiatry, 24,* 551–572.

Golombok, S., & Tasker, F. (1996). Do parents influence the sexual orientation of their children? Findings from a longitudinal study of lesbian families. *Development Psychology, 32,* 3–11.

Green, R. (1978). Sexual identity of 37 children raised by homosexual or transsexual parents. *American Journal of Psychiatry, 135,* 692–697.

Green, R., Mandel., J. B., Hotvedt, M. E., Gray, J., & Smith, L. (1986). Lesbian mothers and their children: A comparison with solo parent heterosexual mothers and their children. *Archives of Sexual Behavior, 15,* 167–184.

Griffith, K. H., & Hebl, M. R. (2002). The disclosure dilemma for gay men and lesbians: "Coming out" at work. *Journal of Applied Psychology, 87,* 1191–1199.

Hare, J., & Richards, L. (1993). Children raised by lesbian couples: Does the context of birth affect father and partner involvement? *Family Relations, 42,* 249–255.

Herek, G. (1988). Heterosexuals' attitudes toward lesbian and gay men: Correlates and gender differences. *Journal of Sex Research, 25,* 451–477.

Herek, G. (1990). The context of anti-gay violence: Notes on cultural and psychological heterosexism. *Journal of Interpersonal Violence, 5,* 316–333.

Herek, G. (2000). The psychology of sexual prejudice. *Current Directions in Psychological Science, 9*(1), 19–22.

Herek, G. (2004). Beyond "homophobia": Thinking about sexual prejudice and stigma in the twenty-first century. *Sexuality Research & Social Policy, 1*(2), 20–21.

Hicks, S. (2000). Good lesbian, bad lesbian: Regulating heterosexuality in fostering and adoption assessments. *Child and Family Social Work, 5,* 157–168.

Hughes, T. L., & Wilsnack, S. C. (1997). Use of alcohol among lesbians: Research and clinical implications. *American Journal of Orthopsychiatry, 67,* 20–36.

Iancu, I., Horesh, N., Lepkifker, E., & Drory, Y. (2003). An epidemiological study of depressive symptomatology among Israeli adults: Prevalence of depressive symptoms and demographic risk factors. *Israeli Journal of Psychiatry and Related Science, 40*(2), 82–89.

Kirkpatrick, M., Smith, C., & Roy, R. (1981). Lesbian mothers and their children: A comparative survey. *American Journal of Orthopsychiatry, 51,* 545–551.

Kreider, R. (2003). *Adopted children and stepchildren: 2000.* Washington, DC: U.S. Department of Commerce, Economics, and Statistics Administration, U.S. Census Bureau.

Lambda Legal. (2005). *Overview of state adoption laws.* Retrieved from www.lambdalegal.org/cgi-bin/iowa/news/resources.html?record=399

Lehmann, J. B., Lehmann, C. U., & Kelly, P. J. (1998). Development and health care needs of lesbians. *Journal of Women's Health, 7,* 379–387.

Lobaugh, E. R., Clements, P. T., Averill, J. B., & Olguin, D. L. (2006). Gay-male couples who adopt: Challenging historical and contemporary social trends toward becoming a family. *Perspectives in Psychiatric Care, 42*(3), 184–195.

Lorant, V., Deliège, D., Eaton, W., Robert, A., Philippot, P., & Ansseau, M. (2003). Socioeconomic inequalities in depression: A meta-analysis. *American Journal of Epidemiology, 157,* 98–112.

Mallon, G. P. (2004). *Gay men choosing parenthood.* New York: Columbia University Press.

Mallon, G. P. (2006). *Lesbian and gay foster and adoptive parents: Recruiting, assessing, and supporting an untapped resource for children and youth.* Washington, DC: Child Welfare League of America.

Mallon, G. P. (2007). Assessing lesbian and gay prospective foster and adoptive families: A focus on the home study process. *Child Welfare, 86*(2), 67–86.

Mallon, G., & Betts, B. (2005). *Recruiting, assessing, and retaining lesbian and gay foster and adoptive families: A good practise guide for social workers.* London: British Association of Adoption and Foster Care.

Maney, D., & Cain, R. (1997). Preservice elementary teachers' attitudes toward gay and lesbian parenting. *Journal of School Health, 67,* 236–242.

Matthews, A. K., Hughes, T. L., Johnson, T., Razzano, L. A., & Cassidy, R. (2002). Prediction of depressive distress in a community sample of women: The role of sexual orientation. *American Journal of Public Health, 92,* 1131–1139.

McGlone, K., Santos, L., Kazama, L., Fong, R., & Mueller, C. (2002). Psychological stress in adoptive parents of special-needs children. *Child Welfare, 81,* 151–171.

Melges, F. T. (1968). Postpartum psychiatric syndromes. *Psychosomatic Medicine, 30,* 95–108.

Mitchell, V. (2008). Lesbian family life, like the fingers of a hand: Underdiscussed and controversial topics. *Journal of Lesbian Studies, 12,* 119–125.

Mooney-Somers, J., & Golombok, S. (2000). Children of lesbian mothers: From the 1970s to the new millennium. *Sexual & Relationship Therapy, 15*(2), 121–126.

Oetjen, H., & Rothblum, E. D. (2000). When lesbians aren't gay: Factors affecting depression among lesbians. *Journal of Homosexuality, 39*(1), 49–73.

O'Hanlan, K. A., Dibble, S. L., Hagan, H.J.J., & Davids, R. (2004). Advocacy for women's health should include lesbian health. *Journal of Women's Health, 13*(2), 227–234.

O'Hara, M.W., & Swain, A. M. (1996). Rates and risk of postpartum depression: A meta-analysis. *International Review in Psychiatry, 8,* 37–54.

O'Hara, M. W., Zekoski, E., Phillips, L. H., & Wright, E. J. (1990). Controlled prospective study of postpartum mood disorders: Comparison of childbearing and non-childbearing women. *Journal of Abnormal Psychology, 99,* 3–15.

Patterson, C. J., & Friel, L. V. (2000). Sexual orientation and fertility. In G. R. Bentley & C.G.N. Mascie-Taylor (Eds.), *Infertility in the modern world: Biosocial perspectives* (pp. 238–260). Cambridge, England: Cambridge University Press.

Ridge, S., & Feeney, J. (1998). Relationship history and relationship attitudes in gay-males and lesbians: Attachment style and gender differences. *Australian and New Zealand Journal of Psychiatry, 32,* 848–859.

Robertson, E., Grace, S., Wallington, T., & Stewart, D. E. (2004). Antenatal risk factors for postpartum depression: A synthesis of recent literature. *General Hospital Psychiatry, 26,* 289–295.

Ross, L. E. (2005). Perinatal mental health in lesbian mothers: A review of potential risk and protective factors. *Women Health, 41,* 113–128.

Ross, L., Epstein, R., Goldfinger, C., Steele, L., Anderson, S., & Strike, C. (2008). Lesbian and queer mothers navigating the adoption system: The impacts on mental health. *Health Sociology Review, 17,* 254–266.

Ross, L. E., Sellers, E. M., Bilbert-Evans, S. E., & Romach, M. K. (2004). Mood changes during pregnancy and the postpartum period: Development of a biopsychosocial model. *Acta Psychiatrica Scandinavica, 109,* 457–466.

Ross, L. E., Steele, L., Goldfinger, C., & Strike, C. (2007). Perinatal depressive symptomatology among lesbian and bisexual women. *Archives of Women's Mental Health, 10*(2), 53–59.

Rothblum, E. D., & Factor, R. (2001). Lesbians and their sisters as a control group: Demographic and mental health factors. *Psychological Science, 12*(1), 63–69.

Ryan, C., & Futterman, D. (1997). Lesbian and gay youth: Care and counseling. *Adolescent Medicine, 8,* 207–374.

Safren, S. A., & Heimberg, R. G. (1999). Depression, hopelessness, suicidality, and related factors in sexual minority and heterosexual adolescents. *Journal of Consulting and Clinical Psychology, 67,* 859–866.

Sandfort, T.G.M., de Graaf, R., Bijl, R. V., & Schnabel, P. (2001). Same-sex sexual behavior and psychiatric disorders: Findings from the Netherlands Mental Health Survey and Incidence Study (NEMESIS). *Archives of General Psychiatry, 58,* 85–91.

Savin-Williams, R. C. (1994). Verbal and physical abuse as stressors in the lives of lesbian, gay male, and bisexual youths: Associations with school problems, running away, substance abuse, prostitution, and suicide. *Journal of Consulting and Clinical Psychology, 62,* 261–269.

Senecky, Y., Agassi, H., Inbar, D., Horesh, N., Diamond, G., Bergman, Y. S., & Apter, A. (2009). Post-adoption depression among adoptive mothers. *Journal of Affective Disorders, 115,* 62–68.

Shaver, P. R., & Hazan, C. (1993). Adult romantic attachment: Theory and evidence. In D. Perlman & W. Jones (Eds.), *Advances in personal relationships* (Vol. 4, pp. 29–70). London: Jessica Kinsley.

Shelley-Sireci, L., & Ciano-Boyce, C. (2002). Becoming lesbian adoptive parents: An explanatory study of lesbian adoptive, lesbian birth, and heterosexual adoptive parents. *Adoption Quarterly, 6*(1), 33–43.

Silverman, J. (2002). AAP stand on gay adoptions angers some members: The AAP found no data suggesting risk to children in family with gay parents (Others urge tolerance). *Pediatric News, 36*(6), 1.

Silverstein, D., & Kaplan, S. (1990). Lifelong issues in adoption. *Adoption Australia,* pp. 24–36.

Smith, D., & Sherwen, C. (1988). *Mothers and their adopted children: The bonding process.* New York: Firsias Press.

Stacey, J., & Biblarz, T. (2001). How does the sexual orientation of parents matter? *American Sociological Review, 66,* 159–183.

Steele, L. S., Ross, L. E., Epstein, R., Strike, C., & Goldfinger, C. (2008). Correlates of mental health service use among lesbian, gay, and bisexual mothers and prospective mothers. *Women & Health, 47*(3), 95–112.

Steele, L. S., & Stratmann, H. (2006). Counselling lesbians about getting pregnant. *Canadian Family Physician, 52,* 605–611.

Strong, C., & Schinfeld, J. S. (1984). The single woman and artificial insemination by donor. *Journal of Reproductive Medicine, 29,* 293–299.

Tasker, F., & Golombok, S. (1997). *Growing up in a lesbian family.* New York: Guilford Press.

Trettin, S., Moses-Kolko, E. L., & Wisner, K. L. (2006). Lesbian perinatal depression and the heterosexism that affects knowledge about this minority population. *Archives of Women's Mental Health, 9,* 67–73.

Trippet, S. E. (1994). Lesbians' mental health concerns. *Health Care for Women International, 15,* 317–323.

Turner, C. S. (1999). *Adoption journeys: Parents tell their stories.* Ithaca, NY: McBooks Press.

van Dam, M. A., Koh, A. S., & Dibble, S. L. (2001). Lesbian disclosure to health care providers and delay of care. *Journal of the Gay & Lesbian Medical Association, 5,* 11–19.

Van Putten, R., & La Wall, J. (1981). Postpartum psychosis in an adoptive mother and in a father. *Psychosomatics, 22,* 1087–1089.

Victoroff, V. (1952). Dynamics and management of para partum neuropathic reactions. *Diseases of the Nervous System, 13,* 291–298.

Chapter 11

Multidisciplinary Roles and Approaches for Treating Postpartum Mood Disorders

Introduction

PMDs are health, mental health, and family dynamics issues. Because of this, there is debate as to who should screen and provide primary treatment, and how managed-care companies should cover costs for care. In countries where health and mental health care are nationalized, an interdisciplinary approach takes precedence, whereas in countries with privatized health care systems, more fragmented treatment approaches are provided. This chapter describes professional roles in treating PMDs, strategies that are most successful for these professionals, and models for more standardized PMD care.

Medical Professionals and Roles

Psychiatrists

The primary roles of psychiatrists are physical and mental health assessment, prescribing medication, and long-term medication management. At times, psychiatrists also provide counseling sessions, but this is less often the case in the United States. When seeking out a psychiatrist, ideally women should find a women's reproductive health psychiatric specialist. The benefit of these specialists is that they are often involved in women's mental health research, up-to-date on the latest prescribing trends, safety of medications during pregnancy or lactation, and have extensive experience in managing PMDs.

Many women receive medication through their primary care physician. Although the benefit of this is that these women receive some kind of care, the cost is that primary care physicians are not specialists in mental health, nor are they specialists in perinatal medication management. It may take some fine-tuning to adjust medications at therapeutic dosages that primary care physicians are not aware of, particularly when a woman is pregnant or nursing. Common results of receiving pharmacotherapy from a primary care physician without a women's reproductive mental health psychiatric consult include the following:

- prescribing medication at lower levels than the woman needs to find relief from symptoms

- prescribing medication that is not as effective as other medications

- taking the woman off or changing medications during pregnancy or lactation

Therefore, it is strongly recommended that women be referred for at least a psychiatric consult prior to being monitored long-term for perinatal mental health conditions by other professionals. For additional guidance, please refer to Wisner et al.'s (2000) article titled "Risk–Benefit Decision Making for Treatment of Depression during Pregnancy," written specifically to guide psychiatrists.

Pediatricians

Pediatricians are one of the most important PMD screening professionals for women. Well-baby and child visits are an excellent portal of entry for mental health care—both during the postpartum year and during the internatal period (the time frame between the birth of one child and the birth of the next) (Feinberg et al., 2006). Pediatricians see postpartum women more frequently than other medical professionals, and are privy to the effect that her mental health may have on infant development (Currie & Rademacher, 2004). In addition, women are more likely to keep medical appointments for their children than for their own medical care (Feinberg et al., 2006).

Most current research sugggests that pediatricians administer PMD assessments in the office at every visit up to one year after delivery. In the Chaudron, Szilagyi, Kitzman, Wadkins, and Conwell (2004) study, slightly less than 50 percent of infant medical records contained standardized postpartum depression assessments. Of these, approximately one in five women was suffering with the disorder. As a result, these women received a referral for social work follow-up. Several researchers have concluded that postpartum depression assessments are easy to integrate into pediatrician visits and do not take a lot of time to implement, and they recommend that pediatricians include postpartum depression screenings as a standard of care for all well-baby visits through the first postpartum year (Chaudron et al., 2004; Freeman et al., 2005).

Despite these recommendations, many pediatricians do not assess for postpartum depression or other PMDs during well-baby visits. This lack of attention is likely caused by several factors, including the following:

◀ Most pediatricians acknowledge the need to identify PMDs but do not assess all women for the disorders. Many rely on a woman's appearance and reported symptoms to warrant an assessment. Given that many mothers do not discuss their symptoms with professionals, this is an ineffective assessment strategy.

◀ The majority of pediatricians (93 percent in Olson et al.'s [2002] study) believe that it is *not* their responsibility to provide postpartum depression intervention due to a lack of time and education.

◀ The majority of pediatricians do not believe in their aptitude to properly diagnose postpartum depression.

◀ Most pediatricians are not interested in learning new postpartum depression assessment methods and applying these new methods to their practice (Olson et al., 2002).

It is important to note that pediatricians do not necessarily need to provide treatment. Simply by assessing and identifying postpartum depression, the pediatrician can make referrals to experts in the community who can consult with these professionals on their assessment findings and provide better treatment (Feinberg et al., 2006).

Family Physicians

Another key medical professional identified in the literature as a "gatekeeper" for PMD assessment and access to care is the family physician. Family physicians are often the primary care doctor for the mother as well as the baby; they may also provide obstetric and gynecological care for the mother and have assisted in the baby's delivery. Because of this extensive involvement in both the mother and child's medical care, they are able to detect even subtle changes in the mother's disposition, appearance, or behaviors, and indicators of infant developmental benchmark concerns. Furthermore, they are privy to the mother's medical and mental health history, from both the biological and personal historical perspectives. Blenning and Paladine's (2005) review article about family physician's follow-up postpartum care recommends that family physicians routinely administer the Edinburgh Postnatal Depression Scale. Family physicians are encouraged to take a proactive approach with their perinatal patients by screening, providing antidepressant treatment, referring to mental health professionals, and initiating these interventions with women prior to delivery should they present as high risk for developing postpartum depression (Blenning & Paladine, 2005; Wisner, Parry, & Piontek, 2002). In addition, should the family physician prescribe an antidepressant, it is recommended that he or she also provide emotional support through the duration of postpartum adjustment and experience of mental health symptoms.

General Practitioners

Women with PMDs are likely to see their primary care physician (general practitioner) as these women often experience somatic symptoms in conjunction with mood condition resulting from the pregnancy. This being the case, there are several ways general practitioners can assist these women. Most frequently, general practitioners will prescribe antidepressant medication or refer to a psychiatrist for the medical management of symptoms. However, other strategies outlined in Chapter 13 are also effective in the general practice setting, particularly if provided in conjunction with medication, as many women wish to talk about their feelings and physical changes instead of or during pharmacotherapy. This balance is often made more difficult because of time constraints and pressures to see a specified number of patients per day. General practitioners may take some extra time, even an extra five to ten minutes, to actively listen, offer encouragement and support through responses to women with PMDs and then offer follow-up listening support from a nurse in the practice.

PMD screening assessments for all women (throughout the first year after delivery) assist staff and the doctor in identifying these women (Davies, Howells, & Jenkins, 2003; Gaynes et al., 2005; Leiferman, Dauber, Heisler, & Paulson, 2008). Not only does this assist in guiding topics for discussion during the appointment, but it may also help the woman identify that she has postpartum depression. Buist et al. (2005) found that general practitioners were able to detect postpartum depression symptoms more frequently than the woman was able to detect in herself.

Should the general practitioner believe pharmacotherapy to be the first option of treatment for an individual woman, it is suggested that the topic be discussed with the woman in detail, with empathy, along with other options, as many women prefer psychosocial assistance over medicinal treatment (Buist et al., 2005). Follow-up appointments to listen to women with postpartum mood changes are extremely valuable (Holden, Sagovsky, & Cox, 1989; Shakespeare, Blake, & Garcia, 2006) and provide additional support and an opportunity to monitor adherence to medication or other treatments being provided. These visits are particularly helpful when the woman's significant other is included in at least some "listening" appointments (Buist et al., 2005).

Obstetricians and Gynecologists

As women who experience PMDs often develop symptoms during pregnancy, these symptoms can be identified and managed throughout the prenatal period by obstetricians and gynecologists. If women are fully engaged in prenatal doctor visits, obstetricians and gynecologists have the opportunity to develop an ongoing relationship with the woman and detect even subtle differences in a woman's appearance, behavior, and thought pattern. This becomes particularly important during the third trimester, as doctor visits increase in frequency and the development of perinatal mood disorders increases significantly compared to the prevalency rates during the first and second trimester. Therefore, obstetricians and gynecologists can provide standardized measurement instruments while women are in the waiting room, discuss her results initially with the nurse, and further discuss symptoms with the doctor (Marcus, Flynn, Blow, & Barry, 2003). Should prenatal mood disorders be determined, the doctor can simultaneously refer or work closely with a psychiatrist and mental health care provider to prevent worsening of mental health symptoms or the development of physical complications, such as preeclampsia, for both the duration of the pregnancy and postpartum period (Marcus et al., 2003). In addition, the obstetrician and gynecologist are best able to monitor the possible side effects of the mood disorder on the developing baby and prepare for possible premature birth, low birth weight, difficult-to-manage temperament, and developmental delays early after delivery (Marcus et al., 2003).

Midwives

Midwives are medical professionals trained to provide ongoing, often female-empowering, support and encouragement throughout pregnancy and delivery. They receive specialized training to deliver infants with or without medical doctor oversight (depending on the state or country). Midwives deliver newborns in family homes, clinics, and hospitals (Midwives Alliance of North America [MANA], 2009). In addition, they are able to provide initial medical care to infants immediately following birth. Because of a midwife's more intimate involvement with the mother and family and the more empowering approach to pregnancy and motherhood, women experiencing perinatal mood changes may be more inclined to discuss these changes with the midwife (Mauthner, 1997). Therefore, midwives are encouraged to visit with mothers daily for a while after delivery to encourage her to talk genuinely about the birthing experience, taking on the motherhood role, mood changes, and concerns (Holden, 1994, Mauthner, 1997).

In the United Kingdom, postpartum midwifery visits occur for two weeks after delivery and may extend up to one month after delivery (Albers & Williams, 2002). Current projects are underway in the United Kingdom to increase midwifery follow-up to one month postpartum, plus a follow-up home visit between 10 and 12 weeks postpartum (MacArthur, Winter, Bick, Henderson, & Knowles, 2005; MacArthur et al., 2002; MacArthur et al., 2003). This expanded follow-up approach improved mental health functioning, including a decrease in postpartum depression symptoms. Others suggest that postpartum discussions be more prescribed, as midwife-guided debriefings in efforts to prevent the development of mood disorders and improve adjustment (Lavender & Walkinshaw, 1998; Raphael-Leff, 1991). However, the empirically based benefits of midwife-guided debriefing has not been supported consistently, with some reporting no difference or more negative perceptions of the delivery (Henderson, Sharp, Priest, Hagan, & Evans, 1998; Priest, Henderson, Evans, & Hagan, 2003; Selkirk, McLaren, Ollerenshaw, McLachlan, & Moten, 2006; Small, Lumley, Donohue, Potter, & Waldenstrom, 2000).

Midwives counsel women, families, and communities about women's health, sexual behavior, reproductive health, and parenting skills (MANA, 2009). During these educational activities, midwives are able to educate mothers and their partners about perinatal mood changes, risk factors for developing these mood changes, and symptoms and emphasize how important it is to talk to the midwife as soon as any mood alterations or behaviors are detected (Mauthner, 1997).

Nurses

Nurses interface with perinatal women depending on their area of specialty and employer. Therefore, nurses are extremely valuable as initial screeners, support or counseling providers and are able to provide referrals or links to external, specialized interventions.

In the office setting, doctors rely on nurses to administer or review standardized PMD assessments as part of routine care (D'Afflitti, 2005). Should nurses detect perinatal mood disorder trends in a significant number of patients, they can initiate additional programs within an office, clinic, or hospital department setting, such as support groups (Tezel & Gözüm, 2006).

Sichel and Driscoll (1999) developed the NURSE model that outpatient nurses can use with postpartum women and suggest using this model to create a strategy to cope with life stressors linked to motherhood. This model can be used across several sessions with women experiencing postpartum depression.

N = nutritional and fluid intake, vitamin/supplements, medications
U = understanding (how does the mother understand her mood symptoms?), may need external counseling to supplement the development of this area
R = relaxation, sleep (quality and quantity)
S = spirituality (how does the mother cope using spiritual strengths and supports?)
E = exercise

Tezel and Gözüm (2006) found that public health nurses in the clinical setting can use the problem-solving model to provide care to women expressing PMD symptoms. Treatments are individualized according to the *Nursing Interventions Classification* (McCloskey & Bulechek, 2000). This combination of the problem-solving model and nursing care strategies decreased depression symptoms more effectively than PMD education alone (Tezel & Gözüm, 2006).

In maternity and delivery wards, maternal–child nurses check on the mother's temperament, attitudes toward self and the baby, self-efficacy for parenting skills, initial mother–baby attachment, and sudden behavioral changes. In the maternity setting, it may be difficult to differentiate the postpartum blues from the development of more serious, longer lasting depression; however, nurses can identify women who initially showed symptoms by using measurement instruments (Driscoll, 2006) and respond in one of four ways:

1. Provide additional educational information to the woman and her family about the normal postpartum blues symptoms, when these symptoms tend to wane, indicators that the blues are transitioning into postpartum depression or anxiety, and what to do should these symptoms start to occur. This form of intervention is recommended within two weeks postpartum (Holden, 1991) and has been shown to decrease postpartum mental health symptoms in Turkish women

(Atici & Gözüm, 2001). Some hospitals have introduced videotaped educational materials about postpartum mood symptoms and what to do should these symptoms arise. These instructional videos are typically available through the televisions in recovery rooms. Nurses can then discuss with the mother and her family any questions they might have about the information they viewed.

2. Provide support and encouragement; encourage the mother to discuss her feelings; delivery and provide referrals to experts in the community where the mother can receive more in-depth care for her symptoms and be monitored more long-term (Driscoll, 2006). In addition, maternal–child care nurses can help to normalize the experience of the role changes linked to new motherhood (Driscoll, 2005, 2006).

3. Contact women by telephone or through a home-visiting nurse, and assess for the worsening of mood symptoms and assess mother-infant bonding and interactions

4. Initiate postpartum support groups linked to the hospital or other medical practices in the community

Home-visiting nurses (as well as home visitors and midwives) are extensively used in most industrialized countries in the world for varying lengths of time. In some countries, home visitors are part of the routine care provided to families from a few weeks postpartum up to one year. During these visits, nurses continually monitor and screen for mental health symptoms (Vik, Aass, Willumsen, & Hafting, 2009), mother–infant bonding and interactions, and the family's ability to manage daily life stressors, social supports, and developmental milestones in the baby. Home-visiting nurses who nurture an encouraging, supportive, ongoing relationship with the mother, child, and family unit have been able to help reduce maternal depression symptoms, increase social networking, and increase healthy mother–child interactions and bonding (Barnard et al., 1988; Navaie-Waliser, Martin, Tessaro, Campbell, & Cross, 2000; Wickberg & Hwang, 1996). In addition to providing therapeutic support, visiting nurses are able to make appropriate referrals and linkages to community resources that can provide additional assistance as needed (Armstrong, Fraser, Dadds, & Morris, 1999).

For more information about nursing care for women with postpartum depression, as well as other educational materials, please refer to Logsdon, Wisner, and Shanahan's (2007) article, "Evidence on Postpartum Depression: 10 Publications to Guide Nursing Practice." Here, nurses will find a "tool kit" that provides basic education about postpartum depression and how to assess, diagnose, and intervene.

Mental Health Professionals and Roles

Social Workers

Similar to nurses, social workers encounter women who are experiencing PMDs across milieus. Perinatal social workers typically work alongside maternity nurses, obstetricians/gynecologists, women's reproductive mental health psychiatrists, and sometimes provide private practice, postpartum follow-up services in the community. In the hospital setting, perinatal social workers assess, diagnose, provide brief interventions, and may encourage doctors to prolong maternity discharge to allow more time for the woman and family to adjust to parenthood roles (Walther, 1997).

School social workers and clinical social workers who work with children experiencing learning, behavioral, or psychological concerns may come into contact with parents who are experiencing or who have experienced difficult postpartum mood changes. Therefore, it is important to conduct a thorough assessment, not only of the child, but also of the mother's pregnancy or delivery and any perinatal mood alterations. When this is the case, the entire family may truly need targeted intervention on role adjustment, perinatal mental health, and social or parenting skills; yet, the child often becomes the identified "problem." Subsequent treatment focuses primarily on changing the child's "problems," when in fact they may be a symptom of, or a reaction to, a family struggling with postpartum mood difficulties.

Social workers who are working in child protection services may be in contact with parents accused of neglecting a child. Research findings indicate postpartum depression as an increased risk factor in child maltreatment (Abrams & Curran, 2007; Buist, 1998; NIH, 2003). Therefore, child protection social workers can routinely assess for perinatal mood disorders, particularly in families with children ages three and under.

Psychologists and Mental Health Counselors

A search for empirical literature was conducted with the EBSCO search engine using these keywords: psychologist, counselor, mental health counselor, and postpartum depression. No information was found that specifically discussed the role of these professionals. Rather, these professionals are alluded to as referral resources for women with PMDs. It is likely that the role of these professionals is similar to that of social workers described above. It is also likely that these professionals use several of the intervention strategies delineated in chapter 13. Yet it is disturbing that no empirically based guidelines were found for these professionals.

Child psychologists and school psychologists may administer diagnostic assessments on children whose parents are currently struggling with a PMD. These children may present with learning disabilities, speech delays, behavioral difficulties, socializing difficulties, or other mental health symptoms. Therefore, even though the primary responsibility may be to assess the child to create an IEP (individualized education program) or to best treat presenting symptoms, the family history of PMDs can shed light on the family dynamics that may play a role in the child's developmental concerns. Psychologists in these positions can assess family members for postpartum mood conditions through retrospective recall or current mood symptoms to assist in family healing.

Supportive Professional Roles

Doulas

Doulas are trained professionals who provide support, encouragement, and education throughout pregnancy, delivery, and postpartum (Middleton, 2003). There are two primary specialties: birthing doulas and postpartum doulas, with some doulas specializing in both. Birthing doulas primarily offer care to women during pregnancy; they are present during the delivery process and for a short time after delivery (Doulas of North America (DONA) International, 2009a). Throughout the prenatal period and delivery, doulas provide education, support, and seek to make women as comfortable as possible. Although they cannot provide medical or mental health intervention, they can advise women and families on medical procedures, explain each step of the pregnancy and delivery, hold a hand, provide comforting massage, and attend to individualized needs throughout the delivery (provide ice chips, prayer).

Postpartum doulas assist the entire family up to three months postpartum. The frequency and duration of postpartum visits depends on the hours set by the doula in his or her practice; some will come at designated times for a specified number of hours, whereas others are available to the family 24 hours a day, seven days a week (DONA, 2009b). The postpartum time period is considered by some as the "fourth trimester," and professionals, family members, and friends often overlook this period (Middleton, 2003). Postpartum doulas are in a unique position—because of the nature of the personal involvement with the mother and family—of attending to the adjustments, role changes, questions, hesitancies, and uncertainties that arise in the home environment (Goldbort, 2002), and that might prevent or decrease PMD symptoms.

During visits, the postpartum doula provides education and support to ensure that the mother is taking care of herself (bathing, eating, drinking fluids, resting, relaxing) and also provides postpartum depression screening (DONA, 2009b; Middleton, 2003). This education and support is not limited to the mother. Doulas educate partners on how to best assist the mother and educate other children in the family on their new roles and ways to assist the mother during this transition. They will also provide additional family support as needed such as watching the child so the mother can have a break, preparing meals, light housework, running errands, baby-proofing the home, offering parenting skill suggestions, and supporting breastfeeding (DONA, 2009b; Goldbort, 2002; Middleton, 2003). These hands-on activities can help decrease depression and anxiety symptoms not only for the woman but also for the entire family (Middleton, 2003). Through one-to-one support and constant attendance, doulas become a member of the woman's support network and are trusted in ways that are traditionally unavailable to medical and mental health professionals (Middleton, 2003).

Educational Support

Early intervention teams are in contact with children who are experiencing developmental delays. These teams typically include a social worker and other specialists who assess the extent of these childhood developmental delays until these children attend school. As these early childhood delays are highly correlated to a parent who is experiencing a PMD, these teams have a prime opportunity to also screen for these disorders and involve maternal postpartum depression treatment conjunctively with the developmental early intervention program created for the child.

Similarly, child day care workers are frequently in contact with children, typically up to or through preschool. Child day care workers are able to identify children who are exhibiting social, behavioral, speech, and other delays. Also, in these settings, early intervention specialists may come to provide extra treatments for developmental delays. Although child care workers are not trained to intervene with parents with a PMD, they can have joint meetings with the early intervention specialists and the parents to provide education and referral services to postpartum specialists in the area.

Once children age out of early intervention programs, the developmental delays may necessitate an IEP to retain additional services through the school district. Although teachers are able to provide continual reports about the child's progress and areas that need ongoing attention, teachers may also be privy to the behavior, appearance, and functioning of the child's parents. During these parent–teacher exchanges, teachers can generally assess for signs that a PMD may be present, particularly if the parent has recently had another baby. Again, teachers are not expected to provide intervention to these parents. However, they can have joint meetings with special education teachers, the school social worker, school psychologist, or school psychiatrist so that the team can provide PMD education to the parents, explain how receiving treatment can assist in their child's improvement, and provide referrals to community supports and treatment options.

Spiritual Support

The research on general depression shows that the more episodes and the greater the intensity of depression an individual has, the less likely these individuals are to trust or believe in a higher power, religious leaders, and congregational members (McConnell, Pargament, Ellison, & Flannelly, 2006; Moreira-Almeida, Neto, & Koenig, 2006; Pargament, 1997; Smith, McCullough, & Poll, 2003). Some individuals with depression report the following: feeling abandoned or punished by God; being judged by one's religious community, which translated to one's perception and relationship to God; and questioning how a loving God could allow pain and sorrow in the world (Dew, Daniel, Goldston, & Koenig, 2008; Galek, 2007). One study of postpartum depressed women found that those who had prior depressive episodes were less likely to want spiritual assistance through postpartum depression than those women whose first depressive episode occurred perinatally (Zittel-Palamara, Cercone, & Rockmaker, 2009).

There are limited studies that broach providing spiritual support to women with PMDs. Those studies have found religious and spiritual involvement to be a protective factor for the development of postpartum depression, particularly for women who experience depression in highly stressful environments (Dankner, Goldberg, Fisch, & Crum, 2000; Felice, Saliba, Grech, & Cox, 2004; Heilemann, Frutos, Lee, & Kury, 2004; Hill & Pargament, 2003; Limlomwongse & Liabsuetrakul, 2006; Mann, McKeown, Bacon, Vesselinov, & Bush, 2008; Moreira-Almeida et al., 2006; Pargament, Smith, Koenig, & Perez, 1998; Seybold & Hill, 2001; Smith et al., 2003; Sorenson, Grindstaff, & Turner, 1995).

Meanwhile, others found that some women with postpartum depression desired, sought out, or were receiving spiritual or religious guidance and support (Zittel-Palamara et al., 2008; Zittel-Palamara, Cercone, & Rockmaker, 2009). It is suggested that religious and spiritual involvement improves social support and coping strategies, changes negative thought processes, provides an inner resilience, provides an environment to express feelings and stress, and promotes healthy lifestyles (Eck, 2002; Eckersley, 2007; Hill et al., 2000; Mann et al., 2008; Moreira-Almeida et al., 2006; Seybold & Hill, 2001). Religious meetings can also provide an environment of forgiveness, love, and hope, which can benefit those who are experiencing mental health conditions (Seybold & Hill, 2001).

Religious leaders, spiritual counselors, and congregations can provide spiritual support and spiritually based support groups (Zittel-Palamara et al., 2009). The types of support most frequently desired by women with postpartum depression include spiritual guidance, counseling, prayer, and support with household and daily activities and responsibilities. Women of all races and ethnicities desired this support. However, in one small study, non-Caucasians appeared to want spiritual support more frequently than their Caucasian counterparts (Zittel-Palamara et al., 2009). Furthermore, those who desired spiritual support did not have access to psychiatric care, therapeutic counseling, or support groups for postpartum depression care; rather, these women represented all of those who were hospitalized for postpartum depression. Therefore, spiritual and religious leaders of congregations or meetings that include diverse populations must be educated about PMDs and provide supportive assistance to these women and families.

Family and Friends

Social support from friends and family is pivotal after delivery. Evidence shows that women who have strong family and social supports experience PMDs less frequently than those who do not (American College of Obstetricians and Gynecologists, 2002; Beck 1996, 1999; Sichel & Driscoll, 1999). In 2000, Logsdon defined four areas of postpartum social supports:

1. Material supports: the provision of day-to-day assistance such as household chores, meal preparation, and child care for other children in the family

2. Emotional supports: nurturing and attending to psychological, emotional, and nurturance needs of the woman through engaging in conversation, offering reassurance, and offering encouragement

3. Informational support: guiding the woman to educational materials, providing answers to questions, and using the self as a role model to guide the woman through the new motherhood roles and responsibilities

4. Comparison support: linking women who are experiencing similar questions, emotional adjustment, and psychological difficulties together in order to provide mutual support through these similarities

When these social supports are lacking in a woman's life, the transition into motherhood can be difficult, leading to PMD symptoms. It is not surprising, therefore, that interventions that seek to improve social supports have been effective in decreasing the intensity of PMD symptoms (Brugha et al., 1998; Logsdon, Birkimer, & Usui, 2000; Séguin, Potvin, St. Denis, & Loisell, 1999). The distinction must be made, however, that not all women need support at similar levels. This would require conducting individualized social-support assessments to identify the types and intensity of social supports needed (Goldbort, 2002; Logsdon, 2000; Logsdon et al., 2000; Richards, 2000; Séguin et al., 1999).

References

Abrams, L. S., & Curran, L. (2007). Not just a middle-class affliction: Crafting a social work research agenda on postpartum depression. *Health & Social Work, 32,* 289–296.

Albers, L., & Williams, D. (2002). Lessons for US postpartum care. *Lancet, 359,* 370–371.

American College of Obstetricians and Gynecologists. (2002). *Clinical Updates in Women's Health Care: Depression in Women. 1*(2), 1–82.

Armstrong, K. L., Fraser, J. A., Dadds, M. R., & Morris, J. A. (1999). A randomized, controlled trial of nurse home visiting to vulnerable families with newborns. *Journal of Paediatrics and Child Health, 35,* 237–244.

Atici, I., & Gözüm, S. (2001). Effect of health education on postpartum problems and anxiety of mothers' at early discharge. *Hacettepe University Journal of the School of Nursing, 8,* 77–91.

Barnard, K. E., Magyary, D., Sumner, G., Booth, C. L., Mitchell, L. K., & Spieker, S. (1988). Prevention of parenting alterations for women with low social support. *Psychiatry, 51,* 248–253.

Beck, C. T. (1996). Postpartum depressed mothers' experiences interacting with their children. *Nursing Research, 45,* 98–104.

Beck, C. T. (1999). *Postpartum depression: Case studies, research, and nursing care.* Symposium developed for AWHONN, The Association of Women's Health, Obstetric and Neonatal Nurses (pp. 1–38), Washington, DC.

Blenning, C. E., & Paladine, H. (2005). An approach to the postpartum office visit. *American Family Physician, 72,* 2491–2496.

Brugha, T. S., Sharp, H. M., Cooper, S. A., Weisender, C., Britto, D., Shinkwin, R., et al. (1998). The Leicester 500 Project: Social support and the development of postnatal depressive symptoms: A prospective cohort survey. *Psychological Medicine, 28*(1), 63–79.

Buist, A. (1998). Childhood abuse, postpartum depression and parenting difficulties: A literature review of associations. *Australian and New Zealand Journal of Psychiatry, 32,* 370–378.

Buist, A., Bilszta, J., Barnett, B., Milgrom, J., Ericksen, K., Condon, J., et al. (2005). Recognition and management of perinatal depression in general practice: A survey of GPs and postnatal women. *Australian Family Physician, 34,* 787–790.

Chaudron, L. H., Szilagyi, P. G., Kitzman, H. J., Wadkins, H. I., & Conwell, Y. (2004). Detection of postpartum depressive symptoms by screening at well-child visits. *Pediatrics, 113,* 551–558.

Currie, M. L., & Rademacher, R. (2004). The pediatrician's role in recognizing and intervening in postpartum depression. *Pediatric Clinics of North America, 51,* 785–801.

D'Afflitti, J. G. (2005). A psychiatric clinical nurse specialist as liaison to OB/GYN practice. *Journal of Obstetric, Gynecological & Neonatal Nursing, 34,* 280–285.

Dankner, R., Goldberg, R. P., Fisch, R. Z., & Crum, R. M. (2000). Cultural elements of postpartum depression: A study of 327 Jewish Jerusalem women. *Journal of Reproductive Medicine, 45,* 97–104.

Davies, B. R., Howells, S., & Jenkins, M. (2003). Early detection and treatment of postnatal depression in primary care. *Journal of Advanced Nursing, 44,* 248–255.

Dew, R. E., Daniel, S. S., Goldston, D. B., & Koenig, H. G. (2008). Religion, spirituality, and depression in adolescent psychiatric outpatients. *Journal of Nervous and Mental Disease, 196,* 247–251.

Doulas of North America (DONA) International. (2009a). *For mothers and families: Birth doula FAQs.* Retrieved from http://www.dona.org/mothers/faqs_birth.php

Doulas of North America (DONA) International. (2009b). *For mothers and families: Postpartum doula FAQs.* Retrieved from http://www.dona.org/mothers/faqs_postpartum.php

Driscoll, J. W. (2005). Recognizing women's common mental health problems: The earthquake assessment model. *Journal of Obstetric, Gynecologic, and Neonatal Nursing, 34,* 246–254.

Driscoll, J. W. (2006). Postpartum depression: How nurses can identify and care for women grappling with this disorder. *AWHONN Lifelines, 10,* 400–409.

Eck, B. E. (2002). An exploration of the therapeutic use of spiritual disciplines in clinical practice. *Journal of Psychology and Christianity, 21*(3), 266–280.

Eckersley, R. M. (2007). Culture, spirituality, religion and health: Looking at the big picture. *Medical Journal of Australia, 186*(10, Suppl.), S54–S56.

Feinberg, E., Smith, M.V., Johnson Morales, M., Claussen, A. H., Smith, D. C., & Perou, R. (2006). Improving women's health during internatal periods: Developing an evidenced-based approach to addressing maternal depression in pediatric settings. *Journal of Women's Health, 15,* 692–703.

Felice, E., Saliba, J., Grech, V., & Cox, J. (2004). Prevalence rates and psychosocial characteristics associated with depression in pregnancy and postpartum in Maltese women. *Journal of Affective Disorders, 82,* 297–301.

Freeman, M. P., Wright, R., Watchman, M., Wahl, R. A., Sisk, D. J., Fraleigh, L., & Weibrecht, J. M. (2005). Postpartum depression assessments at well-baby visits: Screening feasibility, prevalence, and risk factors. *Journal of Women's Health, 14,* 929–935.

Galek, K. (2007). Religious doubt and mental health across the lifespan. *Journal of Adult Development, 14*(1–2), 16–25.

Gaynes, B. N., Gavin, N., Meltzer-Brody, S., Lohr, K. N., Swinson, T., Gartlehner, G., et al. (2005). *Perinatal depression: Prevalence, screening, accuracy, and screening outcomes: Report No. 119.* Research Triangle Park: RTI – University of North Carolina Evidence-Based Practice Center.

Goldbort, J. (2002). Postpartum depression: Bridging the gap between medicalized birth and social support. *International Journal of Childbirth Education, 17*(4), 11–19.

Heilemann, M., Frutos, L., Lee, K., & Kury, F. S. (2004). Protective strength factors, resources, and risks in relation to depressive symptoms among childbearing women of Mexican descent. *Health Care Women International, 25*(1), 88–106.

Henderson, J., Sharp, J., Priest, S., Hagan, R., & Evans, S. (1998, March–April). *Postnatal debriefing: What do women feel about it?* Paper presented at the Perinatal Society of Australia and New Zealand Conference, Alice Springs, Australia.

Hill, P. C., & Pargament, K. I. (2003). Advances in the conceptualization and measurement of religion and spirituality: Implications for physical and mental health research. *American Psychologist 58,* 64–74.

Hill, P. C., Pargament, K. I., Hood, R. W., McCullough, M. E., Swyers, J. P., Larson, D. B., & Zinnbauer, B. J. (2000). Conceptualizing religion and spirituality: Points of commonality, points of departure. *Journal for the Theory of Social Behaviour, 30,* 51–77.

Holden, J. M. (1991). Postnatal depression: Its nature, effects, and identification using the Edinburgh Postnatal Depression Scale. *Birth, 18,* 211–221.

Holden, J. M. (1994). Can non-psychotic depression be prevented? In J. Cox & J. Holden (Eds.), *Perinatal psychiatry: Use and misuse of the Edinburg Postnatal Depression Scale.* London: Gaskell.

Postpartum Mood Disorders

Holden, J. M., Sagovsky, R., & Cox, J. L. (1989). Counseling in a general practice setting: Controlled study of health visitor intervention in treatment of postnatal depression. *British Medical Journal, 298,* 223–226.

Lavender, T., & Walkinshaw, S. (1998). Can midwives reduce postpartum psychological morbidity? A randomised trial. *Birth: Issues in Perinatal Care and Education, 25,* 215–219.

Leiferman, J. A., Dauber, S. E., Hisler, K., & Paulson, J. F. (2008). Primary care physicians' beliefs and practices toward maternal depression. *Journal of Women's Health, 17,* 1143–1150.

Limlomwongse, N., & Liabsuetrakul, T. (2006). Cohort study of depressive moods in Thai women during late pregnancy and 6–8 weeks of postpartum using the Edinburgh Postnatal Depression Scale (EPDS). *Archives of Women's Mental Health, 9,* 131–138.

Logsdon, M. C. (2000). *Social support for pregnant and postpartum women* (Symposium [pp. 1–27]). Washington, DC: Association of Women's Health, Obstetrics and Neonatal Nurses.

Logsdon, M. C., Birkimer, J. C., & Usui, W. M. (2000). The link of social support and postpartum depressive symptoms in African-American women with low incomes. *MCN: The American Journal of Maternal Child Nursing, 25,* 262–266.

Logsdon, M. C., Wisner, K., & Shanahan, B. (2007). Evidence on postpartum depression: 10 publications to guide nursing practice. *Issues in Mental Health Nursing, 28,* 445–451.

MacArthur, C., Winter, H. R., Bick, D. E., Henderson, C., & Knowles, H. (2005). Re-designed community postnatal care trial. *British Journal of Midwifery, 13,* 319–324.

MacArthur, C., Winter, H. R., Bick, D. E., Knowles, H., Lilford, R., Henderson, C., et al. (2002). Effects of redesigned community postnatal care on women's health 4 months after birth: A cluster randomised controlled trial. *Lancet, 359,* 378–386.

MacArthur, C., Winter, H. R., Bick, D. E., Lilford, R. J., Lancashire, R. J., Knowles, H., et al. (2003). Redesigning postnatal care: A randomised controlled trial of protocol-based midwifery-led care focused on individual women's physical and psychological health needs. *Health Technology Assessment, 7*(37), iii–x, 1–86.

Mann, J. R., McKeown, R. E. Bacon, J., Vesselinov, R., & Bush, F. (2008). Do antenatal religious and spiritual factors impact the risk of postpartum depressive symptoms? *Journal of Women's Health, 17,* 745–755.

Marcus, S. M., Flynn, H. A., Blow, F. C., & Barry, K. L. (2003). Depressive symptoms among pregnant women screened in obstetrics settings. *Journal of Women's Health, 12,* 373–380.

Mauthner, N. S. (1997). Postnatal depression: How can midwives help? *Midwifery, 13*(4), 163–171.

McCloskey, J. C., & Bulecheck, G. M. (2000). *Nursing interventions classification (NIC)* (3rd ed.). St. Louis: Mosby.

McConnell, K. M., Pargament, K. I., Ellison, C. G., & Flannelly, K. J. (2006). Examining the links between spiritual struggles and symptoms of psychopathology in a national sample. *Journal of Clinical Psychology, 62,* 1469–1484.

Middleton, W. (2003). Postpartum doulas: Vital members of the maternity care team. *International Journal of Childbirth Education, 18*(2), 8–12.

Midwives Alliance of North America (MANA). (2009). *International definition of a midwife.* Retrieved from http://mana.org/definitions.html

Moreira-Almeida, A., Neto, F. L., & Koenig, H. G. (2006). Religiousness and mental health: A review. *Revista Brasileira de Psiquiatria, 28*(3), 242–250.

National Institutes of Health. (2003). *Women's mental health in pregnancy and the postpartum period.* Retrieved from http://grants.nih.gov/grants/guide/pa-files/PA-03-135.html

Navaie-Waliser, M., Martin, S. L., Tessaro, I., Campbell, M. K., & Cross, A. W. (2000). Social support and psychological functioning among high-risk mothers: The impact of the baby love maternal outreach worker program. *Public Health Nursing, 17,* 280–291.

Olson, A. L., Kemper, K. J., Kelleher, K. J., Hammond, C. S., Zuckerman, B. S., & Dietrich, A. J. (2002). Primary care pediatricians' roles and perceived responsibilities in the identification and management of maternal depression. *Pediatrics, 110,* 1169–1176.

Pargament, K. I. (1997). *The psychology of religion and coping.* New York: Guilford Press.

Pargament, K. I., Smith, B. W., Koenig, H. G., & Perez, L. (1998). Patterns of positive and negative religious coping with major life stressors. *Journal for the Scientific Study of Religion, 37,* 710–724.

Priest, S. R., Henderson, J., Evans, S. F., & Hagan, R. (2003). Stress debriefing after childbirth: A randomised controlled trial. *Medical Journal of Australia, 178,* 542–545.

Raphael-Leff, J. (1991). *Psychological processes of childbearing.* London: Chapman & Hall.

Richards, M. P. (2000). Assessing women's well-being and social and emotional needs in pregnancy and the postpartum period. *Birth: Issues in Perinatal Care, 27*(2), 102–103.

Séguin, L., Potvin, L., St. Denis, M., & Loiselle, J. (1999). Depressive symptoms in the late postpartum among low socioeconomic status women. *Birth, 26,* 157–163.

Selkirk, R., McLaren, S., Ollerenshaw, A., McLachlan, A. J., & Moten, J. (2006). The longitudinal effect of midwife-led postnatal debriefing on the psychological health of mothers. *Journal of Reproductive and Infant Psychology, 24,* 133–147.

Seybold, K. S., & Hill, P. C. (2001). The role of religion and spirituality in mental and physical health. *Current Directions in Psychological Science, 10*(1), 21–24.

Shakespeare, J., Blake, F., & Garcia, J. (2006). How do women with postnatal depression experience listening visits in primary care? A qualitative interview study. *Journal of Reproductive and Infant Psychology, 24,* 149–162.

Sichel, D. A., & Driscoll, J. W. (1999). *Women's moods: What every woman must know about hormones, the brain, and emotional health.* New York: William Morrow.

Small, R., Lumley, J., Donohue, L., Potter, A., & Waldenstrom, U. (2000). Randomised controlled trial of midwife-led debriefing to reduce maternal depression after operative childbirth. *British Medical Journal, 321,* 1043–1047.

Smith, T. B., McCullough, M. E., & Poll, J. (2003). Religiousness and depression: Evidence for a main effect and the moderating influence of stressful life events. *Psychological Bulletin, 129,* 614–636.

Sorenson, A. M., Grindstaff, C. F., & Turner, R. J. (1995). Religious involvement among unmarried adolescent mothers: A source of emotional support? *Sociology of Religion, 56*(1), 71–81.

Tezel, A., & Gözüm, S. (2006). Comparison of effects of nursing care to problem solving training on levels of depressive symptoms in postpartum women. *Patient Education and Counseling, 63,* 64–73.

Vik, K., Aass, I. M., Willumsen, A. B., & Hafting, M. (2009). "It's about focusing on the mother's mental health": Screening for postnatal depression seen from the health visitors' perspective: A qualitative study. *Scandinavian Journal of Public Health, 37,* 239–245.

Walther, V. N. (1997). Postpartum depression: A review for perinatal social workers. *Social Work in Health Care, 24*(3/4), 99–111.

Wickberg, B., & Hwang, C. P. (1996). Counselling of postnatal depression: A controlled study on a population based Swedish sample. *Journal of Affective Disorders, 39,* 209–216.

Wisner, K. L.,. Parry, B. L., & Piontek, C. M. (2002). Clinical practice: Postpartum depression. *New England Journal of Medicine, 347,* 194–199.

Wisner, K. L., Zarin, D. A., Holmboe, E. S., Applebaum, P. S., Gelenberg, A. J., Leonard, H. L., & Frank, E. (2000). Risk–benefit decision making for treatment of depression during pregnancy. *American Journal of Psychiatry, 157,* 1933–1940.

Zittel-Palamara, K., Cercone, S. A., & Rockmaker, J. R. (2009). Spiritual support for women with postpartum depression. *Journal of Psychology & Christianity, 28,* 213–225.

Zittel-Palamara, K., Rockmaker, J. R., Schwabel, K. M., Weinstein, W. L., & Thompson, S. J. (2008). Desired assistance versus care received for postpartum depression: Access to care differences by race. *Archives of Women's Mental Health, 11,* 81–92.

Chapter 12

Medical Interventions

There are extensive medical interventions for PMDs. By and large, these interventions are empirically researched, but relatively new. The most prevalent intervention is medication. Medicinal intervention is most beneficial when coupled with other behavioral changes or supplemental psychosocial intervention. This chapter reviews the medical intervention methods found in the most up-to-date research.

Sleep

When I lecture about helping women and couples with postpartum mood conditions, I often emphasize the underestimated role of sleep deprivation. I typically describe to the audience that sleep deprivation is often used as an interrogation tool. With this being the case, does it not seem ludicrous that society, medical and mental health professionals, family, and friends expect a person, who is providing the majority of infant care, to act or behave at her maximum, baseline mental health capacity? Yet, unfortunately, our society expects just this. A woman has a baby and returns to work, typically within three months. The workload does not diminish; rather, it has most likely piled up over the past three months as coworkers await her return. Add these stressors and the adjustment to the new family dynamics on top of the fact that this person also received little to no sleep from one week up to 15 months postpartum (Romito, Saurel-Cubizolles, & Cuttini, 1994) and you have the perfect storm. It is logical that many people begin feeling hopeless, overwhelmed, anxious, and depressed.

Individuals who have difficulty sleeping, disrupted circadian rhythms, or have alternate sleep pattern due to life situations (such as those who work the "midnight" shift) have higher propensities for mood disorders (Armitage, Hoffmann, & Rush, 1999; Monk, 2005; Üstün et al.,1996; Wirz-Justice, 1995). One biologically based reason for this is that humans are "hard wired" to sleep at night and to engage in daytime activities (Goyal, Gay, & Lee, 2007; Monk, 2005). When biologically programmed sleep patterns are continuously disrupted, sleep deprivation, memory, reactions, and motor skill functions diminish (Goyal et al., 2007; Harrison & Horne, 2000).

During the first six weeks postpartum, women sleep 20 percent less than they did prior to delivery (Coble et al., 1994; Driver & Shapiro, 1992; Hertz et al., 1992; K. A. Lee, Zaffke, & McEnany, 2000; Wolfson, Crowley, Anwer, & Bassett, 2003)—this coincides with the same period when women are most susceptible to postpartum mood changes.

The link between this critical period, sleep deprivation, and the onset of PMDs is, therefore, an etiology intervention or prevention focus for PMDs (Dennis & Ross, 2005; Gay, Lee, & Lee, 2004; Goyal et al., 2007; Horiuchi & Nishihara, 1999; Huang, Carter, & Guo, 2004; D. T. Lee, Yip, Leung, & Chung, 2000; K. A. Lee, Zaffke, & McEnany, 2000; Shinkoda, Matsumoto, & Park, 1999; Swain, O'Hara, Starr, & Gorman, 1997; Wolfson et al., 2003). Goyal et al.'s (2007) study found that the most vulnerable time for mood disorder development, linked to sleep deprivation, is between the third trimester of pregnancy and the third month postpartum, with the most frequent complaint being difficulty falling asleep.

Due to this, one method to assist women with PMDs is sleep intervention. One strategy to improve sleep duration during maternity hospital stays is for nursing staff to assist with night feedings (Kennedy, Gardiner, Gay, & Lee, 2007). Although it is highly promoted and preferable to breast-feed, allowing women to have extended uninterrupted sleep can not only assist in preventing PMDs but also allow the body the amount of sleep needed to mend physically. One of the greatest and most memorable gifts a maternity nurse gave me as I was recovering from my C-section was permission to rest. She said, "Allow yourself every opportunity while you are here to sleep. Let your family, friends, and the nursing staff help you, and stay in the hospital as long as you can. For every other major abdominal surgery, people are permitted time to heal and rest. You just had major abdominal surgery <u>and</u> you are nursing. You are entitled to rest—just like everyone else who has had major abdominal surgery—and who is NOT breastfeeding while they are recovering." My maternity nurse had not received education about this, but she intuitively knew the importance of nurturing the self and allowing women time to recuperate—even if that simply means to sleep. Her response to me was quite different from the one I received when recovering from my first emergency C-section. The maternity nurse was waking me to breast-feed at 4:00 A.M.—after being in labor for 12 hours, being rushed into the operating room, and having had about four hours of sleep over a 36-hour period. "Time to wake up, your little one is hungry." In my groggy, exhausted state, I asked, "Could you feed him this time? I am exhausted." She said, "He needs to eat now. What are you going to do when you go home?" I said, "That's why I have a husband," and rolled over in my bed. She begrudgingly left, and I fought with the guilt for a while the next day. I felt guilt for needing to sleep. In reality, he was just fine. It was one feeding; he still ate, I slept, and was better able to engage with him at the next feeding at 6:00 A.M. Nevertheless, I felt that guilt for a full day, all because I needed two extra hours of sleep.

Another way to assist women while in the hospital is to restructure procedures, assessments, and feedings (as much as possible) to coordinate with a seven- to eight-hour period where the mother can sleep undisturbed (Kennedy et al., 2007). This may include hanging a "DO NOT DISTURB—FAMILY SLEEPING" sign on the door, indicating to visiting friends, family, and staff providing non-emergency or nonessential care to return at another time (Kennedy et al., 2007). A picture of a clock indicating the expected non-sleeping time can also help prepare visitors and staff to know when to return. Also, developing a timed feeding schedule for the mother's partner to help with feedings (Kennedy et al., 2007) allows both partners to receive adequate uninterrupted sleep, which has the potential to ward off mood disturbances due to sleep loss.

A commonsense strategy consists of educating mothers and their partners about expected sleep pattern changes and to plan to sleep at every moment possible (Mercer & Walker, 2006). This education can come from social workers, midwives, doulas, nurses, and doctors, yet often it is not shared. Kennedy et al. (2007), lists several approaches to take by helping professionals provide sleep change interventions.

1. Explain that drastic sleep changes are to be expected but tend to ease up after the first four to six weeks postpartum. These sleep changes include difficulty falling asleep, feeling extremely tired during the day, and, generally, feeling extremely tired no matter what time it is (K. A. Lee & Caughey, 2006; K. A. Lee & Ward, 2005).

2. Explain that when sleep is disrupted or difficult for a prolonged time, it is common for dreams to change (Kennedy et al., 2007).

3. Some women or partners may have a difficult time accepting this and may find it easier to follow a "prescription" for seven to eight hours of uninterrupted sleep at night when possible or to allow for a daytime nap in order to make up for the lost hours of night sleep.

4. Emphasize that these hours of sleep are mandatory for the body to be healthy enough to supply the baby with nutrients (Kennedy et al., 2007).

Sometimes couples need instructions on behaviors that they can change that will help induce sleep rather than prevent it. In other words, take naps when the baby naps, allow others to help watch the baby so that the mother can nap, and stay away from drinking alcoholic beverages prior to sleeping (Kennedy et al., 2007).

The American Academy of Pediatrics (AAP) has specific guidelines for sleeping close to or with one's baby, recommending that newborns do not sleep with parents. Many women opt to sleep with the baby and accidentally fall asleep with the baby while nursing or feeding. Some research shows that mothers who do this sleep better than those who do not (Kennedy et al., 2007; K. A. Lee, Zaffke, & McEnany, 2000; Nishihara & Horiuchi, 1998). This does not mean, however, that this practice is safer for the baby.

Breastfeeding may be a blessing, but may also be an additional stressor. Although nursing is extremely valuable for the infant, it is time consuming and disrupts natural nocturnal sleeping patterns for the mother (Goyal et al., 2007). Although *Healthy People 2010* aims for three in four women to nurse shortly after delivery and for one in two women to nurse through six months (U.S. Department of Health and Human Services, 2000), some women just simply cannot endure the physical demands and constant waking with the baby every two to four hours. This may be one reason why breastfeeding rates decrease by 40 percent from the maternity ward to six months after delivery (Doan, Gardiner, Gay, & Lee, 2007). To sustain milk production, women need to eat well, have a supportive family, and get enough sleep to re-establish their energy, which is expended at each feeding (Cadwell & Turner-Maffei, 2006; Doan et al., 2007; Lewallen et al., 2006).

It is during sleep that the mother will produce the hormone prolactin, which helps to produce breast milk. This hormone also advances deep sleep stages (Doan et al., 2007; Lawrence & Lawrence, 2005). When sleep is not adequate, nursing is sometimes negatively affected, as is cognitive, physical, and mental health functioning (Lee & Caughey, 2006). One way to get around this predicament is to pump breast milk and encourage the woman's partner to feed the baby. Babies who receive breast milk during the evening and late night hours increase the mother and babies sleep intervals by up to 45 minutes (Doan et al., 2007). If unable or opting to not nurse, partners can alternate evening and late night feedings, providing longer durations of uninterrupted sleep for one another. It should be noted, however, that babies tend to sleep for longer durations on breast milk rather than on formula (Doan et al., 2007).

Pharmacological Treatments

Slightly over one in 10, or an estimated 27 million people, in the United States take antidepressant medication (Olfson & Marcus, 2009). Approximately 3.2 million people take antipsychotic medications, 71 percent of which are second-generation antipsychotic agents (the newer ones are medications such as ziprasidone, risperidone, olanzapine, and quetiapine) (Aparasu & Bhatara, 2006). Given these statistics, and that nearly one in two women with a previous mental health history will develop a PMD, it is likely that some women will be taking psychotropic medication when she discovers that she is pregnant.

Historically, once pregnancy is determined, the medical provider stops prescribing medication with good intentions for a healthy pregnancy. However, there are several possible problems with this. First, discontinuing medication immediately may result in bothersome withdrawal symptoms. Second, evidence now shows that women who discontinue use of psychotropic medications at the start of pregnancy are at increased risk to develop perinatal and PMD symptoms. These symptoms are often more severe in nature than previous baseline symptoms. Cohen and colleagues (2006) found that nearly one in two women with a history of depression suffered the re-occurrence of depression symptoms during pregnancy. This same study revealed that over two in three women re-experienced a depressive episode when she discontinued her medication during pregnancy. Women who discontinued lithium during pregnancy (usually prescribed for bipolar disorder) were twice as likely to experience a recurrent bipolar episode as those who continued with medication (Viguera et al., 2000). In addition, the discontinuation of resperidone during pregnancy (usually prescribed for schizophrenia or psychotic symptoms) can result in the onset of postpartum psychosis (Hill et al., 2000). Therefore, depending on the mental health diagnosis and the medication, it might be preferable for the woman to remain on her medication throughout the pregnancy or resume immediately after delivery (Viguera et al., 2000).

The U.S. Food and Drug Administration (FDA) classified all medications for their safety during pregnancy or when breastfeeding. There are five pregnancy safety categories (Merck Manual, 2008):

A. Medications researched with pregnant or nursing women and no risks were found

B. Medications researched in animals that show no risk to the baby but replicated data in humans is limited OR the research in animal studies show some risk but do not appear to show any risk in humans at this point

C. Medications researched in animals that show risk; replicated data in humans is limited, but the benefits of taking the medication outweigh the risks

D. Medications researched in animals *and* in humans that show risk, but the benefits of taking the medication outweigh the risks

E. Medications researched in animals *and* in humans; congenital abnormalities found, but the benefits of taking the medication outweigh the risks

Additional information about many medications and herbal usage during pregnancy may be found on the Organization of Teratology Information Specialists' (OTIS) Web site (www.otispregnancy.org) (Refer to Medication Tables 12-1 and 12-2). In the general population, there is a 3 percent to 5 percent chance of birth defects during each pregnancy—regardless of medication (OTIS, 2008a, 2008b). Studies on the safety of medication during pregnancy look to see if birth defects rise above this 3 percent to 5 percent range.

Antidepressant medication has been used for 50 years in women who are postpartum, nursing, or both (Abreu & Stuart, 2005). The American Psychiatric Association (APA) and the AAP agree that antidepressant medication can be used safely while breastfeeding, but some medications are safer than others (refer to Table 12-1) (AAP Committee on Drugs, 2001; APA, 2000). In an extensive meta-analysis, Einarson et al. (2009) found no detectable patterns of congenital malformations in babies born to mothers who took antidepressant medication during pregnancy compared with babies of mothers who did not take medication. However, clinical trial-based research has not been conducted due to the sensitivity of the population (pregnant, fetus, newborn, long-term risks), so as a rule of thumb, it is better to use medications that are older and have some retrospective data (Lusskin & Turco, 2008).

The most accepted first-line antidepressants to prescribe to nursing women are selective serotonin reuptake inhibitors (SSRIs) or serotonin/norepinephrine reuptake inhibitors (SNRIs); should these medications not produce the expected results, trycyclic antidepressants (TCAs) tend to be the second choice (Abreu & Stuart, 2005; Hines et al., 2004; Lusskin & Turco, 2008). In a study that compared the effectiveness of SSRIs to TCAs to treat postpartum depression, nearly 80 percent of women treated with SSRIs responded positively to the medication compared to two-thirds of women who responded positively to TCAs (Wisner, Peindl, & Gigliotti, 1999). In addition, 80 percent of women who were unresponsive to TCA treatment found relief when their medication was changed to an SSRI.

Some medications are better suited during pregnancy and others are better for postpartum and breastfeeding (see Table 12-1).

Table 12-1 Medications

Benzodiazepines		
Medication/Use	Pregnancy Risk Category	Breastfeeding Risk Category
Alprazolam (Alprazolam Intensol®, Xanax®) *Used* for anxiety, panic attacks, depression, agoraphobia, PMS	D	L3
Chlordiazepoxide (Librium®, Limbitrol®, Limbitrol® DS) *Used* for anxiety, alcohol withdrawal, irritable bowel syndrome	D	L3
Clonazepam (Klonopin®) *Used* for seizures, panic attacks, akathisia, acute catatonia	C	L3
Clorazepate (ClorazeCaps®, ClorazeTabs®, GenXene®, Tranxene®T-TAB®, Tranxene®-SD, Tranxene®-SD Half Strength) *Used* for anxiety, alcohol withdrawal, seizures, irritable bowel syndrome	D	L3
Diazepam (Diazepam Intensol®, Valium®) *Used* for anxiety, panic attacks, seizures, muscle spasms, alcohol withdrawal, irritable bowel syndrome	D	L3 L4 (for those who use consistently)
Lorazepam (Ativan®, Lorazepam Intensol®) *Used* for anxiety, irritable bowel syndrome, epilepsy, insomnia, alcohol withdrawal, nausea/vomiting due to cancer treatment	D	L3
Oxazepam (Serax®) *Used* for anxiety, alcohol withdrawal, irritable bowel syndrome	D	L3
Temazepam (Restoril®)	X	L3

Based on Hale, T. W. (2004). *Medications and mothers' milk: A manual of lactational pharmacology.* Amarillo, TX: Pharmasoft Publishing, L. P.

Anticonvulsants/Mood Stabilizers/Lithium Used for Mental Health		
Medication/Use	Pregnancy Risk Category	Breastfeeding Risk Category
Carbamazepine (Carbatrol®, Epitol®, Equetro®, Tegretol®, Tegretol®-XR) *Used* for seizures, trigeminal neuralgia, bipolar disorder—manic episode, depression, PTSD, alcohol/drug withdrawal, restless leg syndrome, diabetes insipidus, pain syndromes, chorea	C	L2
Lamotrigine (Lamictal®) *Used* for epilepsy, Lennox-Gastaut syndrome, depression, bipolar disorder	C	L3
Lithium carbonate (Cibalith-S®, Eskalith®, Eskalith CR®, Lithane®, Lithobid®, Lithonate®) *Used* for bipolar disorder—treatment and prevention of manic episodes, blood disorders, depression, schizophrenia, impulse control disorders	D	L4
Valproic Acid (Depakote®, Depakote® ER, Depakote® Sprinkle, Depakene®) *Used* for seizure, bipolar disorder—manic episodes, migraine headache prevention, aggressive behaviors in children with attention deficit disorder, chorea, thinking difficulties, learning difficulties, comprehension difficulties	D	L2

Based on Hale, T. W. (2004). *Medications and mothers' milk: A manual of lactational pharmacology.* Amarillo, TX: Pharmasoft Publishing, L. P.

Table 12-1 Medications (*continued*)

Antidepressants: Selective Serotonin Reuptake Inhibitors

Medication/Use	Pregnancy Risk Category	Breastfeeding Risk Category
Citalopram (Celexa®) *Used* for depression, OCD, panic disorder, PMDD, anxiety disorder, PTSD	C	L3
Escitalopram oxalate (Lexapro ®) *Used* for depression, generalized anxiety disorder, panic disorder, social phobia, OCD	C	L3 (for older babies)
Fluoxetine (Prozac®, Prozac® Weekly, Sarafem®) *Used* for depression, OCD, bulimia, PMDD	C	L2 (older babies) L3 (for newborns)
Fluvoxamine (Dumyrox®, Faverin®, Fevarin®, Luvox®) *Used* for OCD, social phobia, depression, panic disorder, agitation from mild dementia	C	L2
Paroxetine (Paxil®, Paxil® CR, Pexeva®) *Used* for depression, panic disorder, social phobia, OCD, generalized anxiety disorder, PTSD, PMDD	D*	L2
Sertraline (Zoloft®) *Used* for depression, OCD, panic attacks, PTSD, social phobia, PMDD, headaches, sexual difficulties	B	L2

Based on Hale, T.W. (2004). *Medications and mothers' milk: A manual of lactational pharmacology.* Amarillo, TX: Pharmasoft Publishing, L. P.
*OBG Management, 2007.

Antidepressants: SNRIs

Medication/Use	Pregnancy Risk Category	Breastfeeding Risk Category
Desvenlafaxine (Pristiq®) *Used* for depression	C*	Not determined
Duloxetine (Cymbalta®) *Used* for depression, anxiety, fibromyalgia, pain conditions linked to diabetes	C*	Not determined
Venlafaxine (Effexor ®, Effexor ® XR) *Used* for depression, generalized anxiety disorder, social anxiety, panic disorder	C	L3

Based on Hale, T.W. (2004). *Medications and mothers' milk: A manual of lactational pharmacology.* Amarillo, TX: Pharmasoft Publishing, L. P.
*The Mayo Clinic, 2009.

Postpartum Mood Disorders

Table 12-1 Medications (continued)

Antidepressants: Trycyclics		
Medication/Use	Pregnancy Risk Category	Breastfeeding Risk Category
Amitriptyline (Elavil®, Endep®, Vanatrip®) *Used* for depression	D	L2
Clomipramine (Anafranil®) *Used* for OCD	C	L2
Desipramine (Norpramin®, Pertofrane®) *Used* for depression	C	L2
Doxepin (Adapin®, Sinequan®) *Used* for depression and anxiety	C	L5
Imipramine (Tofranil®, Tofranil®-PM) *Used* for depression	D	L2
Maprotilene (Ludiomil®) *Used* for depression, anxiety, chronic pain conditions	B	L3
Nortriptyline (Aventyl®, Pamelor®) *Used* for depression	D	L2
Trimipramine (Surmontil®) *Used* for depression	C★	Not determined

Based on Hale, T. W. (2004). *Medications and mothers' milk: A manual of lactational pharmacology.* Amarillo, TX: Pharmasoft Publishing, L. P.
★The Mayo Clinic, 2009

Antidepressants: Others		
Medication/Use	Pregnancy Risk Category	Breastfeeding Risk Category
Bupropion (Wellbutrin ®, Wellbutrin®SR, Wellbutrin ®XL, Zyban®) *Used* for depression, seasonal affective disorder, bipolar disorder–depressive episode, smoking cessasion, attention deficit hyperactivity disorder	C	L3
Mirtazapine (Remeron®, Remeron® SolTab®) *Used* for depression.	C	L3
Nefazodone (Serzone®) *Used* for depression, difficulty falling asleep, anxiety, tremors, chronic pain conditions	C	L4
Nortriptyline (Pamelor ®, Aventyl®) *Used* for depression, panic disorder, post-herpetic neuralgia, smoking cessation	D	L2
Trazodone *Used* for depression, schizophrenia, anxiety, alcohol abuse	C	L2

Based on Hale, T. W. (2004). *Medications and mothers' milk: A manual of lactational pharmacology.* Amarillo, TX: Pharmasoft Publishing, L. P.

Table 12-1 Medications (concluded)

Antipsychotics		
Medication/Use	Pregnancy Risk Category	Breastfeeding Risk Category
First-Generation Antipsychotics		
Chlorpromazine (Thorazine®, Ormazine®) *Used* for schizophrenia, psychotic disorders, bipolar disorder, explosive behavior, aggressive behavior, hyperactivity, nausea/vomiting, hiccups – one month or greater, acute intermittent porphyria, tetanus	C	L3
Clozapine (Clozaril®, FazaClo®) *Used* for schizophrenia, highly suicidal/homicidal behaviors uncontrolled through other means	C	L3
Fluphenazine (Permitil®, Prolixin®) *Used* for schizophrenia and psychotic symptoms (e.g.: delusions, hallucinations, hostility)	C	L3
Haloperidol (Haldol®) *Used* for psychotic disorders, motor tics, verbal tics, Tourette's disorder, explosive behavior, aggressive behavior, hyperactivity, confusion/thinking difficulties	C	L2
Loxapine (Loxitane®) *Used* for schizophrenia	C	L4
Penfluridol (Semap®, Micefal®) *Used* for schizophrenia	Unknown	Unknown
Thioridazine (Mellaril®) *Used* to treat schizophrenia when only when two or more antipsychotic medications have failed to help	C	L4
Thiothixene (Navane®) *Used* to treat schizophrenia	C	L4
Trifluoperazine (Stelazine®, Vesprin®) *Used* for schizophrenia, anxiety (only temporarily and when other medications have not helped)	Unknown	Unknown
Second-Generation Antipsychotics		
Aripiprazole (Abilify®) *Used* for schizophrenia, bipolar disorder, depression	C	L3
Olanzapine (Zyprexa®, Zydis®) *Used* for schizophrenia, bipolar disorder	C	L2
Quetiapine (Seroquel®, Seroquel ®XR) *Used* for schizophrenia, bipolar disorder	C	L4
Risperidone (Risperdal®, Risperdal ®M-TAB®, Risperdal Consta®) *Used* for schizophrenia, bipolar disorder, aggressive behavior, self-injurious behavior	C	L3
Ziprasidone (Geodon®) *Used* for schizophrenia and bipolar disorder	C	L4

Based on Hale, T. W. (2004). *Medications and mothers' milk: A manual of lactational pharmacology.* Amarillo, TX: Pharmasoft Publishing, L. P.

Table 12-2 Herbal Medications

Herbal Supplements		
Medication/Use	Pregnancy Risk Category	Breastfeeding Risk Category
Comfrey (Blackwort, Knitbone, Bruisewort, Russian Comfrey, Slippery Root) *Used* for hemorrhoids and inflammation	X	L5
Echinacea (American Cone Flower, Snakeroot, Achinacea Angustifolia, Black Susan, Echinacea Purpurea) *Used* to improve immune system functioning	Unknown	L3
Evening Primrose Oil *Used* to prevent early term delivery, supports infant brain development, infant eye development, postpartum depression prevention[4]	Unknown	L3
5-Hydroxytryptophan (5-HTP) *Used* for depression, anxiety, sleep disturbances, pain, aggressive behavior, appetite disturbances[1]	Unknown	Unknown
Hypericum perforatum L. (St. John's wort) *Used* for depression, burns/wounds/insect bites, viral infection, sleep difficulties, and cancer	Unknown	L2
Kava-Kava (Awa, Tonga, Kew) *Used* for anxiety, stress, muscle relaxant	Unknown	L5
Matricaria recutita L. (German Chamomile, Wild Chamomile, Sweet False, Hungarian Chamomile) *Used* for insomnia, stress, inflammation, infection, hemorrhoids, mastitis, gastrointestinal discomfort	Unknown	L3
Melatonin *Used* for insomnia	Unknown	L3
Passiflora incarnata L. (Passion Flower) *Used* for insomnia and gastrointestinal-related anxiety symptoms, maintain serotonin blood levels[2]	Unknown	Unknown
Valerian Officinalis (Valerian Root) *Used* for insomnia	Unknown	L3
Zingiber officinale (Ginger Root Tea, Ginger Root Extract) *Used* for nausea, morning sickness[3,5]	Unknown	Unknown

[1]Birdsall, T. C. (1998). 5-Hydroxytryptophan: A clinically-effective serotonin precursor. *Alternative Medicine Review, 3*(4), 271–280.
[2]Natural Standard Monograph (2009) www.naturalstandard.com
[3]Jewsell, D., & Young, G. (2002). Interventions for nausea and vomiting in early pregnancy. *Cochrane Database System Review*, 2002 (1): CD000145.
[4]Gallagher, S. (2004). Omega 3 oils and pregnancy. *Midwifery Today/International Midwife, 69,* 26–31.
[5]Holst, L., Wright, D., Haavik, S., & Nordeng, H. (2009). The use and the user of herbal remedies during pregnancy. *Journal of Alternative and Complementary Medicine, 15,* 787–792.

Recent publicity has surfaced regarding the use of paroxetine during pregnancy, identifying congenital heart anomalies. The risk for the development of these anomalies appears to be greatest during the second half of pregnancy (Chambers et al., 2006). Findings suggest that first trimester exposure to paroxetine increases the risk for heart abnormalities (Bar-Oz et al., 2007; Cuzzell, 2006; FDA, 2006). However, more recent research finds the risk-rate for developing congenital heart anomalies during the first trimester to be similar to that of babies of women who do not take medication during pregnancy (Einarson et al., 2008; OTIS, 2008c). Therefore, paroxetine is not recommended for use during pregnancy or when nursing unless there are extraneous circumstances indicating paroxetine as the best option; however, should the doctor assess that staying on paroxetine be most beneficial for the woman, it appears that the baby is at no more risk for developing congenital heart problems than are other babies (American College of Obstetricians and Gynecologists, 2007; Einarson et al., 2008; Lusskin & Turco, 2008).

Should a woman show signs of mood changes during pregnancy, one strategy is to find a medication that has the fewest risks to the fetus during pregnancy and to the newborn after delivery (for nursing), while providing the greatest benefit to the mother. When possible, it is better to maintain the mother on the same medication throughout pregnancy and postpartum to expose the infant to only one medication.

An estimated one in three babies of mothers who took an antidepressant during pregnancy is born underweight (Oberlander et al., 2007). Babies whose mothers experienced severe mental health difficulties during pregnancy are the most likely to be born underweight (Oberlander et al., 2007). Some babies exposed to antidepressants in utero have experienced what has been termed "poor neonatal adaptation" (Chambers, Johnson, Dick, Felix, & Jones, 1996; FDA, 2006; Laine, Keikkinen, Ekblad, & Kero, 2003; Lusskin & Turco, 2008; Misri et al., 2004; Moses-Kolko et al., 2005; Sivojelezova, Shuhaiber, Sarkissian, Einarson, & Koren, 2005). Symptoms include temporary respiratory distress, shakiness, difficulty eating, difficulty sleeping, jaundice, increased muscle tone, and fluctuations in body temperature. Occasionally, seizures will also occur (Lusskin & Turco, 2008; Oberlander et al., 2007; OTIS, 2008c). These symptoms typically normalize within two days, and there have not been any reported neonatal deaths due to this condition (Lusskin & Turco, 2008).

Another way medication benefits women is through preventing the onset of PMDs, particularly when the woman has had a history of these disorders during past pregnancies (Abreu & Stuart, 2005; Jones & Craddock, 2005; Wisner, Parry, & Piontek, 2002; Wisner & Wheeler, 1994). Prevention can occur in one of two ways: (1) monitor mood changes during pregnancy and administer medication when symptoms become difficult to manage or (2) administer the medication immediately after delivery. When possible, the medication that previously showed positive therapeutic results should be used. When this strategy is used, Wisner and Wheeler (1994) found that only one out of 15 people re-experienced postpartum depression, whereas nearly two in three women who did not take medication had postpartum depression again. Subsequent studies show similar results, indicating that antidepressants (particularly sertraline) can help prevent recurrent postpartum depression (Wisner et al., 2001; Wisner et al., 2004).

Sharma, Smith, and Mazmanian (2006) examined the effectiveness of taking olanzapine immediately after delivery for a minimum of one month to prevent the onset of postpartum psychosis in women with a bipolar disorder diagnosis. Approximately four out of five women who took the medication avoided PMD symptoms; comparatively, slightly more than one in two women who did not take medication wound up having a PMD.

Medication Assessment and Monitoring

When working with women who find out that they are pregnant, social workers and other professionals need to assess several key factors:

- What is the mental health history of the woman and her family? A side note: As when prescribing antidepressants for depression in the general population, make sure to assess for family history and personal history which may indicate bipolarity as antidepressants can accelerate the onset of severe mania—potentially leading to psychosis in postpartum women (Sharma, 2006).

- Is the woman currently taking psychotropic medication? For how long?

- What is the safety of this medication for the fetus or baby?

- What is the preference of the woman's OB/GYN in regard to taking medication throughout pregnancy as a postpartum mood disorder prevention strategy? The woman's preference?

- Discuss having a consultation with a psychiatrist if the woman appears to have significant risk factors in her mental health history (Lusskin & Turco, 2008) or if she is prescribed medication through her primary care physician or other health care provider. Recommend psychiatric consultation prior to discontinuing medication. Encourage the psychiatrist and OB/GYN to work with the woman together to create an optimal plan (Lusskin & Turco, 2008).

- ◀ ADVOCACY! Make sure that all professionals, the woman, and her significant other are aware that women who are taken off psychotropic medication during pregnancy have a high risk of the symptoms returning during the course of the pregnancy and becoming more severe throughout the pregnancy and postpartum period.

- ◀ Encourage the mother to discuss perinatal and postpartum mental health conditions with her friends, family, and significant other (Lusskin & Turco, 2008). Encourage the mother to educate and prepare her support network, to report any mood or behavioral changes that they observe, and to create a plan to address these changes if needed.

Hormone Replacement Therapy

Hormone replacement therapy (HRT) assists perimenopausal women through the often uncomfortable transition symptoms, including mood disorders. The treatment has dramatically relieved depression symptoms during perimenopause (Halbreich, 1997; Soares, Almeida, Joffe, & Cohen, 2001). Yet HRT has received much publicity over the past few years due to findings from the Women's Health Initiative (WHI). WHI findings revealed a slight increase in the development of breast and ovarian cancers, blood clots, stroke, heart disease, and dementia (Beral et al., 2007; Chlebowski et al., 2003; Grodstein, Manson, & Stampfer, 2006; Manson et al., 2003; Prentice et al., 2006; Rossouw et al., 2002; Rossouw et al., 2007; Shumaker et al., 2003; Wassertheir-Smoller et al., 2003). Given these slightly elevated risks, HRT is no longer the first line of treatment for women. However, given hormonally based theoretical underpinnings for perinatal mood disorders, it is logical that symptoms may respond to HRT.

The efficacy of HRT treatment for perinatal and PMDs results vary though. One study found estrogen injections administered just after delivery and conjugated estrogen, orally administered daily for two weeks postpartum, prevented the recurrence of symptoms in women with a history of postpartum psychosis (Hamilton & Sichel, 1992). Subsequent research has supported these findings in women with postpartum depression and psychosis (Ahokas, Aito, & Rimon, 2000; Gregoire, Kumar, Everitt, Henderson, & Studd, 1996; Sichel, Cohen, Robertson, Ruttenberg, & Rosenbaum, 1995). Research that does not show clinically significant changes in postpartum mood symptoms following estradiol treatment suggest that estradiol levels were not at therapeutic doses (C. Kumar et al., 2003). However, higher doses pose greater risks for the negative health risks cited by WHI studies. Therefore, estrogen therapies are only recommended for women experiencing severe postpartum depression (Dennis, Ross, & Herxheimer, 2008).

The majority of HRT research uses estrogen; however, one case study has been reported to have used a combination of estrogen and progesterone to help prevent the onset of postpartum mania with positive mood stabilizing results (Huang, Wang, & Chan, 2008). When used alone, progesterone does not appear to decrease postpartum depression symptoms (van der Meer, Loendersloot, & van Loenen, 1984). When used in long-acting form, progesterone increased postpartum depression rates (Lawrie, Herxheimer, & Dalton, 2000). However, earlier studies on women with previous postpartum depression, found that progesterone treatment prevented re-occurrence of postpartum depression symptoms (Dalton, 1985, 1989). More recent meta-analysis of the available research cautions against the use of synthetic progesterone postpartum and points out that no randomized, placebo-controlled clinical trials have been performed to date on the role of natural progesterone (Dennis, Ross, & Herxheimer, 2008).

Electroconvulsive Treatment

Electroconvulsive treatment (ECT) helps those suffering with severe depression without symptom relief from other less invasive interventions, such as medication. One of the benefits of ECT in women who have PMDs is the relatively quick remission of symptoms, which can improve the mother–baby bond (Forray & Ostroff, 2007). ECT research for PMDs is scant and methodologically lacking. What research is available appears to show benefits for women who are experiencing severe postpartum depression or postpartum psychosis (Forray & Ostroff, 2007; Rabheru, 2001; Reed, Sermin, & Appleby, 1999). One project found that postpartum psychotic symptoms treated with ECT significantly decreased compared to women who had psychotic symptoms unrelated to pregnancy or the postpartum period (Reed et al., 1999). Forray and Ostroff's (2007) small ($n = 5$) study found that women who were exposed to three to six series of ECT treatments experienced remission of PMD symptoms. However, three of the women suffered from brief memory loss resulting from treatment.

ECT is also used during pregnancy (APA, 1993, 1994). Women with severe mental health symptoms, who are unresponsive to medications, or who are unable to continue psychotropic medications due to teratogenic risks to the fetus, are considered for ECT during pregnancy (Rabheru, 2001). Behaviors exhibited by women who suffer from severe mental health impairments include the following: rejecting prenatal care, rejecting food or drink, attempting to self-induce labor, attempting suicide, and being mentally unable to follow medical advice (Rabheru, 2001). These types of behaviors can be potentially harmful to the developing fetus and may indicate the need for ECT. The limited research available shows ECT to be effective during each trimester; however, what is available is methodologically limited and dated (APA, 2001; Bhatia, Baldwin, & Bhatia, 1999; Miller, 1994; Moreno, Munoz, Valderrabanos, & Gutierrez, 1998; Rabheru, 2001; Walker, 1994). Risks of having ECT during pregnancy include miscarriage (especially during the first trimester), premature delivery, insufficient placenta, separation of the placenta from the uterus, and decreased fetal circulation (Moreno et al., 1998; Rabheru, 2001).

Alternative Treatments

Between 1990 and 1997, an estimated one in two women in the United States used alternative medicine instead of or in addition to prescribed medication (Eisenberg et al., 1998); yet less than 40 percent of those who use alternative medicinal products reveal this information to their medical care provider. This is dangerous and will be discussed further in a moment. First, I will discuss reasons why some people use alternative treatments:

1. Increased control over personal health care

2. Seeking to be treated as a person—not as a "pathology"

3. A desire to be viewed holistically rather than simply from the traditional "medical model"

4. A desire for medications with less adverse side effects

5. Alternative medical professionals taking more time listening to the person and creating individualized treatment protocols

6. A desire for an empowerment model of care that is less authoritative and hierarchical in practice (Astin, 1998; Ernst, Rand, & Stevinson, 1998; Tiran & Mack, 2000; Weier & Beal, 2004).

When looking at these factors from a RCT perspective, women's reproductive health has been traditionally viewed by the medical model as pathological. This view lacks equality, mutuality, emotional connectedness and empathy typically sought after by women in order to heal the mind and body. It is not surprising, therefore, that only one in three women with PMDs will seek out assistance from her primary care physician (Lumley et al., 2003). Therefore, women (most frequently those with higher levels of education and those with several health problems) may opt for alternatives to the traditional medical model treatment (Astin, 1998; Weier & Beal, 2004). It is interesting that individuals who suffer with depression and anxiety are also more likely to try alternative methods of treatment (Astin, 1998; Eisenberg et al., 1998; Weier & Beal, 2004). Women who are nursing may also attempt alternative treatments before trying antidepressant medication for symptom relief, due to fears that the medication may harm the baby or necessitate breastfeeding cessation (Weier & Beal, 2004).

Unfortunately, many individuals who use herbal or vitamin strategies to alleviate health or mental health symptoms do not discuss this with traditional health care providers—often attempting to figure out dosing and combinations alone or through reading contemporary books that may not be empirically based (Eisenberg et al., 1998; Weier & Beal, 2004). This can be dangerous as herbal medication principles are the foundation for the creation of patented medication and can cause severe complications when herbs and medications are combined. Similarly, taking high doses of vitamins without proper consultation and monitoring can be dangerous, as certain supplements can build up in the system and cause organ damage and failure. In addition, over-the-counter herbal supplements from India and China have been found to contain high levels of metals, including mercury, arsenic, and lead (Ernst & Coon, 2001; Rai, Kattar, Khatoon, Rawat, & Mehrotra, 2001; Weier & Beal, 2004) and some from the United States have been found to contain pesticides as well as metals (Hugget, Kahn, Allgood, Block, & Schlenk, 2001). Therefore, women who opt for alternative treatments (as those discussed below) should do so only under the direct consult of a naturopath. In addition, medical and mental health practitioners need to include herbal and vitamin supplementation in initial assessments, as well as on a continual basis. The following sections describe some alternative treatments that have been examined in the research literature.

Omega-3 Fatty Acids Supplementation

There is some evidence in the literature that suggests a link between depression and diets insufficient in omega-3 fatty acids (Rees, Austin, & Parker, 2005). In the brain, omega-3 fatty acid appears to affect neurotransmitters and receptors associated with depression (Ikemoto, Nitta, & Furukawa, 2000; Murck, Song, Horrobin, & Uhr, 2004; Rees, Austin, & Parker, 2008; Yehuda, Rabinovitz, Carrasso, & Mostofsky, 1998). International research shows a connection between increased depression symptoms and those who do not include much fish in their diets (Hibbeln, 1998). This negative relationship has also been found in women who experience postpartum depression (Hibbeln, 2002; Hornstra, 2000). However, these findings have been inconsistent, with some studies finding no difference between fish intake or omega-3 fatty acid intake and postpartum depression (Browne, Scott, & Silvers, 2006; Miyake et al., 2006).

During pregnancy, omega-3 fatty acids are naturally depleted from the mother at rates of up to half the mother's baseline levels (Hornstra, 2000). This depletion occurs most during the third trimester (Al et al., 1995)—a time period when mothers are at most risk for depression and anxiety during pregnancy (Rees et al., 2008). Due to this, some researchers have tested omega-3 fatty acid supplementation to prevent the onset of postpartum depression. However, results have varied from showing no differences between groups, slight improvements, to significant improvements (Freeman et al., 2006; Llorente et al., 2003; Marangell, Martinez, Zboyan, Chong, & Puryear, 2005; Rees et al., 2008). The most promising study found that women who took 0.5 g to 2.8 g of omega-3 fatty acids over eight weeks had significant improvement in postpartum depression symptoms, regardless of the dosage (Freeman et al., 2006).

St. John's Wort Supplementation

St. John's wort (hypericum performatum) has gained popularity over the last 10 to 20 years as an alternative treatment for mild to moderate depression. As public interest in this herb has increased, so have the clinical trials, which appear to support the efficacy of St. John's wort to relieve depression symptoms when taken at therapeutic dosages (Bilia, Gallori, & Vincieri, 2002; Gaster & Holroyd, 2000; Kim, Streltzer, & Goebert, 1999; Linde et al., 1996).

There are conflicting reports of the efficacy of St. John's wort compared with antidepressants. Some studies found the herb provided better reduction of depression symptoms and fewer side effects than customary antidepressant medication (Lecrubier, Clerc, Didi, & Kieser, 2002; Linde et al., 1996); yet others show no significant clinical differences (Davidson, 2002; Shelton et al., 2001; Weier & Beal, 2004). Weier and Beal suggested that these differences are most likely due to methodological concerns among studies, with the U.S.-based studies appearing to include more difficult-to-treat depression cases than the European-based studies (which had outcomes that were more positive). Weier and Beal also pointed out that nearly one in three antidepressant research participants typically do not respond positively to the medication (Davidson, 2002), so similar results should be expected with the use of herbal supplementation.

Caution should be used, however, if one chooses herbal supplements to treat health or mental health symptoms, as commercial labeling of these products may not be accurate in the United States (Hendrick, 2003). In addition, care is needed when using St. John's wort with other medications due to the way in which the herb is metabolized in the liver (McIntyre, 2000). When taken in combination with an SSRI, there is a serotonin toxicity risk (McIntyre, 2000; Weier & Beal, 2004). Similar to traditional antidepressants, St. John's wort can influence the onset of a manic episode in individuals with bipolar disorder (Lecrubier et al., 2002; Weier & Beal, 2004). In addition, St. John's wort changes reproductive steroid levels. This can diminish the ability to conceive, alter birth control efficacy, and possibly affect breastfeeding (Hendrick, 2003; Markowitz & DeVane, 2001).

There are no empirically based studies found to date on the use of St. John's wort during pregnancy, on withdrawal symptoms for the newborn, or on longitudinal developmental concerns for the baby. Only one study reported on the symptoms displayed by a baby exposed to St. John's wort during breastfeeding, revealing that the baby was tired, lethargic and had colic (OTIS, 2005b).

Kava-Kava Supplementation

Kava (piper methysticum) is an herb used to reduce symptoms of anxiety, particularly anxiety related to depression, and to help relieve insomnia (Cott, 1999; Kinzler, Kromer, & Lehmann, 1991; Weier & Beal, 2004). Several empirically based studies support these claims (Kinzler et al., 1991; Malsch & Keiser, 2001; Pittler & Ernst, 2000). When compared with benzodiazapine (for example, Valium, Xanax), Kava-kava is as effective in relieving anxiety symptoms, and in some cases more effective than benzodiazapine (Malsch & Keiser, 2001; Weier & Beal, 2004). Moreover, there were no withdrawal symptoms reported following kava treatment (Malsch & Keiser, 2001). However, international case studies have linked kava to liver failure, resulting in the banning of the sale of the herb in many places (Dragull, Yoshida, & Tang, 2003; Weier & Beal, 2004).

There are no empirically based studies that examine the use of kava during pregnancy, withdrawal symptoms in the newborn, longitudinal development of the baby, or in breastfeeding. It is recommended that women do not nurse while using kava (Connor, Davidson, & Churchill, 2001; Weier & Beal, 2004).

Natural Progesterone

Naturopaths and other alternative medical professionals suggest taking natural progesterone for some mental health symptoms linked to women's reproductive health cycles. Although not examined through clinical trial research, the biological mechanisms of natural progesterone suggest that it may help women who are experiencing postpartum depression with anxiety (Hendrick, 2003; Rupprecht & Holsboer, 1999). Although current research suggests synthetically produced progesterone can worsen PMD symptoms, naturally occurring progesterone metabolizes into a steroid that increases the amount of g-aminobutric acid in the central nervous system. The result of this is a decrease in anxiety feelings and an increase in sedation (Hendrick, 2003; Rupprecht & Holsboer, 1999).

Xiong-gui-tiao-xue-yin Supplementation

Xiong-gui-tiao-xue-yin is a Kampo formulation used since the Ming dynasty (1587) for postpartum symptoms, including tearfulness, depression, irritability, decreased verbalization, brooding, and general mental instability (Ushiroyama, Sakuma, & Ueki, 2005). The extract contains the following ingredients: Japanese angelica root (Touki), cnidium rhizome (Senkyu), rehmannia root (Jiou), atractylodes rhizome (Byakujutsu), hoelen (Bukuryou), citrus unshiu peel (Chimpi), cyperus rhizome (Kobushi), moutan bark (Botanpi), lindera root (Uyaku), jujube fruit (Taiso), Siberian Motherwort herb (Yakumoso), ginger rhizome (Shoukyou), and glycyrrhiza root (Kanzo) (Ushiroyama et al., 2005). In their randomized study, Ushiroyama and colleagues examined the effectiveness of 6.0 g of Xiong-gui-tiao-xue-yin on the expression of postpartum depression and maternity blues. They found that women who had taken the extract the day of delivery cried less frequently and expressed fewer symptoms of the maternity blues at three days postpartum than did women who did not take the extract. Three weeks after delivery, only 16 percent of women continued to express mild depression symptoms, whereas twice as many women in the control groups continued to experience depression symptoms. Findings also indicated that Xiong-gui-tiao-xue-yin had decreased symptoms one week postpartum. It should be noted that at this point there is no empirical research that examines the effect of this extract on breastfeeding newborns or their long-term development.

Acupuncture

There are no empirically based studies on the use of acupuncture to relieve mood disorder symptoms during pregnancy or while breastfeeding. However, there is no evidence that acupuncture interferes with medications or herbal or vitamin supplementation. In addition, the practice does not appear to have an effect on lactation (Weier & Beal, 2004).

Massage

Most of the research on postpartum massage involves the mother massaging the infant; resulting in improving the mother–baby bond as well as calming the baby. Although researched to a lesser extent, massage can also benefit mothers suffering with PMDs. One study found that compared with relaxation strategies, 10 massage sessions significantly decreased depression, anxiety, and stress symptoms while improving behavior and increasing cortisol levels in saliva (Field, Grizzle, Scafidi, & Schanberg, 1996; Weier & Beal, 2004).

Light Therapy

Light therapy is traditionally used to treat seasonal affective disorder (SAD), depression symptoms that increase between the months of October and March in the northern hemisphere. It is believed that a lack of exposure to light during these winter months decreases melatonin and tryptophan levels, thereby influencing serotonin synthesis and resulting in the onset of depression (Corral, Wardrop, Zhang, Grewal, & Patton, 2007; Stowe & Nemeroff, 1995). By exposing someone suffering with SAD to specific bright light frequencies (10,000 lux) or dim red light (600 lux) for a designated time period daily (Corral et al., 2007), the body is tricked into producing tryptophan levels similar to those found during summer months when contact with the sun is at its peak (Kasper et al., 2001).

Corral, Kuan, and Kostaras (2000) found light therapy to improve postpartum depression symptoms in two women. Oren et al. (2002) found light therapy to improve depression symptoms in approximately half of the women in the study, similar to the findings in other studies (Corral et al., 2007). Furthermore, no negative side effects on pregnancy or breastfeeding have been examined.

Monitoring and Supporting Assistance

Home Visits

Many countries that have nationalized medicine programs offer women home visits by a public health nurse or midwife through the first postnatal year. Home visits include educational materials about PMD symptoms, skills training, and, at times, psychosocial support and counseling. Women with a child in the Neonatal Intensive Care Unit who received home-visiting education upon hospital discharge show higher self-esteem, better mother-child attachment, better family functioning, and less postpartum depression than women who received customary care (Ahn & Kim, 2004). Health visitors who offer support and guidance for postpartum couples experiencing conflict report a decrease in difficulties (Simons, Reynolds, Mannion, & Morison,

2003). Referrals for PMD treatment increase as a result of these counseling services offered by health visitors and thereby diminish the overall cost of home visitation care (Appleby, Hirst, Marshall, Keeling, et al., 2003).

Day Treatment

Women hospitalized for postpartum psychosis are often recommended to seek day treatment programs upon discharge (Sit, Rothschild, & Wisner, 2006). One problem with this, however, is that in many cases day treatment programs also provide care to chronically mentally ill individuals (Ogrodniczuk & Steinberg, 2005), a population characteristically different from mothers who experience the onset of postpartum mental health symptoms. Being surrounded by chronically mentally ill individuals, who may be in day treatment to maintain their highest level of functioning in the community, has the potential to detrimentally affect women placed in day treatment as a safety net. While these women are in transition to their baseline level of mental health functioning– it is most likely significantly higher than typical day treatment facility users.

Unlike traditional day treatment programs, where seriously and chronically mentally ill individuals receive care for months to years, newer programs are being developed for short-term usage, typically ranging from three to twelve week stints of care (Ogrodniczuk & Steinberg, 2005). Short-term day treatment programs may incorporate other, more transient mental health populations, such as those with obsessive–compulsive disorder, eating disorders, and posttraumatic stress disorder (Ogrodniczuk & Steinberg, 2005). This inclusion of other populations allows day treatment programs to offer other time-effective treatment like cognitive–behavioral therapy.

Although there are not many day treatment programs in the United States that focus specifically on women with PMDs, other countries have developed and researched such programs as the Parent and Baby Day Unit (PBDU) in the United Kingdom (Boath, 1999; Boath, Barnett, Britto, Pryce, & Cox, 1995; Cox, Gerrard, Cookson, & Jones, 1993; Cox, Murray, & Chapman, 1993). The program offers multidisciplinary, high intensity care including psychiatric, nursing, occupational therapy, and nursery. Women are availed of individual, couples, family, and group treatments; art therapy; stress management; assertiveness; parenting and relaxation skills training; yoga classes; and medication management (Boath, Major, & Cox, 2003). When not engaged in these services, women in day treatment spend time interacting with one another, forming support groups or networks, and spend time interacting with their infants in the nursery. Program analysis on the effectiveness of this type of treatment reveals better resolution of depression symptoms compared to routine, follow-up primary care (Boath, Cox, Lewis, Jones, & Pryce, 1999). Further analysis shows the program to be more cost-effective than routine primary care when the cost of medication is factored out (Boath et al., 2003). When reexamined seven years later, it was found that 38 percent of women who attended the day treatment program continued to express symptoms of depression, whereas 70 percent of women who received routine primary care remained depressed. Although there are numerous possible explanations for these differences, the distinction between depression rates is noteworthy.

Hospitalization

Women assessed as a threat to themselves or to others, and who are unable to be managed on medication or by other means, will be hospitalized for protection as well as stabilization. Women admitted with postpartum depression tend to have longer hospital stays than women admitted with postpartum psychosis (Noorlander, Bergink, & van den Berg, 2008). Postpartum depression can last for long periods of time (six months or longer) (Beck, 2002). Women hospitalized with postpartum depression more often have older babies as compared with women hospitalized with postpartum psychosis (Noorlander et al., 2008). This is because the onset of postpartum psychosis can occur so rapidly after delivery that some women move from the maternity ward to the psychiatric ward rather than returning home.

In contrast, however, postpartum depression begins to emerge at least 10 to 12 days after delivery and can intensify in symptoms for up to one year postpartum. For instance, Noorlander et al. (2008), found that hospitalized women with postpartum depression scored higher than women with postpartum psychosis on impaired mother–child bonding, showing feelings of rejection and anger and anxiety about care. This expanse of time can impede the mother–infant bonding process significantly; consequently, more intense intervention may be necessary.

An important concern during the mother's hospitalization is the effect of treatment on mother–infant bonding. It is recommended that women and their infants be hospitalized together (Bell et al., 1994, 1995; Brockington, 1996; Buist et al., 1989; Guscott & Steiner, 1991; R. Kumar, Marks, Platz, & Yoshida, 1995; Poinso, Gay, Glangeaud-Freudenthal, & Rufo, 2002). Some countries and some localities in the United States have created mother–baby inpatient units specifically designed to encourage safe bonding while the mother's postpartum mood condition is treated. Glangeaud-Freudenthal and Barnett (2004) examined the inpatient treatment units created internationally to provide care for mothers and the baby. At the time of their study, they found 30 mother–baby inpatient units in the United Kingdom (Salmon et al., 2003), 15 in France and Belgium (Glangeaud-Freudenthal & Barnett, 2004), and 10 in Australia and New Zealand (Buist, Dennerstein & Burrows, 1989; Milgrom, Burrows, Snellen, Stamboulakis, & Burrows, 1998). Analysis of these programs revealed these multidisciplinary treatments, which include collaboration with social work and social services, to be of great importance to the mother and the baby (Glangeaud-Freudenthal & Barnett, 2004). But this collaborative team is difficult to re-create, possibly because there are no national policies (at the time of Glangeaud-Freudenthal and Barnett's 2004 review) that emphasized or acknowledged the need for both baby and mother to be treated simultaneously on an inpatient basis to support the important mother–baby bond (Buist et al., 2004; Glangeaud-Freudenthal & Barnett, 2004).

Research points to the notion that treatment for the woman alone does not benefit the infant (Forman et al., 2007) and that the only interventions found to positively help the mother and the infant are those that include mother–infant dyads. In other words, simply treating the symptoms of the mother does not benefit the baby or the family system. Mothers who receive inpatient treatment without their baby tend to express guilt and continue to need parenting assistance (Buist et al., 2004; Milgrom, Snellen, Stamboulakis, & Burrows, 1998; Rutter, 1995). When the baby is not included in treatment, the baby remains at risk for developing attachment disorders, emotional and cognitive delays, and behavioral problems. The baby's needs are so important that mother–baby inpatient programs identify the baby as the primary patient and the mother as secondary (Glangeaud-Freudenthal & Barnett, 2004). Characterization of these programs is not generally under the auspices of "psychiatric inpatient" care but rather family treatment centers. These centers most often accept babies up to twelve months old, but some will accept children up to the age of five (Glangeaud-Freudenthal & Barnett, 2004). In addition, the father or partner needs to be involved in the hospital-based treatment, as they can also suffer adjustment and mental health symptoms (Glangeaud-Freudenthal & Barnett, 2004). Treatments offered in mother-baby dyad units include health care, child care, parenting skills, cognitive behavioral therapy, couples counseling, and mother-baby interactive therapy (art, music, dance, and psychodynamic) (Buist et al., 2004).

References

Abreu, A. C., & Stuart, S. (2005). Pharmacologic and hormonal treatments for postpartum depression. *Psychiatric Annals, 35,* 569–576.

AHFS Drug Information. (2008). Drug notebook: Loxapine. Healthline: Connect to better health. Retrieved from http://www.healthline.com/ahfscontent/loxapine

Ahn, Y. M., & Kim, M. R., (2004). The effects of a home-visiting discharge education on maternal self-esteem, maternal attachment, postpartum depression and family function in the mothers of NICU infants. *Taehan Kanho Hakhoe Chi, 34,* 1468–1476.

Ahokas, A., Aito, M., & Rimon, R. (2000). Positive treatment effect of estradiol in postpartum psychosis: A pilot study. *Journal of Clinical Psychiatry, 61,* 166–169.

Al, M.D.M., van Houwelingen, A. C., Kester, A.D.M., Hassaart, T.H.M., De Jong, A.E.P., & Hornstra, G. (1995). Maternal essential fatty acid patterns during normal pregnancy and its relationship with the neonatal essential fatty acid status. *British Journal of Nutrition, 74,* 55–68.

American Academy of Pediatrics Committee on Drugs. (2001). Transfer of drugs and other chemicals into human milk. *Pediatrics, 108,* 776–789.

American College of Obstetricians and Gynecologists (ACOG). (2007). ACOG Practice Bulletin No. 87: Use of psychiatric medications during pregnancy and lactation. *Obstetrics & Gynecology, 110,* 1179–1198.

American Psychiatric Association. (1993). Practice guidelines for major depressive disorder in adults. *American Journal of Psychiatry, 150*(Suppl.), 1–26.

American Psychiatric Association. (1994). Practice guidelines for the treatment of patients with bipolar disorder. *American Journal of Psychiatry, 151*(Suppl.), 1–26.

American Psychiatric Association. (2000). Practice guideline for the treatment of patients with major depressive disorder: Revision. *American Journal of Psychiatry, 157*(4 Suppl.), 1–45.

American Psychiatric Association. (2001). *A task force report on the practice of electroconvulsive therapy: Recommendations for treatment, training, and privileging* (2nd ed.). Washington, DC: Author.

Aparasu, R. R., & Bhatara, V. (2006). Antipsychotic use and expenditure in the United States. *Psychiatric Services, 57,* 1693.

Appleby, L., Hirst, E., Marshall, S., Keeling, F., Brind, J., Butterworth, T., & Lole, J. (2003). The treatment of postnatal depression by health visitors: Impact of brief training on skills and clinical practice. *Journal of Affective Disorders, 77,* 261–266.

Armitage, R., Hoffmann, R. F., & Rush, A. J. (1999). Biological rhythm disturbance in depression: Temporal coherence of ultradian sleep EEG rhythms. *Psychological Medicine, 29,* 1435–1448.

Astin, J. A. (1998). Why patients use alternative medicine: Results of a national study. *JAMA, 279,* 1548–1553.

Bar-Oz, B., Einarson, T., Einarson, A., Boskovic, R., O'Brien, L., Malm, H., et al. (2007). Paroxetine and congenital malformations: Meta-analysis and consideration of potential confounding factors. *Clinical Therapeutics, 29,* 918–926.

Beck, C. T. (2002). Postpartum depression: A metasynthesis. *Quality Health Research, 12,* 453–472.

Bell, A. J., Land, N. M., Milne, S., & Hassanyet, F. (1994). Long-term outcome of post-partum psychiatric illness requiring admission. *Journal of Affective Disorders, 31,* 67–70.

Bell, A. J., Land, N. M., Milne, S., & Hassanyet, F. (1995). Postpartum depression: A specific concept? *British Journal of Psychiatry, 166,* 826–827.

Beral, V., Million Women Study collaborators, Bull, D., Green, J., & Reeves, G. (2007). Ovarian cancer and hormone replacement therapy in the Million Women Study. *Lancet, 369,* 1703–1710.

Bhatia, S. C., Baldwin, S. A., & Bhati, S. K. (1999). Electroconvulsive therapy during the third trimester of pregnancy. *Journal of ECT, 15,* 270–274.

Bilia, A. R., Ballori, S., & Vincieri, F. F. (2002). St. John's wort and depression: Efficacy, safety and tolerability—an update. *Life Science, 70,* 3077–3096.

Birnbaum, C. S., Cohen, L. S., Bailey, J. W., Grush, L. R., Robertson, L. M., & Stowe, Z. N. (1999). Serum concentrations of antidepressants and benzodiazepines in nursing infants: A case series. *Pediatrics, 104,* e11.

Boath, E. (1999). The treatment of postnatal depression. *Marcé Society Newsletter, 7,* 3.

Boath, E., Barnett, B., Britto, D., Pryce, A., & Cox, J. (1995). When the bough breaks: Charles Street Parent and Baby Day Unit. *Journal of Reproductive and Infant Psychology, 13,* 237–240.

Boath, E., Cox, J., Lewis, M., Jones, P., & Pryce, A. (1999). When the cradle falls: The treatment of postnatal depression in a psychiatric day hospital compared with routine primary care. *Journal of Affective Disorders, 53,* 143–151.

Boath, E., Major, K., & Cox, J. (2003). When the cradle falls II: The cost-effectiveness of treating postnatal depression in a psychiatric day hospital compared with routine primary care. *Journal of Affective Disorders, 74,* 159–166.

Brockington, I. F. (1996). *Motherhood and mental health.* Oxford: Oxford University Press.

Browne, J. C., Scott, K. M., & Silvers, K. M. (2006). Fish consumption in pregnancy and omega-3 status after birth are not associated with postnatal depression. *Journal of Affective Disorders, 90,* 131–139.

Buist, A., Dennerstein, L., & Burrows, G. D. (1989). Review of a mother–baby unit in a psychiatric hospital. *Australian and New Zealand Journal of Psychiatry, 24,* 103–108.

Buist, A., Minto, B., Szego, K., Samhuel, M., Shawyer, L., & O'Connor, L. (2004). Mother–baby psychiatric units in Australia: The Victorian experience. *Archives of Women's Mental Health, 7*(1), 81–87.

Cadwell, K., & Turner-Maffei, C. . (2006). *Breastfeeding A-Z terminology and telephone triage.* Sudbury, MA: Jones & Bartlett.

Chambers, C. D., Hernandez-Diaz, S., van Marter, L. J., Werler, M. M., Louik, C., Jones, K. L., & Mitchell, A. A. (2006). Selective serotonin-reuptake inhibitors and risk of persistent pulmonary hypertension of the newborn. *New England Journal of Medicine, 354,* 579–587.

Chambers, C. D., Johnson, K. A., Dick, L. M., Felix, R. J., & Jones, K. L. (1996). Birth outcomes in pregnant women taking fluoxetine. *New England Journal of Medicine, 335,* 1010–1015.

Chlebowski, R. T., Hendrix, S. L., Langer, R. D., Stefanick, M. L., Gass, M., Lane, D., et al. (2003). Influence of estrogen plus progestin on breast cancer and mammography in healthy postmenopausal women: The Women's Health Initiative randomized trial. *JAMA, 289,* 3243–3253.

Coble, P. A., Reynolds, C. F., Kupfer, D. J., Houck, P. R., Day, N. L., & Giles, D. E. (1994). Childbearing in women with and without a history of affective disorder: I. Psychiatric symptomatology. *Comprehensive Psychiatry, 35,* 215–224.

Cohen, L. S., Altshuler, L. L., Harlow, B. L., Nonacs, R., Newport, D. J., Viguera, A. C., et al. (2006). Relapse of major depression during pregnancy in women who maintain or discontinue antidepressant treatment. *JAMA, 295,* 499–507.

Connor, K. M., Davidson, J.R.T., & Churchill, L. E. (2001). Adverse-effect profile of kava. *CNS Spectrums, 6,* 848–853.

Corral, M., Kuan, A., & Kostaras, D. (2000). Bright light therapy's effect on postpartum depression. *American Journal of Psychiatry, 157,* 303–304.

Corral, M., Wardrop, A. A., Zhang, H., Grewal, A. K., & Patton, S. (2007). Morning light therapy for postpartum depression. *Archives of Women's Mental Health, 10,* 221–224.

Cott, J. (1999). Dietary supplements and natural products as psychotherapeutic agents. *Psychosomatic Medicine, 61,* 712–728.

Cox, J. L., Gerrard, J., Cookson, D., & Jones, J. M. (1993). Development and audit of Charles Street Parent and Baby Day Unit, Stoke-on-Trent. *Psychiatric Bulletin, 17,* 711–713.

Cox, J. L., Murray, D., & Chapman, G. (1993). A controlled study of the onset, duration and prevalence of postnatal depression. *British Medical Journal, 163,* 27–31.

Cuzzell, J. Z. (2006). Paroxetine may increase risk for congenital malformations. *Dermatology Nursing, 18*(1), 68.

Dalton, K. (1985). Progesterone prophylaxis used successfully in postnatal depression. *Practitioner, 229,* 507–508.

Dalton, K. (1989). Successful prophylactic progesterone for idiopathic postnatal depression. *International Journal of Prenatal and Perinatal Studies, 1,* 322–327.

Davidson, J.R.T. (2002). Effect of hypericum perforatum (St. John's wort) in major depressive disorder: A randomized controlled trial. *JAMA, 287,* 1807–1815.

Dennis, C. L., & Ross, L. (2005). Relationships among infant sleep patterns, maternal fatigue, and development of depressive symptomatology. *Birth, 32,* 187–193.

Dennis, C. L., Ross, L. E., & Herxheimer, A. (2008). Oestrogens and progestins for preventing and treating postpartum depression. *Cochrane Database Systematic Reviews,* CD001690.

Doan, T., Gardiner, A., Gay, C. L., & Lee, K. A. (2007). Breast-feeding increases sleep duration of new parents. *Journal of Perinatal & Neonatal Nursing, 21,* 200–206.

Dragull, K., & Yoshida, W. Y., & Tang, C. S. (2003). Piperidine alkaloids from Piper methysticum. *Phytochemistry, 63,* 193–198.

Driver, H. S., & Shapiro, C. M. (1992). A longitudinal study of sleep stages in young women during pregnancy and postpartum. *Sleep, 15,* 449–453.

Einarson, A., Jacquelyn, C., Einarson, T. R., & Koren, G. (2009). Incidence of major malformations in infants following antidepressant exposure in pregnancy: Results of a large prospective cohort study. *Canadian Journal of Psychiatry, 54,* 242–246.

Einarson, A., Pistelli, A., DeSantis, M., Malm, H., Paulus, W. D., Panchaud, A., et al. (2008). Evaluation of the risk of congenital cardiovascular defects associated with use of paroxetine during pregnancy. *American Journal of Psychiatry, 165,* 749–752.

Eisenberg, D. M., Davis, R. B., Ettner, S. L., Appel, M. S., Wilkey, S., Van Rompay, M., & Kessler, R. C. (1998). Trends in alternative medicine use in the United States, 1990–1997: Results of a follow-up national survey. *JAMA, 280,* 1569–1575.

Ernst, E., & Coon, J. T. (2001). Heavy metals in traditional Chinese medicine: A systematic review. *Clinical Pharmacology & Therapeutics, 70,* 497–504.

Ernst, E., Rand, J. I., & Stevinson, C. (1998). Complementary therapies for depression: An overview. *Archives of General Psychiatry, 55,* 1026–1032.

Field, T., Grizzle, N., Scafidi, F., & Schanberg, S. (1996). Massage and relaxation therapies' effects on depressed adolescent mothers. *Adolescence, 31,* 903–1002.

Forman, D. R., O'Hara, M. W., Stuart, S., Gorman, L. L., Larsen, K. E., & Coy, K. C. (2007). Effective treatment for postpartum depression is not sufficient to improve the developing mother–child relationship. *Development and Psychopathology, 19,* 585–602.

Forray, A., & Ostroff, R. B. (2007). The use of electroconvulsive therapy in postpartum affective disorders. *Journal of ECT, 23,* 188–193.

Freeman, M. P., Hibbeln, J. R., Wisner, K. L., Brumbach, B. H., Watchman, M., & Glenberg, A. J. (2006). Randomised dose-ranging pilot trial of omega-3 fatty acids for postpartum depression. *Acta Psychiatrica Scandinavica, 113*(1), 31–35.

Gaster, B., & Holroyd, J. (2000). St. John's wort for depression: A systematic review.

Gay, C. L., Lee, K. A., & Lee, S. Y. (2004). Sleep patterns and fatigue in new mothers and fathers. *Biological Research for Nursing, 5,* 311–318.

Glangeaud-Freudenthal, N. M. C., & Barnett, B. E. W. (2004). Mother–baby inpatient psychiatric care in different countries: Data collection and issues—Introduction. *Archives of Women's Mental Health, 7,* 49–51.

Goyal, D., Gay, C. L., & Lee, K. A. (2007). Patterns of sleep disruption and depression symptoms in new mothers. *Journal of Perinatal and Neonatal Nursing, 21,* 123–129.

Gregoire, A. J. P., Kumar, R., Everitt, B., Henderson, A. F., & Studd, J. W. W. (1996). Transdermal oestrogen for treatment of severe postnatal depression. *Lancet, 347,* 930–933.

Grodstein, F., Manson, J. E., & Stampfer, M. J. (2006). Hormone therapy and coronary heart disease: The role of time since menopause and age at hormone initiation. *Journal of Women's Health, 15*(1), 35–44.

Guscott, R. G., & Steiner, M. (1991). A multidisciplinary treatment approach to postpartum psychoses. *Canadian Journal of Psychiatry, 35,* 551–556.

Halbreich, U. (1997). Role of estrogen in post menopausal depression. *Neurology, 48*(Suppl.), S16–S20.

Hale, T. W. (2004). *Medications and mothers' milk: A manual of lactational pharmocology.* Amarillo, TX: Pharmasoft Publishing, L. P.

Hamilton, J. A., & Sichel, D. A. (1992). Prophylactic measures. In J. A. Hamilton & T. N. Harberger (Eds.), *Postpartum psychiatric illness* (pp. 219–224). Philadelphia: University of Pennsylvania Press.

Harrison, Y., & Horne, J. A. (2000). The impact of sleep deprivation on decision making: A review. *Journal of Experimental Psychology: Applied, 6,* 236–249.

Hendrick, V. (2003). Alternative treatments for postpartum depression. *Psychiatric Times, 20*(8), 50–51.

Hertz, G., Fast, A., Feinsilver, S. H., Albertario, C. L., Schulerman, H., & Fein, A. M. (1992). Sleep in normal late pregnancy. *Sleep, 18,* 246–251.

Hibbeln, J. R. (1998). Fish consumption and major depression. *Lancet, 351,* 1213.

Hibbeln, J. R. (2002). Seafood consumption, the DHA content of mothers' milk and prevalence rates of postpartum depression: A cross-national, ecological analysis. *Journal of Affective Disorders, 69,* 15–29.

Hill, R. C., McIvor, R. J., Bach, B.A.O., Wojnar-Horton, R. E., Hackett, L. P., & Ilett, K. F. (2000). Risperidone distribution and excretion into human milk: Case report and estimated infant exposure during breastfeeding. *Journal of Clinical Psychopharmacology, 20,* 285–286.

Hines, R. N., Adams, J., Buck, G. M., Faber, W., Holson, J. F., Jacobson, S. W., et al. (2004). *NTP-CERHR Expert Panel Report on the reproductive and developmental toxicity of fluoxetine.* Research Triangle Park, NC: U.S. Department of Health and Human Services: National Toxicology Program, Center for the Evaluation of Risks to Human Reproduction -Fluoxetine-04.

Horiuchi, S., & Nishihara, K. (1999). Analyses of mother's sleep logs in postpartum periods. *Psychiatry and Clinical Neurosciences, 53,* 137–139.

Hornstra, G. (2000). Essential fatty acids in mothers and their neonates. *American Journal of Clinical Nutrition, 71*(Suppl.), 1262–1269.

Huang, C. M., Carter, P. A., & Guo, J. L. (2004). A comparison of sleep and daytime sleepiness in depressed and non-depressed mothers during the early postpartum period. *Journal of Nursing Research, 12,* 287–296.

Huang, M.-C., Wang, Y.-B., & Chan, C.-H. (2008). Estrogen–progesterone combination for treatment-refractory post-partum mania. *Psychiatry and Clinical Neurosciences, 62,* 126.

Hugget, D. B., Kahn, I. A., Allgood, J. C., Block, D. S., & Schlenk, D. (2001). Organochlorine pesticides and metals in select botanical dietary supplements. *Bulletin of Environmental Contamination and Toxicology, 66,* 150–155.

Ikemoto, A., Nitta, A., & Furukawa, S. (2000). Dietary omega 3 fatty acid deficiency decreases nerve growth factor content in rat hippocampus. *Neuroscience Letters, 285,* 99–102.

Jones, I., & Craddock, N. (2005). Bipolar disorder and childbirth: The importance of recognising risk. *British Journal of Psychiatry, 186,* 453–454.

Kasper, S., Hilger, E., Williet, M., Neumeister, A., Praschal-Reider, N., Heßelmann, B., & Habeler, A. (2001). Drug therapy in seasonal affective disorder: Practice and research. In T. Partonen & A. Magnusson, (Eds.), *Seasonal affective disorder: Practice and research* (pp. 85-94). Oxford, England: Oxford University Press.

Kennedy, H. P., Gardiner, A., Gay, C., & Lee, K. A. (2007). Negotiating sleep: A qualitative study of new mothers. *Journal of Perinatal & Neonatal Nursing, 21*(2), 114–122.

Kim, H. L., Streltzer, J., & Goebert, D. (1999). St. John's wort for depression: A meta-analysis of well-defined clinical trials. *Journal of Nervous & Mental Disease, 187,* 532–538.

Kinzler, E., Kromer, J., & Lehmann, E. (1991). Effect of a special kava extract in patients with anxiety, tension, and excitation states of non-psychotic genesis. *Arzneimittelforschung, 41,* 585–588.

Kumar, C., McIvor, R. J., Davies, T., Brown, N., Papadopoulous, A., Wieck, A., et al. (2003). Estrogen administration does not reduce the rate of recurrence of affective psychosis after childbirth. *Journal of Clinical Psychiatry, 64,* 112–118.

Kumar, R., Marks, M., Platz, C., & Yoshida, K. (1995). Clinical survey of a psychiatric mother and baby unit: Characteristics of 100 consecutive admissions. *Journal of Affective Disorders, 33,* 11–22.

Laine, K., Heikkinen, T., Ekblad, U., & Kero, P. (2003). Effects of exposure to selective serotonin reuptake inhibitors during pregnancy on serotonergic symptoms in newborns and cord blood monoamine and prolactin concentrations. *Archives of General Psychiatry, 60,* 720–726.

Lawrence, R. A., & Lawrence, R. M. (2005). *Breastfeeding: A guide for the medical profession.* Philadelphia: Elsevier Mosby.

Lawrie, T. A., Herxheimer, A., & Dalton, K. (2000). Oestrogens and progestogens for preventing and treating postnatal depression. *Cochrane Database Systematic Reviews, 2*: CD001690.

Lecrubier, Y., Clerc, G., Didi, R., & Kieser, M. (2002). Efficacy of St. John's wort extract 5570 in major depression: A double-blind, placebo-controlled trial. *American Journal of Psychiatry, 159,* 1361–1366.

Lee, D. T., Yip, A. S., Leung, T. Y., & Chung, T. K. (2000). Identifying women at risk of postnatal depression: Prospective longitudinal study. *Hong Kong Medical Journal, 6,* 349–354.

Lee, K. A., & Caughey, A. B. (2006). Evaluating insomnia during pregnancy and postpartum. In H. P. Attarian (Ed.), *Current clinical neurology: Sleep disorders in women: A guide to practical management* (pp. 185-198). Totowa, NJ: Humana Press, Inc.

Lee, K. A., & Ward, T. (2005). Critical components of a sleep assessment for clinical practice settings. *Issues in Mental Health Nursing, 26,* 739–750.

Lee, K. A., Zaffke, M. E., & McEnany, G. (2000). Parity and sleep patterns during and after pregnancy. *Obstetrics & Gynecology, 95,* 14–18.

Lewallen, L. P., Dick, M. J., Flowers, J., Powell, W., Zickefoose, K. T., Wall, Y. G., & Price, Z. M. (2006). Breastfeeding support and early cessation. *Journal of Obstetric, Gynecologic, & Neonatal Nursing, 35,* 166–172.

Linde, K., Ramirez, G., Mulrow, C. D., Pauls, A., Weidnhammer, W., & Melchart, D. (1996). St. John's wort for depression: An overview and meta-analysis of randomised clinical trials. *British Medical Journal, 313,* 253–258.

Llorente, A. M., Jensen, C. L., Voigt, R. G., Fraley, J. K., Berretta, M. C., & Heird, W. C. (2003). Effect of maternal docosahexaenoic acid supplementation on postpartum depression and information processing. *American Journal of Obstetrics and Gynecology, 188,* 1348–1353.

Lumley, J., Small, R., Brown, S., Watson, L., Gunn, J., Mitchell, C., & Dawson, W. (2003). PRISM (Program of Resources, Information, and Support for Mothers): Protocol for a community-randomised trial. *BMC Public Health, 3,* 36–50.

Lusskin, S. I., & Turco, J. (2008). Depression in pregnancy: When doing nothing is not an option. *Contemporary OB/GYN, 53*(2), 48–54.

Malsch, U., & Keiser, M. (2001). Efficacy of kava-kava in the treatment of non-psychotic anxiety, following pre-treatment with benzodiazepines. *Psychopharmacology, 157,* 277–283.

Manson, J. E., Hsia, J., Johnson, K. C., Rossouw, J. E., Assaf, A. R., Lasser, N. L., et al. (2003). Estrogen plus progestin and the risk of coronary heart disease. *New England Journal of Medicine, 349,* 523–534.

Marangell, L. B., Martinez, J. M., Zboyan, H. A., Chong, H., & Puryear, L. J. (2004). Omega-3 fatty acids for the prevention of postpartum depression: Negative data from a preliminary, open-label pilot study. *Depression & Anxiety, 19,* 20–23.

Markowitz, J. S., & DeVane, C. L. (2001). The emerging recognition of herb–drug interactions with a focus on St. John's wort (hypericum perforatum). *Psychopharmacology Bulletin, 35*(1), 53–64.

The Mayo Clinic. (2009). *Drugs and supplements.* Retrieved from http://www.mayoclinic.com/health/drug-information/DrugHerbIndex

McIntyre, M. (2000). A review of the benefits, adverse effects, drug interactions and safety of St. John's wort: The implications with regard to the regulation of herbal medicines. *Journal of Alternative and Complementary Medicine, 6,* 115–124.

Mercer, R. T., & Walker, L. O. (2006). A review of nursing interventions to foster becoming a mother. *Journal of Obstetric, Gynecologic, & Neonatal Nursing, 35,* 568–582.

Merck Manual. (2008). *Gynecology and obstetrics: High-risk pregnancy.* Retrieved from http://www.merck.com/mmpe/sec18/ch262/ch262b.html

Milgrom, J., Burrows, G. D., Snellen, M., Stamboulakis, W., & Burrows, K. (1998). Psychiatric illness in women: A review of the function of a specialist mother–baby unit. *Australian and New Zealand Journal of Psychiatry, 32,* 680–686.

Miller, L. J. (1994). Use of electroconvulsive therapy during pregnancy. *Hospital & Community Psychiatry, 45,* 444–450.

Misri, S., Oberlander, T. F., Fairbrother, N., Carter, D., Ryan, D., Kuan, A. J., & Reebye, P. (2004). Relation between prenatal maternal mood and anxiety and neonatal health. *Canadian Journal of Psychiatry, 49,* 684–689.

Miyake, Y., Sasaki, S., Yokoyama, T., Tanaka, K., Ohya, Y., Fukushima, W., et al. (2006). Risk of postpartum depression in relation to dietary fish and fat intake in Japan: The Osaka Maternal and Child Health Study. *Psychological Medicine, 36,* 1727–1735.

Monk, T. H. (2005). Shiftwork: Basic principles. In M. H. Kryger, T. Roth, & W. C. Dement. (Eds), *Principles and practice of sleep medicine* (4th ed., pp. 673–679). Philadelphia: Elsevier.

Moreno, M. E., Munoz, J. M., Valderrabanos, J. S., & Gutierrez, T. V. (1998). Electroconvulsive therapy in first trimester of pregnancy. *Journal of ECT, 4,* 251–254.

Moses-Kolko, E. L., Bogen, D., Perel, J., Bregar, A., Uhl, K., Levin, B., & Wisner, K. L. (2005). Neonatal signs after late in-utero exposure to serotonin reuptake inhibitors: Literature review and implications for clinical applications. *JAMA, 293,* 2372–2383.

Murck, H., Song, C., Horrobin, D. F., & Uhr, M. (2004). Ethyleicosapentaenoate and dexamethasone resistance in therapy-refractory depression. *International Journal of Neuropsychopharmacology, 7,* 341–349.

Nishihara, K., & Horiuchi, S. (1998). Changes in sleep patterns of young women from late pregnancy to postpartum: Relationships to their infants' movements. *Perceptual & Motor Skills, 87,* 1043–1056.

Noorlander, Y., Bergink, V., & van den Berg, M. P. (2008). Perceived and observed mother–child interaction at time of hospitalization and release in postpartum depression and psychosis. *Archives of Women's Mental Health, 11,* 49–56.

Oberlander, T. F., Reebye, P., Misri, S., Papsdorf, M., Kim, J., & Grunau, R. E. (2007). Externalizing and attentional behaviors in children of depressed mothers treated with a selective serotonin reuptake inhibitor antidepressant during pregnancy. *Archives of Pediatric & Adolescent Medicine, 161,* 22–29.

OBG Management. (2007). SSRIs in pregnancy: How they stack up. *OBG Management, 19*(9), 24–32. Retrieved from http://www.obgmanagement.com/pdf/1909/1909OBGM_Evidence1.pdf

Ogrodniczuk, J. S., & Steinberg, P. I. (2005). A renewed interest in day treatment. *Canadian Journal of Psychiatry, 50,* 77.

Olfson, M., & Marcus, S. C. (2009). National patterns in antidepressant medication treatment. *Archives of General Psychiatry, 66,* 848–856.

Oren, D. A., Wisner, K. L., Spinelli, M., Epperson, C. N., Peindl, K. S., Terman, J. S., & Terman, M. (2002). An open trial of morning light therapy for treatment of antepartum depression. *American Journal of Psychiatry, 159,* 666–669.

Organization of Teratology Information Specialists (OTIS). (2005b). *St. John's wort (hypericum perforatum) and pregnancy.* Retrieved from http://www.otispregnancy.org/pdf/stjohnswort

Organization of Teratology Information Specialists (OTIS). (2008a). *Bupropion (Wellbutrin®) and pregnancy.* Retrieved from http://www.otispregnancy.org/pdf/bupropion

Organization of Teratology Information Specialists (OTIS). (2008b). *Citalopram/escitalopram (Celexa®/Lexapro®) and pregnancy.* Retrieved from http://www.otispregnancy.org/pdf/citalopram

Organization of Teratology Information Specialists (OTIS). (2008c). *Paroxetine (Paxil®) and pregnancy.* Retrieved from http://www.otispregnancy.org/pdf/paroxetine

Parker, G. B., Gibson, N., Brotchie, H., Heruc, G., Rees, A. M., & Hadzi-Pavolvic, D. (2006). Omega-3 fatty acids and mood disorders. *American Journal of Psychiatry, 163,* 969–978.

Pittler, M. H., & Ernst, E. (2000). Efficacy of kava extract for treating anxiety: Systematic review and meta-analysis. *Journal of Clinical Psychopharmacology, 20,* 84–89.

Poinso, F., Gay, M. P., Glangeaud-Freundenthal, & Rufo, M. (2002). Care in a mother–baby psychiatric unit: Analysis of separation at discharge. *Archives of Women's Mental Health, 5,* 49–58.

Prentice, R. L., Langer, R. D., Stefanick, M. L., Howard, B.V., Pettinger, M., Anderson, G. L., et al. (2006). Combined analysis of Women's Health Initiative observational and clinical trial data on postmenopausal hormone treatment and cardiovascular disease. *American Journal of Epidemiology, 163,* 589–599.

Rabheru, K. (2001). The use of electroconvulsive therapy in special patient populations. *Canadian Journal of Psychiatry, 46,* 710–719.

Rai, V., Kattar, P., Khatoon, S., Rawat, A.K.S., & Mehrotra, S. (2001). Heavy metal accumulation in some herbal drugs. *Pharmaceutical Biology, 39,* 384–387.

Reed, P., Sermin, N., & Appleby, L. (1999). A comparison of clinical response to electroconvulsive therapy in puerperal and non-puerperal psychoses. *Journal of Affective Disorders, 54,* 255–260.

Rees, A. M., Austin, M. P., & Parker, G. (2005). Role of omega-3 fatty acids in the treatment of depression in the perinatal period. *Australian and New Zealand Journal of Psychiatry, 39,* 274–281.

Rees, A. M., Austin, M. P., & Parker, G. B. (2008). Omega-3 fatty acids as a treatment for perinatal depression: Randomized double-blind placebo-controlled trial. *Australian and New Zealand Journal of Psychiatry, 42,* 199–205.

Postpartum Mood Disorders

Romito, P., Saurel-Cubizolles, M. J., & Cuttini, M. (1994). Mothers' health after the birth of the first child: The case of employed women in an Italian city. *Women's Health, 21,* 1–23.

Rossouw, J. E., Anderson, G. L., Prentice, R. L., LaCroix, A. Z., Kooperberg, C. L., Stefanick, M. L., et al. (2002). Risks and benefits of estrogen plus progestin in healthy postmenopausal women: Principal results from the Women's Health Initiative randomized controlled trial. *JAMA, 288,* 321–333.

Rossouw, J. E., Prentice, R. L., Manson, J. E., Wu, L-L., Barad, D., Barnabei, V. M., et al. (2007). Postmenopausal hormone therapy and risk of cardiovascular disease by age and years since menopause. *JAMA, 297,* 1465–1477.

Rupprecht, R., & Holsboer, F. (1999). Neuropsycho-pharmacological properties of neuroactive steroids. *Steroids, 64*(1–2), 83–91.

Rutter, M. (1995). Clinical implications of attachment concepts: Retrospect and prospect. *Journal of Child Psychology and Psychiatry, 36,* 549–571.

Salmon, M., Abel, K., Cordingley, L., Friedman, T., & Appleby, L. (2003). Clinical and parenting skills outcomes following joint mother–baby psychiatric admission. *Australian & New Zealand Journal of Psychiatry, 37,* 556–562.

Sharma, V. (2006). A cautionary note on the use of antidepressants in postpartum depression. *Bipolar Disorder, 8,* 411–414.

Sharma, V., Smith, A., & Mazmanian, D. (2006). Olanzapine in the prevention of postpartum psychosis and mood episodes in bipolar disorder. *Bipolar Disorder, 8,* 400–404.

Shelton, R. C., Keller, M. B., Gelenberg, A., Dunner, D. L., Hirschfeld, R., Thase, M. E., et al. (2001). Effectiveness of St. John's wort in major depression: A randomized controlled trial. *JAMA, 285,* 1978–1986.

Shinkoda, H., Matsumoto, K., & Park, Y. M. (1999). Changes in sleep-wake cycle during the period from late pregnancy to puerperium identified through the wrist actigraph and sleep logs. *Psychiatry & Clinical Neurosciences, 53*(2), 133–135.

Shumaker, S. A., Legault, C., Rapp, S. R., Thal, L., Wallace, R. B., Ockene, J. K., et al. (2003). Estrogen plus progestin and the incidence of dementia and mild cognitive impairment in postmenopausal women: The Women's Health Initiative memory study: A randomized controlled trial. *JAMA, 289,* 2651–2662.

Sichel, D. A., Cohen, L. S., Robertson, L. M., Ruttenberg, A., & Rosenbaum, J. F. (1995). Prophylactic estrogen in recurrent postpartum affective disorder. *Biological Psychiatry, 38,* 814–818.

Simons, J., Reynolds, J., Mannion, J., & Morison, L. (2003). How the health visitor can help when problems between parents add to postnatal stress. *Journal of Advanced Nursing, 44,* 400–411.

Sivojelezova, A., Shuhaiber, S., Sarkissian, L., Einarson, A., & Koren, G. (2005). Citalopram use in pregnancy: Prospective comparative evaluation of pregnancy and fetal outcome. *American Journal of Obstetrics & Gynecology, 193,* 2004–2009.

Sit, D., Rothschild, A. J., & Wisner, K. L. (2006). A review of postpartum psychosis. *Journal of Women's Health, 15,* 352–368.

Soares, C. N., Almeida, O. P., Joffe, H., & Cohen, L. S. (2001). Efficacy of estradiol for the treatment of depressive disorders in perimenopausal women: A double-blind, randomized, placebo-controlled trial. *Archives of General Psychiatry, 58,* 529–534.

Stoner, S. C., Sommi, R. W. Jr., Marken, P. A., Anya, I., & Vaughn, J. (1997). Clozapine use in two full-term pregnancies. *Journal of Clinical Psychiatry, 58,* 364–365.

Stowe, Z. N., Cohen, L. S., Hostetter, A., Ritchie, J. C., Owens, M. J., & Nemeroff, C. B. (2000). Paroxetine in human breast milk and nursing infants. *American Journal of Psychiatry, 157,* 185–189.

Swain, A. M., O'Hara, M. W., Starr, K. R., & Gorman, L. L. (1997). A prospective study of sleep, mood, and cognitive function in postpartum and non-postpartum women. *Obstetrics & Gynecology, 90,* 381–386.

Tiran, D., & Mack, S. (Eds.). (2000). *Complementary therapies for pregnancy and childbirth* (2nd ed.). New York: Bailliére Tindall.

U.S. Food and Drug Administration. (2006). *SSRIs and treatment challenges of depression in pregnancy.* Retrieved from http://www.fda.gov/Safety/MedWatch/SafetyInformation/SafetyAlertsforHumanMedicalProducts/ucm150749.htm

U.S. Department of Health and Human Services. (2000). Maternal, infant, and child health, objective 19: Increase the proportion of mothers who breastfeed their babies. In *Health People 2010* (2nd ed.). Washington, DC: U.S. Government Printing Office.

Ushiroyama, T., Sakuma, K., & Ueki, M. (2005). Efficacy of the Kampo medicine Xiong-gui-tiao-xue-yin (Kyuki-chouketsu-in), a traditional herbal medicine, in the treatment of maternity blues syndrome in the postpartum period. *American Journal of Chinese Medicine, 33*(1), 117–126.

Üstün, T. B., Privett, M., Lecrubier, Y., Weiller, E., Simon, G., Korten, A., et al. (1996). Form, frequency and burden of sleep problems in general health care: A report from the WHO collaborative study on psychological problems in general health care. *European Psychiatry, 11*(Suppl. 1), 5s–10s.

van der Meer, Y. G., Loendersloot, E. W., & van Loenen, A. C. (1984). Effect of high dose progesterone in postpartum depression. *Journal of Psychosomatic Obstetrics Gynaecology, 3,* 67–68.

Viguera, A., Nonacs, R., Cohen, L., Tondo, L., Murray, A., & Baldessarini, R. (2000). Risk of recurrence of bipolar disorder in pregnant and nonpregnant women. *American Journal of Psychiatry, 157,* 179–184.

Walker, R., & Swartz, C. M. (1994). Electroconvulsive therapy during high-risk pregnancy. *General Hospital Psychiatry, 16,* 348–353.

Wassertheir-Smoller, S., Hendrix, S., Limacher, M., Heiss, G., Kooperberg, C., Baird, A., et al. (2003). Effect of estrogen plus progestin on stroke in postmenopausal women: The Women's Health Initiative: A randomized trial. *JAMA, 289,* 2673–2684.

Weier, K. M., & Beal, M. W. (2004). Complementary therapies as adjuncts in the treatment of postpartum depression. *Journal of Midwifery & Women's Health, 49*(2), 96–104.

Wirz-Justice, A. (1995). *Biological rhythms in mood disorders.* New York: Raven Press.

Wisner, K. L., Parry, B. L., & Piontek, C. M. (2002). Clinical practice: Postpartum depression. *New England Journal of Medicine, 347,* 194–199.

Wisner, K. L., Peindl, K. S., & Gigliotti, T. V. (1999). Tricyclics vs SSRIs for postpartum depression. *Archives of Women's Mental Health, 1,* 189–191.

Wisner, K. L., Perel, J. M., Peindl, K. S., Hanusa, B. H., Findling, R. L., & Rapport, D. (2001). Prevention of recurrent postpartum depression: A randomized clinical trial. *Journal of Clinical Psychiatry, 62,* 82–86.

Wisner, K. L., Perel, J. M., Peindl, K. S., Hanusa, B. H., Piontek, C. M., & Findling, R. L. (2004). Prevention of postpartum depression: A pilot randomized clinical trial. *American Journal of Psychiatry, 161,* 1290–1292.

Wisner, K. L., & Wheeler, S. B. (1994). Prevention of recurrent postpartum major depression. *Hospital Community Psychiatry, 45,* 1191–1196.

Wolfson, A. R., Crowley, S. J., Anwer, U., & Bassett, J. L. (2003). Changes in sleep patterns and depressive symptoms in first-time mothers: Last trimester to 1-year postpartum. *Behavioral Sleep Medicine, 1,* 54–67.

Yehuda, S., Rabinovitz, S., Carrasso, R. L., & Mostofsky, D. I. (1998). Fatty acids and brain peptides. *Peptides, 19,* 407–419.

Chapter 13

Psychosocial Interventions

Introduction

Grace
~ Brangwynne Purcell

What if we knew the future
at birth
and the sky spelled out lines and paths to follow
into the quiet
and fear of death

What if when we fell
it was into feathers
of geese, curled and downy
Not into cliffs
and the sea
that pulls us out
to live as mermaids
imprisoned by scales

What if demons kept quiet
allowing the hollows of
passion and delight
to reign, run wild
know no boundary

What would we do then
What path could we choose
Would pain then cease and
disillusionment fade

Could meaning
be found skin deep
like a scratch and sniff sticker
or would there still be longing

What if
after all that
there was still longing
and unabridged desire
for more
or less
or maybe just greener grass
What then

What if
without fear or tremor
we accepted grace
What if mercy
flowed through us
to the other side
and on into
the person behind
and in front
through a door we open or close

Maybe then we would quiet
the soul quicken
and demons could find a place
among passions
and geese among cliffs
and there could be blessing
through the disguise
of dreams

Psychological interventions are as effective as medical treatments, yet specialists tend to be difficult to find in the United States. The administration of cognitive behavioral therapy, interpersonal psychotherapy, and medication have been found by Elkin et al. (1989) to be equally effective in alleviating the symptoms of depression, and others have found similar results specifically for postpartum depression (Appleby, Warner, Whitton, & Faragher, 1997; Cooper & Murray, 1997). However, few medicinal, psychotherapeutic, or supportive models aimed at reducing maternal depression alter the interactions between the mother and the baby or the developmental consequences of maternal depression on the infant (Clark, Tluczek, & Wenzel, 2003). Therefore, applying psychotherapeutic, psychosocial support or pharmacotherapy is most advantageous when combined with a mother–child therapeutic component.

Psychosocial interventions are of particular interest to women who have a perinatal mood disorder, as many prefer options other than medication. Although adverse effects of medications during the perinatal period have been minimal, many women prefer to limit unknown risks to the developing fetus. This chapter will describe the evidence-based psychotherapeutic interventions that have had positive results, as well as other support and encouragement options.

Support and Encouragement Strategies

Education and Debriefing

One strategy to prevent or "soften" the onset of postpartum mood changes is to debrief the woman and her family following delivery. Debriefing is a time for medical staff to discuss the details of delivery and a time for women and families to share their experience of the events that took place during the delivery. Further, the medical staff has the opportunity to explain normal reactions to deliveries that were traumatic or did not go as originally planned. Although posttraumatic delivery debriefing is reported to be welcomed and appreciated, it has not consistently been shown to preclude the onset of postpartum mental health symptoms (Cooke & Stacey, 2003; Gamble et al., 2005; Priest, Henderson, Evans, & Hagan, 2003; Small, Lumley, Donohue, Potter, & Waldenström, 2000; Wessely, Rose, & Bisson, 2000). It is proposed that the full effects of the traumatic delivery have not had enough time to incorporate into the psyche within days after the event, thereby lessening the effectiveness of debriefing to prevent the onset of postpartum mood disorder (PMD) symptoms (Gamble et al., 2005; Horowitz, 1993). At times, unfortunately, debriefing for posttraumatic stress is actually more harmful than helpful (Rose, Bisson, & Wessely, 2003).

Gamble et al.'s (2005) posttraumatic delivery debriefing study did show a decrease in trauma-related symptoms, stress, depression, and self-blame. The 40- to 60-minute debriefing intervention, administered by midwives, included nine main topic areas:

1. Develop a nonjudgmental and accepting relationship with the mother.

2. While listening, encourage the mother to continue sharing as she recalls her birthing experience.

3. Use open-ended questions and reflective responses as the mother shares.

4. Nonjudgmentally, but honestly, respond to the mother's questions or misperceptions.

5. Assess how the mother is integrating her emotional and behavioral reactions to the traumatic delivery, while recognizing grief or loss issues. Therapeutically confront cognitive misperceptions related to the trauma (examples provided by the authors—self-blame, feeling inadequate)

6. Carefully and considerately discuss possible ways the labor process could have gone differently, while remaining unconditionally supportive and nonjudgmental.

7. Assess and provide socioemotional support education. Suggest ways that other women have used to cope with traumatic birth experiences.

8. Positively reinforce self-helping strategies that the mother plans and discusses.

9. Plan and establish socioemotional supports from experts, other women who have experienced traumatic deliveries, and friends and family.

Support Groups

Support groups for postpartum depression are online, offered through hospitals and health or mental health clinics and sometimes arise through word of mouth in a community. Support groups allow women to meet other women experiencing similar situations, thereby normalizing PMDs (Scrandis, 2005). Through normalization and socialization, some women find it easier to manage symptoms. In 1992, Fleming, Klein, and Corter assessed the effectiveness of social support groups on mothers' postpartum depression symptoms. Although depression symptoms did not decrease, interaction with their child increased when compared to the interaction levels of women in a control group. In Taiwan, a brief support group (four sessions) provided training on stress management skills, communication skills, and life planning skills and discussed issues related to the transition to motherhood (Chen, Tseng, Chou, & Wang, 2000). Results showed less depression, less perceived stress, and improved social support.

Nondirective Counseling

Nondirective counseling is parallel to providing encouragement and support to women with postpartum depression. Cooper et al. (2003) examined the effectiveness of nondirective counseling based on the work of Holden, Sagovsky, and Cox (1989). Holden et al.'s (1989) study found that women who received nondirective counseling reported a decrease in postpartum depression symptoms two times more often than women who did not receive any counseling for their symptoms. These findings were replicated by a similar study in 1996 (Wickberg & Hwang, 1996).

Using this strategy, women are encouraged to talk about current difficulties with taking care of their babies; financial concerns; and interactions with their significant other, family, and friends. Results showed that nondirective counseling reduced the mother's symptoms of postpartum depression. The infant's emotional and behavioral responses improved as well, and more receptive mother–baby contact was observed (Murray et al., 2003). This reduction in postpartum depression symptoms continued at 4.5 months; however, it did not prevent the re-occurrence of postpartum depression in later pregnancies (Cooper et al., 2003). Mothers who received nondirective counseling continued to have difficulty developing secure attachment with their babies and had difficulty addressing early problematic behaviors (Murray et al., 2003).

Psychotherapeutic Interventions

Cognitive Behavioral Therapy

Cognitive behavioral therapy (CBT) takes the premise that thoughts lead to feelings, feelings lead to behaviors, behaviors lead to consequences, and consequences reinforce thoughts. CBT strategies intervene by changing this pattern at any point. Relative to PMDs, the majority of research looks at changing cognitive distortions (negative thought processes) and teaching new behaviors. Currently, CBT interventions which include ways to manage parent–infant interactions and stress are the most effective. Milgrom, Ericksen, McCarthy, and Gemmill's (2006) small study found that mothers who received three months of CBT focused on relieving depression symptoms failed to be relieved of parenting stress, whereas mothers who received direct parent–infant treatment saw more rapid relief from depression symptoms.

In Prendergast and Austin's (2001) study, *Early Childhood Nurses* with community nursing, midwifery, and basic counseling education, provided CBT counseling to women identified with postpartum depression under the supervision of a psychiatrist. The early childhood nurses were trained to provide the following CBT-based counseling:

1. Education about postpartum depression

2. Cognitive monitoring assignments

3. Anxiety management skills

4. Assertiveness skills

5. Self-esteem changing assignments

6. "Pleasant-event" planning

7. Diary-keeping

The protocol was administered to women with postpartum depression over a six-week period at home. Seven in ten women who received CBT counseling stated that contact with the early childhood nurse was a key reason why their depression symptoms improved. Interestingly, only 45 percent of women in the comparison group (who received 20- to 60-minute emotionally supportive weekly sessions in a clinic setting) went to all of their appointments, whereas 100 percent of women in the home-visit CBT group completed all six sessions. Women in the control group who did not keep all appointments stated that the sessions were not helpful, the location was not convenient or was not a hospitable environment, and too much attention was given to the baby. Immediate and six-month follow-up results revealed similar improvements in depression symptoms.

Cognitive behavioral techniques based on the work of Hawton, Salkovskis, Kirk, and Clark (1989) and McDonough (1993) focus on the interaction between the mother and infant. In this situation, reduction of postpartum depression symptoms is considered a secondary benefit from the CBT treatment (Cooper, Murray, Wilson, & Romaniuk, 2003). Mothers identify difficulties experienced while taking care of the baby such as getting the baby to sleep or eat. Mother–infant interactions are observed, and concerns are identified and then addressed. Women receive individualized education, interaction skills modeling, and positive reinforcement for changes in their interactions with the baby. Results show that CBT was effective not only in changing the quality of mother-infant interactions, but also in reducing the mother's symptoms of postpartum depression (Cooper et al., 2003). Further analysis showed improved emotional responses and behaviors from the infants and more receptive mother–baby contact (Murray, Cooper, Wilson, & Romaniuk, 2003). At a five-year follow-up, children showed slightly better emotional and behavioral adjustment than did children of mothers who did not receive counseling; however, this difference was not statistically significant. Analysis from the five-year follow-up also showed that postpartum depressed women with social difficulties also had children with greater emotional and behavioral difficulties (Murray et al., 2003). Therefore, CBT was unable to address factors related to social adversities. The reduction in postpartum depression symptoms continued at 4.5 months; however, the intervention did not prevent the reoccurrence of postpartum depression in later pregnancies. Furthermore, the mothers continued to have difficulty managing their baby's early-onset behavior problems and difficulty developing secure attachment with the baby (Murray et al., 2003).

Combinations of cognitive behavioral techniques to assist women with postpartum posttraumatic disorder are presented in Ayers, McKenzie-McHarg, and Eagle's (2007) case reports. Woman #1 was asked to discuss her postpartum trauma. The authors identified faulty beliefs and thought patterns and gave Woman #1 a homework assignment geared toward changing these faulty beliefs or thoughts: Have 16 people the woman did not know complete a survey that assessed their personal opinions about a person who had survived the trauma that the woman had experienced. The survey results tangibly showed her the way others would "judge" her situation, thereby altering the way that she internalized the experience and changed her thoughts about herself. Next, Woman #1 was guided through the traumatic experience step-by-step. Key troublesome moments were identified, and strategies such as role playing were used to address these moments, resulting in resolution of hyperemotional reactivity. In addition, Woman #1 was taught visualization techniques to use when experiencing a flashback. At the end of 10 sessions, Woman #1 no longer experienced posttraumatic symptoms and had replaced faulty beliefs about herself and others with more realistic and healthy perceptions.

In another case report, faulty beliefs about the postpartum posttraumatic event and subsequent avoidance behaviors were identified in Woman #2, who attended counseling with her partner (Ayers et al., 2007). The couple received education about how the events evolved into symptoms of posttraumatic stress and depression and about identified faulty beliefs, which led to feelings of anger, low self-esteem, and avoidance behaviors. Woman # 2 was guided through the trauma that was audiotaped. She was instructed to listen to the audiotape repeatedly at designated times until she became emotionally desensitized to the event through the use of cognitive reappraisal skills. Simultaneously, Woman # 2 exercised and attended couples counseling sessions. Following twelve weeks of treatment, Woman #2's posttraumatic stress symptoms ceased, her depression symptoms decreased, and her relationship with her partner recovered.

Psychodynamic Therapy

Psychodynamic therapy provides an environment for people to discuss concerns. Through these discussions, clients learn the development of current behaviors or reactions based on the individual's past history. From this new understanding, clients are supported through addressing unresolved issues arising from past history that are affecting the individual's current quality of life and interactions with others. This strategy has been success-fully used to assist women with postpartum depression (Cooper et al., 2003; Cramer et al., 1990; Stern, 1995). One study using this model had a thera-pist engage mothers in a discussion about their personal development and early attachment history with their family of origin. The therapist linked the mother's attachment style, baby interactions, and symbolic meaning of the infant to the mother's past attachment experiences. Results showed that psychodynamic therapy significantly reduced postpartum depression symptoms up to nine months. Follow-up analysis revealed that the baby showed improved emotional and behavioral responsiveness and improved mother-baby interactions (Murray et al., 2003). However, psychodynamic therapy did not prevent the reoccurrence of postpartum depression in later pregnancies. In addition, it did not improve the mother's ability to man-age difficult behavioral problems, and it did not improve secure attachment with the baby (Murray et al., 2003). At the five-year follow-up, children of women who received psychodynamic therapy and who also experienced social hardships had slightly worse emotional and behavioral functioning than did children of women who received no counseling, CBT treatment, or nondirective counseling; although these differences were not statistically significant (Murray et al., 2003).

Interpersonal Psychotherapy

Developed over 30 years ago by Klerman and Weissman, interpersonal psy-chotherapy has been used to successfully treat depression (Elkin et al., 1989; Weissman & Markowitz, 1994). One benefit of using this therapy is that the method is in a manual format, making application more reliable and standardized. In addition, the modality is reasonably easy to learn and can be used by medical doctors, nurses, social workers, and psychologists across a variety of settings (Segre, Stuart, & O'Hara, 2004).

Interpersonal psychotherapy has been used, with positive results, to assist women who are depressed during pregnancy as a strategy to reduce the reoccurrence of depression postpartum, as well as a strategy to improve the development of the fetus (Grote, Bledsoe, Swartz, & Frank, 2004b). It has also been beneficial to low-income and nonwhite perinatally depressed women (Grote et al., 2004a, 2004b). To improve access to care in these populations, Grote et al. (2004a) suggested offering treatment in public care obstetric and gynecologic clinics, providing an option to receive treatment over the phone, offering flexible treatment times, and assisting in gaining access to social services in the woman's community.

Treatment is categorized into four phases:

1. Pretreatment assessment
2. Initial treatment
3. Intermediate treatment
4. Treatment conclusion (Klerman et al., 1984, Segre et al., 2004; Stuart & Robertson, 2003)

Treatment addresses four depression-related factors:

1. Relational disagreements or arguments
2. Role transition
3. Grief and loss
4. Relational sensitivity (Klerman et al., 1984, Segre et al., 2004; Stuart & Robertson, 2003)

Based on Grote et al.'s work, researchers have tested the efficacy of using interpersonal psychotherapy to assist women with perinatal depression, with positive results (O'Hara, Stuart, Gorman, & Wenzel, 2000; Spinelli & Endicott, 2003). In the pretreatment phase, women are diagnostically assessed for postpartum depression, typically using standardized measurement instruments, clinical interview, and ruling out somatic symptoms of the perinatal period (Segre et al., 2004). Adding an ethnographic interview combined with psycho-education generally improves engagement of nonwhite women in the interpersonal therapeutic process (Grote et al., 2004a).

The initial session begins following a positive assessment for perinatal depression. During these sessions, women are taught that postpartum depression is a medical condition. The depression diagnosis is defined from an interpersonal perspective, based on a thorough assessment of the women's current interpersonal relationships and history. Then connections between the women's interpersonal relationships and depression symptoms are brought to light. These identified connections, based on the four depression-related factors become the foundation for the development of therapeutic goals and a therapeutic contract (O'Hara et al., 2000; Segre et al., 2004). The most commonly identified goals included the following:

- Relational arguments or disagreements (primarily with one's significant other or family members): baby care needs, family visitation, and sexual intimacy

- Role-related transition: changes in independence and activities with friends, parenting skill concerns, changes in work-related roles

- Grief and loss: death of a parent, other family member, or infant; spontaneous or elective abortion; and losses related to abandonment and abuse concerns

- Relational sensitivity (no clear descriptions were provided in the empirical literature) (O'Hara et al., 2000; Segre et al., 2004)

Intermediate sessions strongly examine communication patterns, emotional reactions, and the use of conjoint sessions (Segre et al., 2004). In concluding treatment sessions, women's progress, strengths, resilience, and ability to prevail over depression are emphasized, and women are prepared with steps to take should the depression return in the future (O'Hara et al., 2000; Segre et al., 2004). Segre et al.'s (2004) article provides an excellent, detailed description of each step in the interpersonal psychotherapeutic process for assisting women during the perinatal period if you are interested in learning more about this modality.

Group Counseling

Although women with postpartum depression more often opt for counseling over medication (Cooper et al., 2003), it is reported that women more often shy away from group treatment as opposed to individual counseling (Cooper et al., 2003; Seeley, Murray, & Cooper, 1996). This may be due to the stigma attached to mental health problems and, more specifically, to the misperception that all mothers with mental health conditions are unfit to be a parent. Nonetheless, group counseling may be a preferred model as it can address the difficulties often experienced by women with postpartum depression such as marital discord, life stresses, limited social supports, lack of social skills, and distorted negative thoughts (Meager & Milgrom, 1996). Exposure to peers experiencing similar difficulties has the potential to more rapidly dissolve myths about motherhood and to create a conducive environment for RCT components such as mutual empathy, mutual empowerment, and emotional connectedness (previously described in chapter 2) (Lane, Roufeil, Williams, & Tweedie, 2001).

Several studies examine different theoretical foundations on the effectiveness of group counseling for women with postpartum depression. The majority of these studies have small sample sizes, making results difficult to generalize, yet group therapy has been successful in most of these trials. One 10-week group treatment program for women with postpartum depression, showed significant reduction in depression and stress related to parenting, as compared to women in a waiting list group (Meager & Milgrom, 1996).

In 1997, Morgan, Matthey, Barnett and Richardson found women exposed to psycho-educational group treatment experienced significantly fewer depressed symptoms at the end of treatment.

Group counseling has also been used to assist women experiencing postpartum posttraumatic stress disorder following an emergency cesarean section. In Sweden, mental health workers who specialize in maternity and child welfare collaborate to provide postpartum group counseling for women who have had an emergency C-section (Alfvén, Henning, & Holmertz, 1996). These groups meet soon after delivery, and sometimes meet several times during the first year postpartum (Ryding, Wirén, Johansson, Ceder, & Dahlström, 2004). By and large, empirical evaluation of these groups has not been conducted to determine effectiveness. Despite positive reception from the women involved in two small Swedish studies that did evaluate group counseling effectiveness, results indicated that the intervention did not have any impact on posttraumatic stress symptoms (Ryding et al., 2004; Ryding, Wijma, & Wijma, 1998).

Bioecological Model

This model has primarily been applied to adolescents with postpartum moods. Adolescent females with postpartum depression present a unique challenge due to developmental needs, focus on social approval, the environment in which they live, experience with violence, and the extent to which they have developed self-esteem and resiliency (Harrykissoon, Rickert & Weimann, 2002; Logsdon, Hertweck, Ziegler, & Pinto-Folz, 2008; Meadows-Oliver, Sadler, Swartz, & Ryan-Krause, 2007; Sadler et al., 2007).

Research on treating this population stresses the importance of providing social supports as evidence shows health, mental health, and social function improvements with these supports (Logsdon, Birkimer, Ratterman, Cahill, & Cahill, 2002; Logsdon et al., 2008; Polomeno, 1996). Logsdon et al. (2008) examined a bioecological model to provide postpartum depression treatment for adolescent females. Similar to the micro, mezzo, and macro levels in social work, this model focuses primarily on the adolescent's environmental surroundings, the adolescent's ability to use skills to negotiate this environment, and peer supports, with the premise that the interaction of these factors affects the adolescent's development (Bronfenbrenner & Ceci, 1994; Logsdon et al., 2008).

Based on this model, the way that postpartum adolescents viewed stress predicted postpartum depression (Logsdon et al., 2008). Many of the adolescent females in this study had experienced or witnessed violence. In addition, nearly 40 percent of adolescents in this study expressed depression symptoms. Intervention focus should be on increasing these youth's self-esteem (Logsdon et al., 2008).

Mother–Infant Dyad Intervention

As previously mentioned, many intervention strategies aimed at the mother's mental health symptoms are often effective in reducing depression symptoms. However, they have not been as helpful in improving the mother–infant relationship and interaction, thereby keeping these babies at risk for developmental difficulties from infancy through adolescence. The most promising family-focused interventions to date are ones that incorporate the child into the treatment plan.

Mother–infant interventions that show the greatest promise incorporate traditional and nontraditional strategies. Tiffany Field, Maria Hernandez-Reif, and Miguel Diego, and their team at the Touch Research Institute, have accumulated over 30 peer-reviewed articles that discuss mothers with PMDs, mother–infant interactions, and therapeutic strategies to improve both the mother's symptoms and the infant's outcomes. Several of these articles discuss the effectiveness of music therapy and mother-initiated massage with her infant (Field, Hernandez-Reif, & Diego, 2006; Hernandez-Reif, Diego, & Field, 2006). Results indicate that mothers became significantly more relaxed and that depressed mood and anxiety also decreased. Moreover, providing massage to the infant decreased depression, anxiety, and stress for the mother. These findings were also supported by observed physiological changes in salivary cortisol levels, changes in serotonin and dopamine levels, and EEG/EKG changes (Feijo et al., 2006; Field, 1997; Field, Hernandez-Reif, Diego, Schanberg, & Kuhn, 2005; Hernandez-Reif et al., 2006).

Massage during pregnancy has also been shown to reduce the onset of maternal and paternal prenatal depression, reduce pain during pregnancy, and improve newborn behaviors (Field, Diego, & Hernandez-Reif, 2009; Field, Figueiredo et al., 2008). More notably, massage provided during pregnancy appears to protect against premature delivery, improve immune system functioning, and improve infant growth rates and has shown an increase in temperature of preterm babies placed in incubators, a decrease in stress-related behaviors, and a decrease in infant motor delays often associated with depression during pregnancy (Diego, Field, & Hernandez-Reif, 2008; Diego et al., 2007; Diego et al., 2009; Field, Diego, & Hernandez-Reif, 2006, 2007; Hernandez-Reif, Diego, & Field, 2007).

Another mother–infant dyad treatment strategy was evaluated by Clark, Tluczek, and Wenzel (2003) in which three interventions were applied:

1. Mothers received peer support and therapy in a group setting.

2. While mothers were attending individual or group treatment, infants received developmental therapy with other infants in a group setting focusing on emotional regulation and social interaction.

3. After the mothers and infants received individual group treatment, the mother–infant dyads met in a group setting together, where mothers receive instruction and reinforcement for sensitive and responsive interactions with their infant.

In addition to these three mother–infant interventions, fathers attended two group sessions. Results of this innovative treatment strategy revealed decreased postpartum depression symptoms in the mother, improved maternal perceptions of the baby, and improved maternal ability to sensitively interact with her baby. However, the results for the infant showed no significant developmental changes after the study, however, this may be due to a small sample size.

In Zürich, Germany, Pedrina (2004) has been working on a new form of psychoanalytic group treatment program that includes infants in the group setting. Although reported findings are from a small sample size (nine mother–infant dyads and four fathers who attended sporadically), this work represents an interesting departure from more traditional highly structured group treatment protocols. Group sessions were held every other week for 90 minutes for one year and two months. Sessions ended as the infants were able to walk. Goals were defined by the group and focused on dependence and autonomy conflict in relationship to the baby, father, and significant others, dependence and aggression conflict, and role identity conflict. The underlying issues that were elucidated about the dependence and autonomy conflict revealed unproductive "interactive, nonverbal communication circles" in which the women would become stuck. In other words, the women would repeatedly try to resolve issues (for example, the baby is crying) by using skills that did not work in the past. They were unable to think of other skills to use, thereby feeling trapped. The result of this reoccurring cycle increased the mother's stress level and decreased her ability to believe that when the situation arose again in the future, she would be able to successfully manage it—again—feeling trapped.

Dependence and aggression conflict discussions focused on how dissatisfaction with the baby's father resulted in aggressive or impatient interactions with the infant. Over time, the group began to reveal episodes of exposure to violence and aggressive behaviors from their family of origin. Two main types of reactions surfaced:

1. Women who had an aggressive family of origin growing up were fearful of aggressive behaviors occurring in their new family, which would result in destroying the family.

2. Women who did not have this history were confident that aggressive feelings and disagreements would eventually fade, creating a stronger relationship within the family.

Several role conflicts surfaced for the women about how to manage competing demands for her time and focus, including her various roles as mother, wife, daughter, employee, and friend, all while trying to maintain her sense of self. Group discussions about role conflicts became more interesting when fathers joined the group. In these joint parent sessions, it became apparent that couples were trying to define the "mother role" and "father role" in an alternate way than their families of origin had, searching for a solution that best fit their circumstances. Through group discussions, the couples were able to express their role choices and were able to change these choices in cases where the original role expectations or choices were not working as successfully as they had originally hoped . In essence, the group gave permission for couples to change previous role arrangements. In other cases, the group acted as a "watchdog" by providing couples with feedback when one partner was expecting too much from the other. This allowed couples to make non–intimidating choices that benefited the family without overly stressing one partner over the other.

Children played an interesting role in the group structure. Initially, mother–infant interaction difficulties were apparent. However, over time, mothers were able to tighten up or loosen up their interactions with their infant through modeling of other, more effective interaction strategies from other group members. As the infants matured, they began to interact with other infants and other parents. This provided a nurturing environment for the infants to gain autonomy in a healthy way. In addition, the infants would mimic the moods and behaviors of the mother, which was noted by the entire group and became a learning tool during sessions.

Although not all of the women who participated were assessed to be clinically depressed, all experienced some form of mental health–related dissatisfaction. All infants involved expressed behavioral, psychological, or physical disturbances including intense crying episodes, sleep disturbances, "neurodermatitis," and vomiting episodes. At the end of group treatment, infants no longer experienced the above-described symptoms and women no longer reported mental health disturbances with the exception of two women who also had a personality disorder diagnosis.

Postpartum depression symptoms that do not improve after counseling may be indicative of other underlying phenomena beyond the postpartum onset of mental health symptoms. Researchers found that several "immature defenses" exist, such as possessing a significant number of dysfunctional attitudes, difficulty with object relations, difficulty regulating emotions, maladaptive reactivity, insecure attachment style, high interpersonal sensitivity, and poor ego development (Bond, 2004; Hamilton & Dobson, 2002; Magalhães et al., 2007; McMahon, Barnett, Kowalenko, & Tennant, 2005; Valbak, 2004). There is some indication that these factors are related to adverse childhood events that resulted in insecure attachments and difficulties regulating emotions experienced as an adult, thereby leading to the development of depression (West, Rose, Spreng, Verhoef, & Bergman, 1999). The combination of the experience of adverse childhood events, reactions to these events, and relationship difficulties as an adult influence the length of the postpartum depression—sometimes lasting up to three or four years (McLennan, Kotelchuck, & Cho, 2001; McMahon et al., 2005; McMahon, Trapolini, & Barnett, 2008). In one study, women with insecure attachment styles due to childhood trauma were seven times more likely to experience longer postpartum depression episodes (McMahon et al., 2008). These individuals will most likely need more long-term psychotherapeutic treatments (Magalhães et al., 2007).

There are limited researched psychotherapeutic interventions to address postpartum posttraumatic stress, obsessive–compulsive disorder, and psychosis.

References

Alfvén, M., Henning, E., & Holmertz, V. (1996). *Kejsarsnittsboken (The cesarean section book)*. Stockholm: Cordia.

Appleby, L., Warner, R., Whitton, A., & Faragher, B. (1997). A controlled study of fluoxetine and cognitive-behavioral counseling in the treatment of postnatal depression. *British Medical Journal, 314,* 932–936.

Ayers, S., McKenzie-McHarg, K., & Eagle, A. (2007). Cognitive behaviour therapy for postnatal post-traumatic stress disorder: Case studies. *Journal of Psychosomatic Obstetrics & Gynecology, 28*(3), 177–184.

Bond, M. (2004). Empirical studies of defense style: Relationships with psychopathology and change. *Harvard Review of Psychiatry, 12,* 263–278.

Bronfenbrenner, U., & Ceci, S. J. (1994). Nature–nurture reconceptualized in developmental perspective: A bioecological model. *Psychological Review, 101,* 568–586.

Chen, C. H., Tseng, Y. F., Chou, F. H., & Wang, S.Y. (2000). Effects of support group intervention in postnatally distressed women: A controlled study in Taiwan. *Journal of Psychosomatic Research, 49,* 395–399.

Clark, R., Tluczek, A., & Wenzel, A. (2003). Psychotherapy for postpartum depression: A preliminary report. *American Journal of Orthopsychiatry, 73,* 441–454.

Cooke, M., & Stacey, T. (2003). Differences in the evaluation of postnatal midwifery support by multiparous and primiparous women in the first two weeks after birth. *Australian Midwifery, 16*(3), 18–24.

Cooper, P. J., & Murray, L. (1997). The impact of psychological treatment of postpartum depression on maternal mood and infant development. In P. J. Cooper & L. Murray (Eds.), *Postpartum depression and child development* (pp. 201–220). New York: Guilford Press.

Cooper, P. J., Murray, L., Wilson, A., & Romaniuk, H. (2003). Controlled trial of the short- and long-term effect of psychological treatment on post-partum depression, 1: Impact on maternal mood. *British Journal of Psychiatry, 182,* 412–419.

Cramer, B., Robert-Tissot, C., Stern, D., Serpa-Rusconi, S., DeMuralt, M., Besson, G., et al. (1990). Outcome evaluation in brief mother–infant psychotherapy: A preliminary report. *Infant Mental Health Journal, 11,* 278–300.

Diego, M., Field, T., & Hernandez-Reif, M. (2008). Temperature increases in preterm infants during massage therapy. *Infant Behavior & Development, 31*(1), 149–152.

Diego, M., Field, T., Hernandez-Reif, M., Deeds, O., Ascencio, A., & Begert, G. (2007). Preterm infant massage elicits consistent increases in vagal activity and gastric motility that are associated with greater weight gain. *Acta Pædiatrica, 96,* 1588–1591.

Diego, M. A., Field, T., Hernandez-Reif, M., Schanberg, S., Kuhn, C., & Gonzalez-Quintero, V. H. (2009). Prenatal depression restricts fetal growth. *Early Human Development, 85* (1), 65–70.

Elkin, I., Shea, M. T., Watkins, J. T., Imber, S. D., Sotsky, S. M., Collins, J. F., et al. (1989). National Institute of Mental Health Treatment of Depression Collaborative Research Program: General effectiveness of treatments. *Archives of General Psychiatry, 46,* 971–982.

Feijo, L., Hernandez-Reif, M., Field, T., Valley-Gray, S., Simco, E., & Burns, W. (2006). Mothers' depressed mood and anxiety levels are reduced after massaging their preterm infants. *Infant Behavior & Development, 29,* 476–480.

Field, T. (1997). The treatment of depressed mothers and their infants. In L. Murray & P. J. Cooper (Eds.), *Postpartum depression and child development* (pp. 221–236). New York: Guilford Press.

Field, T., Diego, M., & Hernandez-Reif, M. (2006). Prenatal depression effects on the fetus and newborn: A review. *Infant Behavior & Development, 29,* 445–455.

Field, T., Diego, M., & Hernandez-Reif, M. (2007). Massage therapy research. *Developmental Review, 27,* 75–89.

Field, T., Diego, M., & Hernandez-Reif, M. (2009). Depressed mothers' infants are less responsive to faces and voices. *Infant Behavior & Development, 32,* 239–244.

Field, T., Figueiredo, B., Hernandez-Reif, M., Diego, M., Deeds, O., & Ascencio. A. (2008). Massage therapy reduces pain in pregnant women, alleviates prenatal depression in both parents and improves their relationships. *Journal of Bodywork & Movement Therapies, 12*(2), 146–150.

Field, T., Hernandez-Reif, M., & Diego, M. (2006). Intrusive and withdrawn depressed mothers and their infants. *Developmental Review, 26,* 15–30.

Field, T., Hernandez-Reif, M., Diego, M., Schanberg, S., & Kuhn, C. (2005). Cortisol decreases and serotonin and dopamine increase following massage therapy. *International Journal of Neuroscience, 115,* 1397–1413.

Fleming, A. S., Klein, E., & Corter, C. (1992). The effects of a social support group on depression, maternal attitudes and behavior in new mothers. *Journal of Child Psychology and Psychiatry, 33,* 685–698.

Gamble, J., Creedy, D., Moyle, W., Webster, H., McAllister, M., & Dickson, P. (2005). Effectiveness of a counseling intervention after a traumatic childbirth: A randomized controlled trial. *Birth, 32,* 11–19.

Grote, N. K., Bledsoe, S. E., Swartz, H. A., & Frank, E. (2004a). Culturally relevant psychotherapy for perinatal depression in low-income OB/GYN patients. *Clinical Social Work Journal, 32,* 327–347.

Grote, N. K., Bledsoe, S. E., Swartz, H. A., & Frank, E. (2004b). Feasibility of providing culturally relevant, brief interpersonal psychotherapy for antenatal depression in an obstetrics clinic: A pilot study. *Research on Social Work Practice, 14,* 397–407.

Hamilton, K. E., & Dobson, K. S. (2002). Cognitive therapy and depression: Pretreatment patient predictors of outcome. *Clinical Psychology Review, 22,* 875–893.

Harrykissoon, S. D., Rickert, V. I., & Weimann, C. M. (2002). Prevalence and patterns of intimate partner violence among adolescent mothers during the postpartum period. *Archives of Pediatric & Adolescent Medicine, 156,* 325–330.

Hawton, K., Salkovskis, P., Kirk, J., & Clark, D. M. (1989). *Cognitive behavioural approaches to adult psychiatric disorders.* Oxford, England: Oxford University Press.

Hernandez-Reif, M., Diego, M., & Field, T. (2006). Instrumental and vocal music effects on EEG and EKG in neonates of depressed and nondepressed mothers. *Infant Behavior & Development, 29,* 518–525.

Hernandez-Reif, M., Diego, M., & Field, T. (2007). Preterm infants show reduced stress behaviors and activity after 5 days of massage therapy. *Infant Behavior & Development, 30,* 557–561.

Holden, J., Sagovsky, R., & Cox, J. L. (1989). Counseling in a general practice setting: A controlled study of health visitor intervention in the treatment of postnatal depression. *British Medical Journal, 298,* 223–226.

Horowitz, M. J. (1993). Stress-response syndromes: A review of post-traumatic stress and adjustment disorders. In J. P. Wilson & B. Raphael (Eds.), *International handbook of traumatic stress syndromes* (pp. 49–60). New York: Plenum Press.

Klerman, G. L., Weissman, M. M., Rounsaville, B. J., & Chevron, E. S. (1984). *Interpersonal psychotherapy of depression.* New York: Basic Books.

Lane, B., Roufeil, L. M., Williams, S., & Tweedie, R. (2001). It's just different in the country: Postnatal depression and group therapy in a rural setting. *Social Work Health and Mental Health, 34*(3/4), 333–348.

Logsdon, M. C., Birkimer, J. C., Ratterman, A., Cahill, K., & Cahill, N. (2002). Social support in pregnant and parenting adolescents: Research, critique, and recommendations. *Journal of Child and Adolescent Psychiatric Nursing, 15,* 75–83.

Logsdon, M. C., Hertweck, P., Ziegler, C., & Pinto-Folz, M. (2008). Testing a bioecological model to examine social support in postpartum adolescents. *Journal of Nursing Scholarship, 40*(2), 116–123.

Magalhães, P.V.S., Pinheiro, R. T., Faria, A. D., Osório, C. M., da Silva, R. A., & Botella, L. (2007). Impact of defense style on brief psychotherapy of postpartum depression. *Journal of Nervous and Mental Disease, 195,* 870–873.

McDonough, S. (1993). Interaction guidance: Understanding and treating early infant–caregiver relationship disorders. In C. Zeanah (Ed.), *Handbook of infant mental health* (pp. 414–426). New York: Guilford Press.

McLennan, J., Kotelchuck, M., & Cho, H. (2001). Prevalence, persistence and correlates of depressive symptoms in a national sample of mothers and toddlers. *Journal of the American Academy of Child & Adolescent Psychiatry, 40,* 1316–1323.

McMahon, C., Barnett, B., Kowalenko, N., & Tennant, C. (2005). Psychological factors associated with persistent postnatal depression: Past and current relationships, defense styles and the mediating role of insecure attachment style. *Journal of Affective Disorders, 84,* 15–24.

McMahon, C., Trapolini, T., & Barnett, B. (2008). Maternal state of mind regarding attachment predicts persistence of postnatal depression in the preschool years. *Journal of Affective Disorders, 107*(1–3), 199–203.

Meadows-Oliver, M., Sadler, L. S., Swartz, M. K., & Ryan-Krause, P. (2007). Sources of stress and support and maternal resources of homeless teenage mothers. *Journal of Child & Adolescent Psychiatric Nursing, 20,* 116–125.

Meager, I., & Milgrom, J. (1996). Group treatment for postpartum depression: A pilot study. *Australian and New Zealand Journal of Psychiatry, 30,* 852–860.

Milgrom, J., Ericksen, J., McCarthy, R., & Gemmill, A. W. (2006). Stressful impact of depression on early mother–infant relations. *Stress and Health, 22,* 229–238.

Morgan, M., Matthey, S., Barnett, B., & Richardson, C. (1997). A group programme for postnatally depressed women and their partners. *Journal of Advanced Nursing, 26,* 913–920.

Murray, L., Cooper, P. J., Wilson, A., & Romaniuk, H. (2003). Controlled trial of the short- and long-term effect of psychological treatment of post-partum depression, 2: Impact on the mother-child relationship and child outcome. *British Journal of Psychiatry, 182,* 420–427.

O'Hara, M. W., Stuart, S., Gorman, L. L., & Wenzel, A. (2000). Efficacy of interpersonal psychotherapy for postpartum depression. *Archives of General Psychiatry, 57,* 1039–1045.

Pedrina, F. (2004). Group therapy with mothers and babies in postpartum crises: Preliminary evaluation of a pilot project. Translated from German by P. Schmid-Tomlinson. *Group Analysis, 37*(1), 137–151.

Polomeno, V. (1996). Social support during pregnancy. *International Journal of Childbirth Education, 11,* 14–21.

Prendergast, J., & Austin, M. P. (2001). Early childhood nurse-delivered cognitive behavioural counseling for post-natal depression. *Australasian Psychiatry, 9*(3), 255–259.

Priest, S., Henderson, J., Evans, S., & Hagan, R. (2003). Stress debriefing after childbirth: A randomised controlled trial. *Medical Journal of Australia, 178,* 542–545.

Rose, S., Bisson, J., & Wessely, S. (2003). Psychological debriefing for preventing post traumatic stress disorder (PTSD). *Cochrane Database of Systematic Reviews,* 2. Oxford, England: Update Software, 2003.

Ryding, E. L., Wijma, K., & Wijma, B. (1998). Postpartum counseling after an emergency cesarean. *Clinical Psychology and Psychotherapy, 5,* 231–237.

Ryding, E. L., Wirén, W., Johansson, G., Ceder, B., & Dahlström, A-M. (2004). Group counseling for mothers after emergency cesarean section: A randomized controlled trail of intervention. *Birth, 31,* 247–253.

Sadler, L. S., Swartz, M. K., Ryan-Krause, P., Seitz, V., Meadows-Oliver, M., Grey, M., & Clemmens, D. A. (2007). Promising outcomes in teen mothers enrolled in a school-based parent support program and child care center. *Journal of School Health, 77,* 121–130.

Scrandis, D.A. (2005). Normalizing postpartum depressive symptoms with social support. *Journal of the American Psychiatric Nurses Association, 11,* 223–230.

Seeley, S., Murray, L., & Cooper, P. J. (1996). The outcome for mothers and babies of health visitor intervention. *Health Visitor, 69,* 135–138.

Segre, L. S., Stuart, S., & O'Hara, M. W. (2004). Interpersonal psychotherapy for antenatal and postpartum and postpartum depression. *Primary Psychiatry, 11*(3), 52–56, 66.

Small, R., Lumley, J., Donohue, L., Potter, A., & Waldenström, U. (2000). Randomised controlled trial of midwife led debriefing to reduce maternal depression after operative childbirth. *British Medical Journal, 321,* 1043–1047.

Spinelli, M. G., & Endicott, J. (2003). Controlled clinical trial of interpersonal psychotherapy versus parenting education program for depressed pregnant women. *American Journal of Psychiatry, 160,* 555–562.

Stern, D. (1995). *The motherhood constellation.* New York: Basic Books.

Stuart, S., & Robertson, M. (2003). *Interpersonal psychotherapy: A clinician's guide.* London, England: Edward Arnold Ltd.

Valbak, K. (2004). Suitability for psychoanalytic psychotherapy: A review. *Acta Psychiatrica Scandinavica, 109,* 164–178.

Weissman, M. M., & Markowitz, J. C. (1994). Interpersonal psychotherapy: Current status. *Archives of General Psychiatry, 51,* 599–606.

Wessely, S., Rose, S., & Bisson, J. A. (2000). A systematic review of brief psychological interventions ("debriefing") for the treatment of immediate trauma related symptoms and the prevention of post traumatic stress disorder. *The Cochrane Library, 4.*

West, M., Rose, S., Spreng, S., Verhoef, M., & Bergman, J. (1999). Anxious attachment and severity of depressive symptomatology in women. *Women's Health, 29,* 47–56.

Wickberg, B., & Hwang, C. (1996). Counselling of postnatal depression: A controlled study on a population based Swedish sample. *Journal of Affective Disorders, 39,* 209–216.

Chapter 14

Access to Postpartum Mental Health Care

Introduction

Access to care for women with PMDs will be discussed in this chapter from three perspectives: primary (micro level), secondary (mezzo level), and tertiary (macro level). Access to care at the primary level examines factors within women, the secondary level examines factors in care providers and professions, and the tertiary level examines policies and programs (refer to Figure 14-1).

Figure 14-1   Access to Postpartum Mood Disorder Care Levels

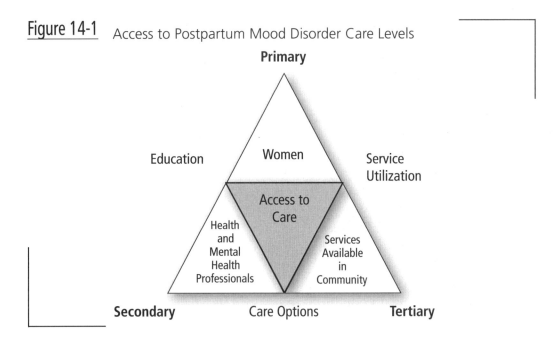

Primary Level

Some women are able to identify a few mental health changes; others are unable to recognize postpartum mental health changes in themselves as they attempt to minimize, hide or normalize their symptoms (Abrams, Dornig, & Curran, 2009; Sealy, Fraser, Simpson, Evans, & Hartford, 2009). Rather than attribute mood changes to depression, postpartum women may consider mood changes a result of sleep deficiency or baby-related concerns such as excessive crying or difficulty feeding. (Boath, Bradley, & Henshaw, 2004; Buist et al., 2007; Carter et al., 2005; McIntosh, 1993; Ugarriza, 2002; Whitton, Warner, & Appleby, 1996). This inability to recognize symptoms is often reinforced by others who tell the mother that her symptoms are a normal reaction and who say that mothers who are performing their role appropriately do not feel depressed (Abrams et al., 2009).

Those who are able to recognize mood alterations often have a disinclination to discuss symptoms with medical or mental health professionals, significant others, or their support systems (Buist et al., 2007). In one study, less than 33 percent of women conferred with a medical provider (Lumley et al., 2003), while another found that 2 percent of women spoke to a mental health practitioner (Kendell, Chalmers, & Platz, 1987). Talking to a professional about mental health changes after delivery appears to differ by symptoms. In one study, nearly two in three women who experienced postpartum depression symptoms consulted with a medical professional, whereas only two in five women who experienced postpartum anxiety symptoms (without depression) consulted with a professional (Woolhouse, Brown, Krastev, Perlen, & Gunn, 2009).

When surveyed, women indicate that their silence is related to several factors: the stigma affixed to mental health conditions, the fear of being labeled a "bad mother" or "crazy," and the fear that their child would be removed from their care (Abrams et al., 2009; Dennis & Chung-Lee, 2006). Women report feeling guilt for failing to achieve the idealized role of motherhood; as a result, these women may not share their feelings with a professional (Amankwaa, 2003; Beck, 2002). These feelings of guilt and shame for being unable to easily take on the role of motherhood are observed across cultures (Dennis & Chung-Lee, 2006; Edge, Baker, & Rogers, 2004; Kim & Buist, 2005; Nahas, Hillege, & Amasheh, 1999); yet some cultures do not even have the language to describe PMD symptoms, making it even more difficult to seek out assistance and supplemental support.

Women who recognize postpartum mood changes often indicate difficulty receiving care. In one study, approximately 16 percent stated they had no knowledge of who to speak to or where to locate aide (Zittel-Palamara,

Rockmaker, Schwabel, Weinstein, & Thompson, 2008). Access to care is further problematic for ethnic minorities, who not only have higher prevalency rates, but who also have a greater propensity to be living in lower socio-economic situations or in isolated neighborhoods, which makes traveling to find insurance-covered care difficult (Alvidrez & Azocar, 1999; Rosen, Tolman, & Warner, 2004).

Ethnic minorities in the United States are more likely to distrust the medical and mental health care systems; therefore, it is understandable that this population is less likely to engage or seek out medical and mental health care, than their white counterparts (Kurz, 2005; Song, Sands, & Wong, 2004; U.S. Department of Health and Human Services [HHS], 2001a). Zittel-Palamara et al.'s (2008) study found that despite desiring medical and mental health care, low income, ethnic minorities living in urban areas were less likely to receive the care they wanted than were their white counterparts. It is interesting that Latina women in the United States are encouraged to rely on the family for care unless outside assistance is encouraged by the husband, or patriarchal family head, whereas African American women are encouraged to remain strong, self-reliant, and to "tough it out" (Abrams et al., 2009).

Culturally based avoidance of medical and mental health care by women with postpartum mood conditions is also thematic in other countries around the world (Abrams et al., 2009). Rather than a reliance on medicine or other therapeutic strategies, international ethnic minorities tend to prefer culturally traditional options or spiritual support (Abrams et al., 2009). Family and friends, many times, will steer women with postpartum mood disturbances away from professional practices and can end up reinforcing this avoidance (Abrams et al., 2009; Chan, Levy, Chung, & Lee, 2002; Dennis & Chung-Lee, 2006; Nahas et al., 1999; Templeton, Velleman, Persaud, & Milner, 2003; Teng, Blackmore, & Stewart, 2007).

A recent Canadian study in Toronto examined barriers to postpartum depression care for women who are immigrants to the country. This study found that two main barriers to care exist—practical and cultural. Practical barriers include speaking a foreign language, a lack of knowledge about existent care, and ways to access these services (Teng et al., 2007). Cultural barriers can be the stigma attached to postpartum depression or the denial by family or friends of a woman's clinical symptoms. In addition, professionals attempting to provide care for immigrant women's postpartum depression needs found it difficult to do so for several reasons: inability to understand the woman's primary language, social or cultural preference and context; screening tools that were not in the woman's primary language; and not feeling competent to assist (Teng et al., 2007). This is similar to results found in immigrants living in Australia (Small, Rice, Yelland, & Lumley, 1999). Despite

Canada's universal health care system and use of different strategies to follow-up on postpartum mood changes in women, these barriers appear similar to those experienced by other underserved groups in the United States.

Those women who were able to discuss postpartum mental health changes reported disappointing responses from medical or mental health care providers. These women felt patronized, not taken seriously, and reported not having enough time to discuss the symptoms with a professional (Abrams et al., 2009; Wood & Meigan, 1997). Too often, women were given a prescription without further discussion of medicinal side effects or other treatment options (Wood & Meigan, 1997), despite reports that women often consider medicine a last choice option (Abrams et al., 2009; Buist et al., 2007; Holopainen, 2002; Whitton, Warner, & Appleby, 1996). In some cases, medical care was not timely, with some women waiting up to six months for an appointment (Wood & Meigan, 1997). The responses from medical and mental health providers further exacerbate postpartum mood symptoms and the feelings of being marginalized, helpless, and hopeless.

When working one-to-one with a woman experiencing a PMD, with a group, or with the entire family, professional, multidisciplinary teams can proactively advocate throughout the process of screening, diagnosis, treatment, and follow-up care. Advocacy on behalf of the client may take several forms such as speaking up for the appropriate care needed from community-based agencies, educating child protection workers about PMDs, and teaching clients how to advocate on their own behalf within the social service or mental health care systems (Lagan, Knights, Barton, & Boyce, 2009). Should child protective services conclude that the child is unsafe and alternative living arrangements for the child are necessary, the multidisciplinary team can step in to provide additional guidance, grief and loss counseling, and acute crisis support through child protective service and legal involvement while maintaining focus on improving the mother's mental health (Lagan et al., 2009). In addition, professionals may need to educate and confront managed care companies to approve monetary reimbursement for the mother, child, and family. In the advocacy role, it is simply not enough to hand a woman a prescription or outside referral name and phone number. Professionals may need to set up the appointment, call the client to encourage and support keeping the appointment, discuss how the appointment went, and make sure that the care provided was suitable (Lagan et al., 2009). If the treatment was unsatisfactory, then professionals need to assist the woman, child, or family in obtaining treatment that is more suitable. In the meantime, professionals can continually offer support and education until proper treatment and protocol are obtained from external resources in the community (Lagan et al., 2009).

Advocacy also includes skilled, global assessment of common high-stress factors that often co-occur with PMDs such as finances, living environment, transportation, child care, communication difficulties within the family system, and limited support systems (Lagan et al., 2009). Therefore, referrals for PMD care are not limited to improving mental health symptoms. Rather, a full treatment plan needs to include several referrals to programs that can help provide respite care, affordable child care, transportation to appointments, public assistance/WIC as needed, alternative living arrangements, parenting skills training, support groups, social skills training, anger management training, early intervention for child developmental needs, and a safe environment to heal emotional and mental health needs. The sooner these referrals, supports, and treatments are provided to the mother and the family, the better the prognosis.

Mezzo Level

One of the barriers to PMD care is the limited education and assessment skills that medical and mental health professionals receive about the conditions (Logsdon, Wisner, Billings, & Shanahan, 2006). Medical and mental health providers face a three-pronged obstacle to provide PMD care:

1. Inadequate diagnostic education
2. Minimal intervention training
3. Limited referral options in the community

In the United Kingdom, a small number of mental health professionals receive specialized PMD training (Oates, 2000). The traditional medical education model inadequately prepares medical professionals to treat PMD (Lloyd & Hawe, 2003). Nearly one in two pediatricians reported receiving little or no instruction on postpartum depression, and a similar number were not aware of the prevalence rates of postpartum depression (Wiley, Burke, Gill, & Law, 2004). In addition, only 7 percent of pediatricians on one project knew of postpartum depression screening instruments, even though 51 percent of them believed that they could integrate screening into customary practice.

In a study of primary care physicians, 40 percent did not assess for postpartum depression and only one in three provided referrals for the condition (Leiferman, Dauber, Heisler, & Paulson, 2008). Apparently, many medical and mental health providers do not assess for PMD, stating it is unethical to diagnose a condition for which care cannot adequately be provided (Logsdon et al., 2006). Buist et al. (2007) suggested that medical professionals receive training in the following perinatal areas:

1. Diagnosis of mental health conditions during and after pregnancy
2. Perinatal mental health management
3. How to administer screening tools to perinatal women—and if not instituting a universal screening policy—how to identify those women that should be screened
4. Side effects of medications to treat perinatal mental health
5. Other treatments that can be integrated into general practice
6. Information about referrals available for perinatal women with mental health symptoms

Screening

The most commonly used screening tool is the Edinburgh Postnatal Depression Scale (EPDS). The EPDS has been extensively researched across countries and languages and has been shown to have good reliability and validity (Cox & Holden, 2003; Cox, Holden, & Sagovsky, 1987). The EPDS can be found at http://www.fresno.ucsf.edu/pediatrics/downloads/edinburghscale.pdf.

Established in Australia in 2001, one multidisciplinary, national program, BeyondBlue, instituted a routine screening program for all perinatal women (Buist et al., 2007). With the support of the Royal Australian College of General Practitioners, the Division of Primary Mental Health Care coordinators, and the Division of General Practice coordinators, the program was widely publicized. The program was integrated into public hospitals and private sector services and included general practitioners, obstetricians, midwives, maternity and child health nurses. Findings generally revealed a positive experience for both medical professionals and perinatal women if the information from the screening led to supportive care and referrals to have specific needs met. In addition, women valued perinatal mental health educational materials that were provided in conjunction with the screenings. However, the authors stated that providers who are willing to screen, treat, and refer these women for care also needed more policies to support these efforts, education, and continuing supervision.

These screening efforts face several barriers in the United States. First, there are no existing mandates for screening all perinatal women. Second, no screening tools are available that reliably predict PMD symptoms; current methods are, at best, capable of detecting individuals who are already experiencing symptoms (Austin & Lumley, 2002; Buist et al., 2007). Finally, once detected, there are few treatment options available in most areas across the country.

Future Possibilities

One possible way to address the needs of the perinatal family is to consolidate care through one family-based perinatal care agency, which could be duplicated in areas around the country. This would take the Australian developed hospital-based mother–child unit to treat severe postpartum (Buist et al., 2004) and the Australian screening program (Buist et al, 2007), for examples, to the outpatient community and provide additional ancillary, multidisciplinary support services. Ideally, this agency would be multidisciplinary in scope, accept insurance, provide a sliding fee scale for those without insurance, and offer a myriad of programs and specialists to provide holistic and comprehensive care. An agency such as this would require medical professionals, mental health providers, and other paraprofessionals.

Medical practitioners would consist of psychiatrists, family physicians, obstetricians and gynecologists, perinatal nurses, lactation consultants, home health care providers, midwives, and student interns enrolled in like programs. Mental health practitioners would comprise social workers, psychologists, marriage and family counselors, and higher education student interns. Paraprofessionals include doulas, birthing instructors, spiritual advisors or clergy, child care providers, and student interns. The inclusion of student interns will reinforce experiential learning with didactic specialized training.

Services provided in the agency at the medical level would include examinations, standardized mental health assessments during pregnancy and up to one-year postpartum, follow-up services in the home and in the agency setting, breastfeeding support, and personalized supportive care throughout the perinatal period. Education about the birthing process, nutrition, exercise, and mental health would be provided from conception through one year postpartum. Should PMD be detected, psychiatric consultation and follow-up would be scheduled and the psychiatrist would provide education on medications, risks and benefits and refer to mental health providers for additional intervention options.

Services provided by mental health practitioners would include biopsychosocial history assessments, family and support system assessments, family education about pregnancy and mental health risks, symptoms, and prevention strategies throughout the perinatal period. Barriers to care would be assessed and addressed prior to delivery; methods to prepare for these barriers would be developed. Following delivery, women would receive standardized PMD assessments and intervention options, and education would be provided. Intervention options would include individual, couple, family, or group counseling; short-term respite care; and a sleep clinic (where women could receive eight hours of uninterrupted sleep while a child care worker would engage and watch the child. Early intervention for the child would be provided to address cognitive or developmental delays. Services provided by paraprofessionals would include doula support throughout the perinatal period, child care while the woman or couple receives treatment, and religious or spiritual consultation for support and encouragement.

Using one location for multidisciplinary treatment would improve primary, micro-level care. Women and families will know where to go for education, care, and follow-up. Through community knowledge about the agency, stigmatization may be defused as women could go to the agency for care that is unrelated to mental health. Women would be able to find relief through child care, respite services, and sleep, thereby reducing the feeling of being hopeless. Furthermore, women would be cared for by trained professionals, and in so doing, negative responses by practitioners could be decreased.

Macro-Level Access to Care Concerns

Despite efforts to improve treatment options, decrease stigma, and educate the community to identify PMDs through communitywide public health campaigns, research shows available educational materials are written at levels far advanced for the lay population and Web-based information is often incorrect (Logsdon & Hutti, 2006; Sealy et al., 2009; Schanie, Pinto-Folz, & Logsdon, 2008; Summers & Logsdon, 2005).

Although numerous empirical intervention strategies documented in the research literature, many medical and mental health providers generally have little or no professional training on diagnosing PMD; these providers also lack information on how to treat these conditions. Given this, many providers want to refer women to others who specialize in perinatal mood disorders. One study found that family physicians and female doctors were more likely to intervene by referring women to social workers or other mental health professionals, than were older doctors and those who were obstetricians and gynecologists (Thomas, Sleath, Jackson, West, & Gaynes, 2008).

In this situation, appropriate protocol is to refer to specialists in the community to intervene. Frustratingly, most communities in the United States have few specialists to provide interventions. One study of PMD specialists posted online found only 384 care providers in the United States; seven states had no PMD specialists listed (Zittel-Palamara et al., 2009). Although there certainly are many more professionals who have experience in providing treatment to women with PMDs (Springate & Chaudron, 2006), many are not making this specialty known via the Internet. Given that women may attempt to find education and specialists in their community through online searches, professionals need to make this specialty public. Rather, it appears that there is an "underground network" of specialists in the community. This presents professionals with a conundrum of wanting to assist but having no recourse other than referral for or prescribing psychotropic medicine.

Professional Curriculum

Logsdon et al.'s (2005) research on these areas concludes that a PMD curriculum needs to be developed and included in all medical and mental health programs. This curriculum ought to include symptoms, screening, diagnosis, treatments, effect on the family, effect on childhood development, strategies to successfully link women to care, locating referrals in the community, and making programs available in one's practice (as applicable). As many professionals lack this curricular education, continuing education programs can provide professional training on PMDs, with a primary focus on postpartum depression. Several brief continuing educational programs are available online, whereas more extensive, hands-on training can be obtained through Postpartum Support International (http://postpartum.net/). Unfortunately, there are limited online continuing education programs that provide information about the effects on children and strategies to manage this.

Organizational Statements

Several professional organizations have a stated position to improve perinatal mood disorder research and treatments. In 1999, the Association of Women's Health, Obstetric and Neonatal Nurses promoted the institution of postpartum depression screening to all mothers with newborns, as well as patient education about the possibility of mood changes during pregnancy or after birth (Nursing for Women's Health, 2007).

In 2005, the Registered Nurses Association of Ontario, Canada, created a best practice protocol to treat postpartum depression. A multidisciplinary group of professionals from multiple practice locations orchestrated the development of this protocol (for example, hospitals, universities, clinical practice). This team paid particular attention to the most successful and up-to-date research and treatment findings (McQueen & Dennis, 2007) and integrated these with women's reported treatment preferences, the experience of medical and mental health professionals, and available resources (Field & Lohr, 1990; McQueen & Dennis, 2007; Oosterhuis, Bruns, Watine, Sandberg, & Horvath, 2004). The group concluded that careful orchestration of multidisciplinary care is imperative for women and families suffering from PMDs as the diagnosis involves medical, psychological, cognitive, developmental, emotional, and access-to-care (finances, transportation, child care) components (McQueen & Dennis, 2007). The full 95-page document can be read (http://www.rnao.org/Storage/11/600_BPG_Post_Partum_Depression.pdf).

Although social work organizations have not made a formal statement about professional responsibilities regarding perinatal mood disorders, Abrams and Curran (2007) presented a compelling argument for the profession to do so. Ethically, social workers are required to provide sound, evidence-based care to all high-risk populations, with careful attention given to culture and those who are marginalized and underserved. Clearly, the entire nature of this book identifies perinatal mood disorders and the effect of these disorders on the entire family within the auspices of the National Association of Social Workers' code of ethical responsibility.

Policies

Given the magnitude of preventing and treating perinatal depression, the effects of these disorders on childhood development and family functioning make the need to create new policies to improve care a human rights issues (Dhanda & Narayan, 2007; Gill, Pande, & Malhotra, 2007; Mirza & Jenkins, 2004; Patel, Saraceno, & Kleinman, 2006). The United Nations Population, United Nations Convention on the Rights of Persons with Disabilities, World Health Organization (WHO), and International Covenant of Economic, Social and Cultural Rights have proposed advancing the intervention and treatment of perinatal depression through all-inclusive, international efforts— that intervention and treatment for health and mental health disorders is a human right and allows people to have the highest quality of life possible. The neglect of perinatal mood disorders is that prevalent (Chisholm et al., 2007; Prince et al., 2007; Saxena, Thornicroft, Knapp, & Whiteford, 2007). Others clarify that perinatal mental health intervention need not only be relegated to clinical disorders but, rather, should also focus on the mother's ability to cope and adapt to motherhood and all the stressors that coincide (Rahman, Patel, Maselko, & Kirkwood, 2008). In 2008, the WHO identified eight maternal mental health goals. More than half of these goals pertain to perinatal mental health for the mother and the family and encourage the international development of strategies to address these areas:

1. Universal screening

2. Treatment protocols

3. Affordable psychotropic medications

4. Education

5. Psychosocial support

6. Mother–infant interventions

7. Educating fathers on ways to equally support in child care and other household activities

8. Social support structures for women

9. Development of culturally relevant intervention strategies (Engle, 2009).

The Mental Health and Addiction Equity Act of 2008 stipulates that individuals have the right to receive coverage for mental health conditions similar to coverage received for physical health conditions. Prior to the passing of this act, insurance companies could deny mental health services to perinatal women suffering with mental health symptoms (Sobey, 2002). Furthermore, perinatal mental health is categorized as a combined health and mental health concern. This also caused difficulty in receiving insurance coverage as separate departments could argue: Health insurance will not cover the cost of treatment because this is a mental health concern and mental health insurance will not cover the cost of treatment because this is a health concern. The end result is gaps in coverage for women. Hopefully, with the passage of the Mental Health Parity Act, these trends will begin to diminish.

In 2001, the H.R.-20 Bill: Melanie Stokes Postpartum Depression Research and Care Act was presented to Congress to provide funding to the National Institutes of Health for research on the etiology, epidemiology, development of diagnostic instruments, and new interventions and to provide informational and educational programs for the general public as well as for medical and mental health professionals (Washingtonwatch.com, 2008). Prior to 2010, the act was passed by Congress and has been held up in the Senate HELP Committee due to an added clause supporting medication as the primary source of assistance. It is uncertain if concerns about this clause have been resolved.

In 2007, Senators Robert Menendez (NJ), Durbin (IL), Snowe (ME), Brown (OH), Dodd (CT), and Lautenberg (NJ) introduced the MOTHERS Act to the U.S. Senate for the second time. The MOTHERS Act (Mom's Opportunity to Access Help, Education, Research, and Support for Postpartum Depression Act) would provide funding to states through grant money to assist women during the first postpartum year (110th Congress, 2007). This funding will provide education and screening for women for PMDs as well as PMD medical care as needed to women and their families. In addition, the act would designate funding for epidemiological, diagnostic, and intervention research to improve the disparities that currently exist for PMD care in the United States (110th Congress, 2007).

As of June 2010, Senator Menendez, in conjunction with Bobby Rush U.S. Representative of Illinois and actress Brooke Shields, announced the passing of the Melanie Blocker Stokes MOTHERS Act. The act, passed by Congress in March 2010, is included in President Obama's health insurance reform plan. This is an excellent step in the right direction; however, it remains to be seen how the policy will be implemented.

The state of New Jersey instituted a Postpartum Screening Bill by Governor Jon Corzine in 2006, making perinatal postpartum depression screening universal (Geoghegan, 2006). This bill allots $4.5 million for universal screening as well as PMD educational materials that must be provided to all families (Mental Health Weekly, 2006). These materials include information about symptoms, intervention, and referral resources. Reports on the effectiveness of this bill are yet unavailable.

International Protocols

Victoria, Australia, implemented new legislation to guide maternity care (Victorian Government of Human Services, 2004). As a part of this legislation, provisions were made, based on several survey research data on women's needs and desires for care, to increase public health maternity care—including PMD care. The inspiration for this project came from the care provided by general practice physicians and midwives through a suburban Melbourne hospital and adjoining clinics that served many non-English-speaking, immigrant, and impoverished women. Some women received care from the hospital only, the clinic only, or a combination of the two locations. Women only seen by hospitals reported the least satisfaction with antenatal care, whereas women who received care through a birth center and who saw the same medical professional throughout pregnancy reported better satisfaction, less waiting time, feeling that there was adequate time to discuss concerns, and feeling that their concerns were taken seriously (Brown & Bruinsma, 2006). These positive perinatal care findings were reported most frequently by women who received continuity of care from a midwife. Brown and Bruinsma (2006) stated that the care desired by women in Victoria, Australia, may be difficult to integrate into existent systems and difficult to fund. Nevertheless, these new systems are the most beneficial for women's perinatal health and mental health outcomes. The system of postpartum care provided in Victoria, Australia, has been found to vary significantly from unit to unit across the area. Two commonalities, however, are that postpartum care is provided in hectic, disorganized environments and that there is difficulty getting efficient care. This results in the mother having a difficult rest and recovery period after delivery (McLachlan, Forster,

Yelland, Rayner, & Lumley, 2008). In reaction to these findings, McLachlan et al. (2008) proposed that the provision of postpartum care become more standardized according to best-practice guidelines rather than organizational structural guidelines.

Sweden provides child health clinics for children from birth to preschool age, commonly reaching just under 100 percent of the total population (Jansson, Isacsson, & Nyberg, 1998; Swedish National Board of Health and Welfare, 1981). The care provided in these clinics include PMD screening, parental support, and some therapeutic treatment, parenting skills training, childhood development assessment, healthy-child visits, immunizations, and preventive care education (Swedish National Board of Health and Welfare, 1981). Parenting classes are offered throughout the first postpartum year to all parents and provide education on infant development, care, nursing, nutrition, physical health, preventing accidents, mother/father roles, and maintaining the couple's relationship (Fabian, Rådestad, Waldenström, 2006). Typically, these ancillary services are administered by child health nurses who provide emotional, expert, and empathetic medical and some mental health care (Arborelius & Bremberg, 2003; Fägerskiöld, Timpka, & Ek, 2003; Jansson, Isacsson, Kornfält, & Lindholm, 1998; Örtenstrand & Waldenström, 2005). Overall, the majority of Swedish mothers are satisfied with child health clinic services (Sitzia & Wood, 1997; van Teijlingen, Hundley, Rennie, Graham, & Fitzmaurice, 2003). It is interesting that those who are more dissatisfied with the care are depressed or anxious mothers and parents with infants who had feeding difficulties. The women who felt dissatisfied desired more attention to their mental health symptoms over the attention that was provided to the child (Örtenstrand & Waldenström, 2005). In addition, most of the women who did not access the parenting education services were immigrants (non-Swedish-speaking), had newborns with significant health problems, smoked throughout the pregnancy, achieved low levels of education, were admitted to the hospital, or found the timing of their pregnancy inopportune (Fabian et al., 2006).

In the United Kingdom, most women receive care during pregnancy from a general practitioner or midwife, whereas postpartum care is typically delivered by midwives and health visitors (also known as public health nurses) (Alder et al., 2008). This postpartum care is provided to all new mothers from two weeks after delivery through the first postpartum year, including at-home visits to the mother and newborn (Sobey, 2002). Since 1996, Scotland instituted universal postpartum depression screening, and the use of the EPDS was suggested (CRAG Working Group on Maternity Services, 1996). This was expanded in 1999 to include management of identified postpartum depression (Scottish Executive, 2001b), and again in 2001 to include multidisciplinary early identification of symptoms, interventions, and referrals for care (Alder et al., 2008; Scottish Executive, 2001a). Despite these efforts, however, between 47% and 68% of providers follow Intercollegiate Guidelines (Alder et al., 2008).

Research Funding

Despite WHO predictions that depression will become one of the top three causes of death by 2030 and that PMDs could become the top cause of death for women in the United States, there remains limited funding opportunities to improve screening, best-practice models, and treatment protocols and provide full access to care in the United States (Goodrum, Hankins, Jermain, & Chanaud, 2003; Lindahl et al., 2005; Mathers & Loncar, 2006). Historically, several national-level efforts have been made to include pregnant women in research protocols. In 1985, the report of the U.S. Public Health Service Task Force on Women's Health Issues concluded that more consideration be placed on women's inclusion in health-related research (Mastroianni, Faden, & Federman, 1994). Five years later, the National Institutes of Health initiated the Office for Research on Women's Health to spotlight women's health in research projects (Mastroianni, Faden, & Federman, 1994b; Merkatz, 1998). It was not until 1997 that new guidelines were delineated to include pregnant women in health research activities (Mastroianni et al., 1994a, 1994b; HHS, 1998, 2001a). By 2000, HHS, the FDA, and the National Institutes for Child Health and Human Development convened to improve research on drugs commonly used during pregnancy and lactation, including psychopharmaceuticals used to treat perinatal mood disorders. As a result of these meetings, a drug registry was developed to monitor the effects of psychopharmaceutical medication on the fetus, infant, and mother if used during pregnancy and lactation (HHS, FDA, Center for Drug Evaluation and Research, and Center for Biologics Evaluation and Research, 1999). Due to delays in these research activity policies and policy changes, empirically researched articles that guide medical and mental health practice have not been completely and uniformly integrated into professional curriculum or into clinical practices. This results in a twofold reaction: Doctors are not versed in the latest research on psychopharmaceutical use during pregnancy or while breastfeeding and discontinue these medications during pregnancy or do not prescribe these medications during pregnancy or when a mother is nursing (Addis & Koren, 2000; Pole, Einarson, Pairaudeau, Einarson, & Koren, 2000).

Women fear that taking medication during pregnancy or while nursing will negatively affect her child and may opt to suffer needlessly through debilitating mental health conditions, which in all likelihood could be more detrimental to the fetus and newborn's development than possible medication side effects (Goodrum et al., 2003; Koren, Bologa, Long, Feldman, & Shear, 1989; Pole et al., 2000).

Current federal proposals to address these gaps in funding, research, and clinical application of findings are the Safe Motherhood Act for Research and Treatment and the National Children's Study of Environmental Effects on Child Health and Development (S. 2328/H. R. 4602, 2003; Branum et al., 2003; Harkin, 2002). The primary goals of these proposals are to improve communication between agencies and improve dissemination of information to professionals working with perinatal women (Goodrum et al., 2003). Although these federally initiated statements and task forces are an excellent start, enforcement of these statements and funding to promote strategic plans need continual support and follow-through from the highest levels (Goodrum et al., 2003).

References

110th Congress. (2007). *Text of S. 1375 [110th]: Mom's Opportunity to Access Health, Education, Research, and Support for Postpartum Depression Act.* Retrieved from Govtrack.us: A Civic Project to Track Congress Web site: http://www.govtrack.us/congress/billtext.xpd?bill=s110-1375

Abrams, L. S., & Curran, L. (2007). Not just a middle-class affliction: Crafting a social work research agenda on postpartum depression. *Health & Social Work, 32,* 289–296.

Abrams, L. S., Dornig, K., & Curran, L. (2009). Barriers to service use for postpartum depression symptoms among low-income ethnic minority mothers in the United States. *Quality Health Research, 19,* 535–551.

Addis, A., & Koren, G. (2000). Safety of fluoxetine during the first trimester of pregnancy: A meta-analytical review of epidemiological studies. *Psychological Medicine, 30,* 89–94.

Alder, E. M., Reid, M., Sharp, L. J., Cantwell, R., Robertson, K., & Kearney, E. (2008). Policy and practice in the management of postnatal depression in Scotland. *Archives of Women's Mental Health, 11,* 213–219.

Alvidrez, J., & Azocar, F. (1999). Distressed women's clinic patients: Preferences for mental health treatments and perceived obstacles. *General Hospital Psychiatry, 21,* 340–347.

Amankwaa, L. C. (2003). Postpartum depression among African-American women. *Issues in Mental Health Nursing, 24*(3), 297–317.

Arborelius, E., & Bremberg, S. (2003). Supportive and nonsupportive qualities of child health nurses' contacts with strained infant mothers. *Scandinavian Journal of Caring Science, 17,* 169–175.

Austin, M-P., & Lumley, J. (2002). Antenatal screening for postnatal depression: A systematic review. *Acta Psychiarica Scandinavica, 106,* 1–8.

Beck, C.T. (2002). Postpartum depression: A metasynthesis. *Qualitative Health Research, 12,* 453–472.

Boath, E., Bradley, E., & Henshaw, C. (2004). Women's views of antidepressants in the treatment of postnatal depression. *Journal of Psychosomatic Obstetrics and Gynecology, 25,* 221–233.

Branum, A. M., Collman, G. W., Correa, A., Keim, S. A., Kessel, W., Kimmel, C. A., et al. (2003). The National Children's Study of environmental effects on child health and development. *Environmental Health Perspectives, 111,* 642–646.

Brown, S. J., & Bruinsma, F. (2006). Future directions for Victoria's public maternity services: Is this "what women want"? *Australian Health Review, 30*(1), 56–64.

Buist, A., Ellwood, D., Brooks, J., Milgrom, J., Hayes, B. A., Sved-Williams, A., et al. (2007). National program for depression associated with childbirth: The Australian experience. *Best Practice & Research Clinical Obstetrics and Gynaecology, 21*(2), 193–206.

Buist, A., Minto, B., Szego, K., Samhuel, M., Shawyer, L., & O'Connor, L. O. (2004). Mother–baby psychiatric units in Australia: The Victorian Experience. *Archives of Women's Mental Health, 7,* 81–87.

Carter, F. A., Carter, J. D., Luty, S. E., Wilson, D. A., Frampton, C. M., & Joyce, P. R. (2005). Screening and treatment for depression during pregnancy: A cautionary note. *Australia and New Zealand Journal of Psychiatry, 39,* 255–261.

Chan, S. W. C., Levy, A., Chung, T., & Lee, D. (2002). A qualitative study of the experiences of a group of Hong Kong Chinese women diagnosed with postnatal depression. *Issues and Innovations in Nursing Practice, 39,* 571–579.

Chisholm, D., Flisher, A. J., Lund, C., Patel, V., Saxena, S., Thornicroft, G., & Tomlinson, M. (2007). Scale up services for mental disorders: A call for action. *Lancet, 370,* 1241–1252.

Cox, J., & Holden, J. (2003). Using the EPDS in clinical settings: research evidence. In *Perinatal mental health: A guide to the Edinburgh Postnatal Depression Scale (EDPS).* Glasgow, United Kingdom: Royal College of Psychiatrists (Bell & Bain Ltd).

Cox, J., Holden, J., & Sagovsky, R. (1987). Detection of postnatal depression: Development of the 10-item Edinburgh Postnatal Depression Scale. *British Journal of Psychiatry, 150,* 782–786.

CRAG Working Group on Maternity Services. (1996). *Report on detection and early intervention in postnatal depression.* Edinburgh: NHS Quality Improvement Scotland.

Dennis, C. L., & Chung-Lee, L. (2006). Postpartum Depression help-seeking barriers and maternal treatment preferences: A qualitative systematic review. *Birth: Issues in Perinatal Care, 33,* 323–331.

Dhanda, A., & Narayan, T. (2007). Mental health and human rights. *Lancet, 370,* 1197–1198.

Edge, D., Baker, D., & Rogers, A. (2004). Perinatal depression among black Caribbean women. *Health Social Care Community, 12,* 430–438.

Engle, P. L. (2009). Maternal mental health: Program and policy implications. *American Journal of Clinical Nutrition, 89*(Suppl.), 963S–966S.

Fabian, H. M., Rådestad, I. J., & Waldenström, U. (2006). Characteristics of primiparious women who are not reached by parental education classes after childbirth in Sweden. *Acta Pædiatrica, 95,* 1360–1369.

Fägerskiöld, A., Timpka, T., & Ek, A. C. (2003). The view of the child health nurse among mothers. *Scandinavian Journal of Caring Science, 17,* 160–168.

Field, M. J., & Lohr, K. N. (1990). *Guidelines for clinical practice: Directions for a new program.* Washington, DC: Institutes of Medicine, National Academy Press.

Geoghegan, A. H. (2006). Not just an option: Postpartum depression screening becomes law in the state of New Jersey. *Nursing Spectrum, 18a*(20), NJ/NY8–NJ/NY12.

Gill, K., Pande, R., & Malhotra, A. (2007). Women deliver for development. *Lancet, 370,* 859–887.

Goodrum, L. A., Hankins, G. D. V., Jermain, D., & Chanaud, C. M. (2003). Conference report: Complex clinical, legal, and ethical issues of pregnant and postpartum women as subjects in clinical trials. *Journal of Women's Health, 12,* 857–867.

Harkin, T. (2002). Safe Motherhood Act for Research and Treatment. *Journal of the American Medical Women's Association, 57*(3), 144, 158.

Holopainen, D. (2002). The experience of seeking help for postnatal depression. *Australian Journal of Advanced Nursing, 19*(3), 39–44.

Jansson, A., Isacsson, Å., Kornfält, R., & Lindholm, L. (1998). Quality in child healthcare: The views of mothers and public health nurses. *Scandinavian Journal of Caring Science, 12,* 195–204.

Jansson, A., Isacsson, Å., & Nyberg, P. (1998). Help-seeking patterns among parents with a newborn child. *Public Health Nursing, 15,* 319–328.

Kendell, R. E., Chalmers, J. C., & Platz, C. (1987). Epidemiology of puerperal psychoses. *British Journal of Psychiatry, 150,* 662–673.

Kim, J., & Buist, A. (2005). Postnatal depression: A Korean perspective. *Australasian Psychiatry, 13*(1), 68–71.

Koren, G., Bologa, M., Long, D., Feldman, Y., & Shear, N. H. (1989). Perception of teratogenic risk by pregnant women exposed to drugs and chemicals during the first trimester. *American Journal of Obstetrics and Gynecology, 160*(5 pt 1), 1190–1194.

Kurz, B. (2005). Depression and mental-health service utilization among women in WIC. *Journal of Ethnic & Cultural Diversity in Social Work, 14*(3/4), 81–102.

Lagan, M., Knights, K., Barton, J., & Boyce, P. M. (2009). Advocacy for mothers with psychiatric illness: A clinical perspective. *International Journal of Mental Health Nursing, 18,* 53–61.

Leiferman, J. A., Dauber, S. E., Heisler, K., & Paulson, J. F. (2008). Primary care physicians' beliefs and practices toward maternal depression. *Journal of Women's Health, 17,* 1143–1150.

Lindahl, V., Pearson, J. L., & Colpe, L. (2005). Prevalence of suicidality during pregnancy and the postpartum. *Archives of Women's Mental Health, 8,* 77–87.

Lloyd, B., & Hawe, P. (2003). Solutions forgone? How health professionals frame the problem of postnatal depression. *Social Science Medicine, 57,* 1783–1795.

Logsdon, M. C., & Hutti, M. (2006). Readability: An important issue impacting healthcare for women with postpartum depression. *American Journal of Maternal/Child Nursing, 11,* 350–355.

Logsdon, M. C., Wisner, K., Billings, D. M., & Shanahan, B. (2006). Raising the awareness of primary care providers about postpartum depression. *Issues in Mental Health Nursing, 27,* 59–73.

Lumley, J., Small, R., Brown, S., Watson, L., Gunn, J., Mitchell, C., & Dawson, W. (2003). PRISM (Program of Resources, Information, and Support for Mothers): Protocol for a community-randomised trial. *BMC Public Health, 3,* 36–50.

Mastroianni, A. C., Faden, R., & Federman, D. (Eds.). (1994a). *Legal considerations.* Washington, DC: National Academy Press.

Mastroianni, A. C., Faden, R., & Federman, D. (Eds). (1994b). *Women's participation in clinical studies.* Washington, DC: National Academy Press.

Mathers, D. C., & Loncar, D. (2006). Projections of global morality and burden of disease from 2002 to 2030. *PLoS Medicine, 3*(11), e442. doi:10. 137/ journal.pmed.0030442 Retrieved from http://medicine.plosjournals.org/ archive/1549-1676/3/11/pdf/10.1371_journal.pmed.0030442-L.pdf

McIntosh, J. (1993). Postpartum depression: Women's help-seeking behaviour and perceptions of cause. *Journal of Advanced Nursing, 19,* 178–184.

McLachlan, H. L., Forster, D. A., Yelland, J., Rayner, J., & Lumley, J. (2008). Is the organisation and structure of hospital postnatal care a barrier to quality care? Findings from a state-wide review in Victoria, Australia. *Midwifery, 24,* 358–370.

McQueen, K., & Dennis, C. L. (2007). Development of a postpartum depression best practice guideline: A review of the systematic process. *Journal of Nursing Care Quality, 22*(3), 199–204.

Mental Health Weekly. (2006). New Jersey enacts postpartum screening law. *Mental Health Weekly, 16*(41), 7.

Merkatz, R. B. (1998). Inclusion of women in clinical trials: A historical overview of scientific, ethical, and legal issues. *Journal of Obstetrics, Gynecology, and Neonatal Nursing, 27,* 78–84.

Mirza, I., & Jenkins, R. (2004). Risk factors, prevalence and treatment of anxiety and depressive disorders in Pakistan: Systematic review. *British Medical Journal, 328,* 794–979.

Nahas, V., Hillege, S., & Amasheh, N. (1999). Postpartum depression: The lived experience of Middle Eastern migrant women in Australia. *Journal of Nurse-Midwifery, 44,* 65–74.

Nursing for Women's Health. (2007). AWHONN news and views: Conquering postpartum depression: AWHONN supports the MOTHERS Act. *Nursing for Women's Health, 11,* 422–423.

Oates, M. (2000). *Perinatal maternal mental health services 2000.* London: Royal College of Psychiatrists.

Oosterhuis, W. P., Bruns, D. E., Watine, J., Sandberg, S., & Horvath, A. R. (2004). Evidence-based guidelines in laboratory medicine: Principles and methods. *Clinical Chemistry, 50,* 806–818.

Örtenstrand, A., & Waldenström, U. (2005). Mothers' experiences of child health clinic services in Sweden. *Acta Pædiatrica, 94,* 1285–1294.

Patel, V., Saraceno, B., & Kleinman, A. (2006). Beyond evidence: The moral case for international mental health. *Psychiatry, 163,* 1312–1314.

Pole, M., Einarson, A., Pairaudeau, N., Einarson, T., & Koren, G. (2000). Drug labeling and risk perceptions of teratogenicity: A survey of pregnant Canadian women and their health professionals. *Journal of Clinical Pharmacology, 40,* 573–577.

Prince, M., Patel, V., Saxena, S., Maj, M., Maselko, J., Phillips, M., & Rahman, A. (2007). No health without mental health. *Lancet, 370,* 859–887.

Rahman, A., Patel, V., Maselko, J., & Kirkwood, B. (2008). The neglected "m" in MCH programs: Why mental health of mothers is important for child nutrition. *Tropical Medicine & International Health, 13,* 579–583.

Registered Nurses Association of Ontario. (2005). *Interventions for postpartum depression.* Toronto: Registered Nurses Association of Ontario. Retrieved from http://www.rnao.org/Storage/11/600_BPG_Post_Partum_Depression.pdf

Rosen, D., Tolman, R. M., & Warner, L. A. (2004). Low-income women's use of substance abuse and mental health services. *Journal of Health Care for the Poor and Underserved, 15*(2), 206–219.

Safe Motherhood Act for Research and Treatment (Smart Mom Act), S. 2328/H. R. 4602, 2–21, 107th Cong. (2003).

Saxena, S., Thornicroft, G., Knapp, M., & Whiteford, H. (2007). Resources for mental health: Scarcity, inequity and inefficiency. *Lancet, 370,* 878–889.

Schanie, C. L., Pinto-Folz, M. D., & Logsdon, M. C. (2008). Analysis of popular press articles concerning postpartum depression: 1998–2006. *Issues in Mental Health Nursing, 29,* 1200–1216.

Scottish Executive. (2001a). *Framework for maternity services.* Scotland: Edinburgh Scottish Executive.

Scottish Executive (2001b). *Our national health: A plan for action a plan for change.* Scotland: Edinburgh Scottish Executive.

Sealy, P. A., Fraser, H., Simpson, J. P., Evans, M., & Hartford, A. (2009). Community awareness of postpartum depression. *Journal of Obstetric, Gynecologic, & Neonatal Nursing, 38,* 121–133.

Sitzia, J., & Wood, N. (1997). Patient satisfaction: A review of issues and concepts. *Social Science Medicine, 45,* 1829–1843.

Small, R., Rice, P. L., Yelland, J., & Lumley, J. (1999). Mothers in a new country: The role of culture and communication in Vietnamese, Turkish and Filipino women's experiences of giving birth in Australia. *Women & Health, 28*(3), 77–101.

Sobey, W. S. (2002). Barriers to postpartum depression prevention and treatment: A policy analysis. *Journal of Midwifery & Women's Health, 47,* 331–336.

Song, D., Sands, R. G., & Wong, Y. L. I. (2004). Utilization of mental health services by low income pregnant and postpartum women on medical assistance. *Women & Health, 39*(1), 1–23.

Springate, B. A., & Chaudron, L. H. (2006). Mental health providers' self-reported expertise and treatment of perinatal depression. *Archives of Women's Mental Health, 9,* 60–61.

Summers, A. L., & Logsdon, M. C. (2005). Web site for postpartum depression: Convenient, frustrating, incomplete, and misleading. *MCN: American Journal of Maternal/Child Nursing, 30*(2), 88–94.

Swedish National Board of Health and Welfare. (1981). *Health care for mothers and children within the primary health care system* (Allmänna råd från Socialstyrelsen, 4). Stockholm: Socialstyrelsen.

Templeton, L., Velleman, R., Persaud, A., & Milner, P. (2003). The experience of postnatal depression in women from black and minority ethnic communities in Whiltshire, UK. *Ethnicity and Health, 8,* 207–221.

Teng, L., Blackmore, E. R., & Stewart, D. E. (2007). Healthcare worker's perceptions of barriers to care by immigrant women with postpartum depression: An exploratory qualitative study. *Archives of Women's Mental Health, 10,* 93–101.

Thomas, N., Sleath, B. L., Jackson, E., West, S., & Gaynes, B. (2008). Survey of characteristics and treatment preferences for physicians treating postpartum depression in the general medical setting. *Community Mental Health Journal, 44,* 47–56.

Ugarriza, D. N. (2002). Postpartum depressed women's explanation of depression. *Journal of Nursing Scholarship, 34*(3), 227–233.

U.S. Department of Health and Human Services. (1998). Additional DHHS protections for pregnant women, human fetuses, and newborns involved as subjects in research, and pertaining to human in vitro fertilizations. *Federal Regulations, 63,* 27793.

U.S. Department of Health and Human Services. (2001a). Additional protections pertaining to research, development, and related activities involving fetuses, pregnant women, and related activities involving fetuses, pregnant women, and human in vitro fertilization. *Federal Regulations, 45,* 56780.

U.S. Department of Health and Human Services. (2001b). *Mental health: Culture, race, and ethnicity—A supplement to mental health: A report of the surgeon general.* Rockville, MD: U.S. Department of Health and Human Services, Substance Abuse and Mental Health Services Administration, Center for Mental Health Services. Retrieved from http://mentalhealth. samhsa.gov/cre/toc.asp

U.S. Department of Health and Human Services, Food and Drug Administration, Center for Drug Evaluation and Research, & Center for Biologics Evaluation and Research. (1999). *Guidance for industry: Establishing pregnancy registries. Federal Regulations, 24,* 201.63.

van Teijlingen, E. R., Hundley, V., Rennie, A. M., Graham, W., & Fitzmaurice, A. (2003). Maternity satisfaction studies and their limitations: "What is, must still be best." *Birth, 30,* 75–82.

Victorian Government Department of Human Services. (2004). *Future directions for Victoria's maternity services.* Melbourne: Metropolitan Health and Aged Care Services, Victorian Department of Human Services.

Washingtonwatch.com. (2008). *H.R. 20, The Melanie Blocker-Stokes Postpartum Depression Research and Care Act.* Retrieved from http://www. washingtonwatch.com/bills/show/110_HR_20.html

Whitton, A., Warner, R., & Appleby, L. (1996). The pathway to care in postnatal depression: Women's attitudes to post-natal depression and its treatment. *British Journal of General Practice, 46,* 427–428.

Wiley, C. C., Burke, G. S., Gill, P. A., & Law, N. E. (2004). Pediatricians' views of postpartum depression: A self-administered survey. *Archives of Women's Mental Health, 7,* 231–236.

Wood, A. F., & Meigan, M. (1997). The downward spiral of postpartum depression. *American Journal of Maternal/Child Nursing, 22,* 308–316.

Woolhouse, H., Brown, S., Krastev, A., Perlen, S., & Gunn, J. (2009). Seeking help for anxiety and depression after childbirth: Results of the Maternal Health Study. *Archives of Women's Mental Health, 12,* 75–83.

World Health Organization, United Nations Population Fund. (2008). *Maternal mental health and child survival, health, and development in resource-constrained settings: Essential for achieving the millennium development goals.* Geneva: Author.

Zittel-Palamara, K., Lawrence, S. A., Cercone, S. Hitchcock, J., Colman, M. E., Rockmaker, J. R., & Wilson-Wolff, K. (2009). *Access to postpartum mood disorder care.* Unpublished manuscript.

Zittel-Palamara, K., Rockmaker, J. R., Schwabel, K. M., Weinstein, W. L., & Thompson, S. J. (2008). Desired assistance versus care received for postpartum depression: Access to care differences by race. *Archives of Women's Mental Health, 11*(2), 81–92.

Appendix

Checklist of Postpartum Mood Disorder Risk Factors: Factors Obtained through the Empirical Literature

Note: This list may not be all-inclusive and is not meant to diagnose.
PICU = pediatric intensive care unit.
NICU = neonatal intensive care unit.

	Baby Blues	Postpartum Depression	Postpartum Anxiety	Postpartum Panic	Postpartum Posttraumatic Stress	Postpartum Obsessive-Compulsive Disorder	Postpartum Psychosis
Adolescence		X					
Antenatal anxiety	X	X	X				
Antenatal depression		X	X				
Antenatal obsessions						X	
Antenatal panic				X			
Antenatal sleep difficulty		X					
Autoimmune system activation		X					
Baby – health problems at delivery	X	X	X	X	X		X
Baby – in PICU or NICU	X	X	X		X		
Baby blues	X	X	X				
Cesarean section		X	X		X		X
Childhood abuse or trauma		X	X		X		
Conflicts with significant other	X	X	X	X	X	X	X
Criticized for infant care		X	X				
Criticized for household care		X	X				
Delivery complications		X	X		X		
Difficult pregnancy		X					
Difficulty adapting into motherhood role	X	X	X	X	X	X	X
Difficulty remembering delivery events					X		

	Baby Blues	Postpartum Depression	Postpartum Anxiety	Postpartum Panic	Postpartum Posttraumatic Stress	Postpartum Obsessive-Compulsive Disorder	Postpartum Psychosis
Distrust of medical staff during delivery					X		
Domestic violence during pregnancy		X					
Domestic violence postpartum		X					
Elective abortion history	X	X	X				
Employment stress	X	X	X	X			
Exaggerated sense of responsibility for baby	X	X	X	X		X	
Exhaustion	X	X	X	X			
Exposure to life-threatening situation(s)		X	X		X		
Extreme euphoria about baby							X
Extreme life event stressors during pregnancy	X	X	X				
Family history of bipolarity		X	X				X
Family history of postpartum depression	X	X	X				
Family history of postpartum psychosis							X
Family stress	X	X	X	X			
Fear of childbirth					X		
Fear for baby's health			X		X	X	
Fear for baby's safety			X		X	X	
Financial stress		X	X	X			
Grief	X	X					
Having many children		X					
Health problems		X		X			
History of delivery complications					X		
History of coping difficulties	X	X	X				

	Baby Blues	Postpartum Depression	Postpartum Anxiety	Postpartum Panic	Postpartum Posttraumatic Stress	Postpartum Obsessive-Compulsive Disorder	Postpartum Psychosis
History of prenatal anxiety	X	X	X			X	
History of prenatal bipolarity	X						X
History of prenatal depression	X	X	X			X	
History of prenatal obsessive-compulsive disorder						X	
History of prenatal panic attacks				X			
History of prenatal personality disorders		X					
History of prenatal psychiatric hospitalization							X
History of prenatal schizophrenia							X
History of poor attachment		X	X				
History of postpartum mood disorder	X	X	X	X	X	X	X
Hormone imbalance	X	X	X	X	X	X	X
Hormone sensitivity	X	X	X	X	X	X	X
Hypomanic symptoms days after delivery							X
Infant – difficult temperament		X					
Infant – colic		X					
Isolating self		X		X		X	
Limited social supports	X	X	X	X	X	X	X
Limited support partner	X	X	X	X	X	X	X
Low-birthweight baby							X
Low-income		X					
Low self-esteem		X					
Marital discord	X	X	X	X	X	X	X
Menstrual cycle dysfunction	X	X					

Risk Factor	Baby Blues	Postpartum Depression	Postpartum Anxiety	Postpartum Panic	Postpartum Posttraumatic Stress	Postpartum Obsessive-Compulsive Disorder	Postpartum Psychosis
Minority/Immigrant	X	X	X				
Minimal to no sleep for days after delivery							X
Miscarriage(s)		X	X				
Nutritional deficiencies		X					
Over age 35		X					
Physical limitations		X					
Poor communication with medical professionals during delivery					X		
Postpartum sleep difficulties		X	X				
Premature delivery		X	X		X		X
Premenstrual dysphoric disorder	X	X	X				
Primary language other than that of residing country	X	X					
Resents pregnancy or baby	X	X					
Sense of loss	X	X					
Single parent		X					
Trauma during pregnancy					X		
Trauma during delivery					X		
Thyroid dysfunction		X					
Unplanned pregnancy	X						
Unwanted pregnancy	X	X	X	X			
Weaning from nursing				X			
Witnessing a violent crime		X			X		

Checklist of Postpartum Mood Disorder Risk Factors

Checklist of Postpartum Mood Disorder Symptoms: Symptoms Obtained through the Empirical Literature

Note: This list may not be all-inclusive and is not meant to diagnose.

Symptom	Baby Blues	Postpartum Depression	Postpartum Anxiety	Postpartum Panic	Postpartum Posttraumatic Stress	Postpartum Obsessive-Compulsive Disorder	Postpartum Psychosis
Abdominal pain		X					
Actions to harm others							X
Actions to harm self		X					X
Agitation		X			X	X	X
Anxiety	X	X	X	X	X	X	X
Appetite changes		X					X
Avoidance behaviors		X	X	X	X	X	X
Backaches		X					
Compulsive behaviors						X	X
Compulsive thoughts		X	X	X		X	X
Cognitive distortions		X	X	X	X	X	X
Confusion	X	X					X
Decreased attentiveness	X	X			X		X
Decreased sexual desire		X					
Delusions							X
Depersonalization							X
Depressed mood		X			X		
Diarrhea			X				
Difficulty coping		X	X	X	X	X	X
Difficulty concentrating		X	X		X	X	X
Disoriented							X

Symptom	Baby Blues	Postpartum Depression	Postpartum Anxiety	Postpartum Panic	Postpartum Posttraumatic Stress	Postpartum Obsessive-Compulsive Disorder	Postpartum Psychosis
Dizzy			X	X			
Exaggerated responses to "normal" stimuli				X	X		
Excessive activity							X
Excessive talking							X
Fear – for baby's health and safety			X	X	X	X	X
Fear – in general			X	X	X		X
Fear – of being alone			X	X		X	
Fear – of being a "bad mom"		X	X	X	X	X	X
Fear – of caretaking for baby		X	X	X	X	X	X
Fear – of leaving the house			X	X			
Feeling angry		X	X		X		
Feeling decreased independence	X	X					
Feeling despair		X			X		
Feeling disconnected to others		X	X	X	X	X	X
Feeling guilt		X	X		X	X	
Feeling hopeless		X			X		
Feeling inadequate		X	X		X	X	X
Feeling numb					X		
Feeling out of control		X	X	X	X		X
Feeling rage		X			X		
Feeling trapped		X	X	X	X	X	
Feeling vulnerable	X	X	X	X	X	X	X
Grandiose thoughts							X
Grief/loss	X	X					

Symptom	Baby Blues	Postpartum Depression	Postpartum Anxiety	Postpartum Panic	Postpartum Posttraumatic Stress	Postpartum Obsessive-Compulsive Disorder	Postpartum Psychosis
Hallucinations							X
Headaches		X					
Heart palpitations			X	X			
Hot/cold flashes				X			
Hyperactive							X
Hyperventilating			X	X			
Impatient							X
Impulsive							X
Irrational fears		X	X	X	X	X	X
Irritability	X	X	X		X		X
Lack of interest in baby		X			X		X
Lack of interest in general		X			X		X
Lost touch with reality							X
Mood swings	X	X			X		X
Muscle tension			X	X	X		
Nausea			X				
Nightmares					X		
Numbing sensations					X		
Obsessions		X	X		X	X	X
Odd/bizarre behavior						X	X
Paranoid thoughts						X	X
Perceived threats to safety					X	X	X
Rapid heartbeat			X	X	X		
Religious preoccupation						X	X

Symptom	Baby Blues	Postpartum Depression	Postpartum Anxiety	Postpartum Panic	Postpartum Posttraumatic Stress	Postpartum Obsessive-Compulsive Disorder	Postpartum Psychosis
Re-living delivery trauma					X		
Repeated disturbing images of delivery					X		
Repeated ruminations that cause distress					X	X	X
Restlessness			X		X		X
Sadness	X	X					
Short temper		X					X
Shortness of breath			X	X			
Sleep changes	X	X	X		X		X
Sweating				X	X		
Tearful	X	X			X		
Thoughts to harm others						X	X
Thoughts to harm self		X				X	X
Tingling sensations			X	X	X		
Trembling				X	X		
Vomiting			X				
Withdrawal from others		X	X	X	X	X	X
Worried	X	X	X	X	X	X	X

Referral Resources for Postpartum Mood Disorders

A Lighter Shade of Blue: Postpartum Adjustment, Depression, and Anxiety Support
   http://www.angelfire.com/oh3/alightershadeofblue/index.html
   24-hr hotline: (513) 225-7284
   E-mail questions or comments: hopejoysweetness@yahoo.com

Barry Brown Health Education Center
   106 Carnie Blvd., Suite 104
   Voorhees, NJ 08043
   (856) 745-8847

Jennifer Mudd Houghtaling Postpartum Depression Foundation
   200 E. Delaware Apt. 3D
   Chicago, IL 60611
   (312) 867-7239
   E-mail: info@ppdchicago.org
   24-hour hotline for Chicago area: (866) 364-MOMS (6667)

MedEdPPD.org (with support from the National Institutes of Mental Health)
   Mothers and Others
   http://www.mededppd.org/mothers/default.asp

Men and Postpartum Depression
   Dr. Will Courtenay
   2811 College Avenue, Suite 1
   Berkeley, CA 94705
   (415) 346-6719
   www.postpartummen.com

Mother to Mother: Postpartum and Pregnancy Telephone Support
   7225 Manchester Rd, Floor 2
   Maplewood, MO 63143
   (314) 644-7001
   (877) 644-7001
   http://www.mothertomothersupport.org/index.html

Online PPD Support Group

http://www.ppdsupportpage.com/index.html
Administrator: Jessica Banas
821 S. Avenida Del Oro E
Pueblo West, CO 81007

Out of the Valley Ministries, Inc.

Christian Postpartum Depression Support for Women and Their Families
http://www.christianppdsupport.org/
For information, questions, and prayer requests: tara@outofthevalley.org

Postpartum Depression Alliance of Illinois

PPD Illinois Helpline: (847) 205-4455

Postpartum Experience

Located in Virginia
http://www.postpartumexperience.com/index.html

Postpartum Progress

http://postpartumprogress.typepad.com/weblog/

Postpartum Resource Center of New York, Inc.

109 Udall Road
West Islip, NY 11795
(631) 422-2255
http://www.postpartumny.org

Postpartum Stress Center, LLC

http://www.postpartumstress.com/index.html
1062 Lancaster Avenue
Rosemont Plaza, Suite 2
Rosemont, PA 19010
(610) 525-7527

Postpartum Support International

P.O. Box 60931
Santa Barbara, CA 93160
(805) 967-7636
http://www.postpartum.net
Helpline: (800) 944-4PPD (4773)
support@postpartum.net

PPD Hope – Family Mental Health Institute
1050 17th Street NW
Suite 600
Washington, DC 20036
(202) 496-4977
E-mail: info@ppdhope.org
www.PPDHope.org

**Ruth Rhoden Craven Foundation for
Postpartum Depression Awareness**
http://www.ppdsupport.org/index.htm
Chairman: Helena Bradford
(843) 881-2047
buzerhel@aol.com

Terminology

Adjustment disorders: Coping difficulties that occur for no less than three months and no more than six months—in other words, transient in nature—not long-term coping difficulties. The coping difficulties occur in response to extreme life stressors such as a divorce, death, or other crisis. More information about adjustment disorders may be found through the Mayo Clinic (http://www.mayoclinic.com/health/adjustment-disorders/DS00584).

Adrenal cortex: The adrenal gland is positioned at the top of a person's kidneys. The adrenal cortex is the external part of the adrenal gland. The adrenal cortex manages the metabolism of fat and carbohydrates through the release of steroid hormones. It will also adjust the equilibrium of salt and water in the body through the release of mineralocorticoid hormones.

Adrenal glands: Adrenal glands are located at the upper portion of each kidney. Refer to Adrenal cortex.

Adrenocorticotropic hormone: When this hormone is released by the pituitary gland, the adrenal cortex activates to synthesize cortisol and other hormones.

Agoraphobia: Is a fear of being out in public or open spaces. Usually, the fear is in relation to areas where the person feels trapped or where help would be difficult to find. In response to this fear, the person avoids these public or open spaces, for example, by refusing to leave the home. An online support group for those suffering with, or supports of someone with, agoraphobia can be found through MDJunction (http://www.mdjunction.com/agoraphobia).

Androgen: Androgens are male sex hormones. There are several types, testosterone being the most common.

Antenatal: The time between conception through delivery. This period is divided into the first, second, and third trimesters of pregnancy.

Antisocial personality disorder: Characteristically, antisocial personality disorder behavior is seen prior to age 15 and remains through adulthood. Common symptoms of antisocial personality disorder include impulsiveness, poor academic and/or job performance, thoughtless behavior, feeling bored, difficulty feeling intimacy, and perceiving oneself as a victim. These symptoms form a pattern of behavior and view of the world. As a result, individuals with antisocial personality disorder discount the boundaries and rights of others and behave in ways contradictory to social norms. Consequently, these individuals are often in trouble with law enforcement and involved in the judicial system. More information and support can be found through PsychCentral (http://psychcentral.com/disorders/sx7t.htm).

APGAR score: An APGAR score is assigned to babies upon delivery as a method to assess the health status of the newborn. Health areas assessed by an APGAR score include the baby's heart and respiration rates, skin and muscle tone, and reactiveness to catheterization of the nostril. APGAR scores range from 0 to 10; the higher the score, the more healthy the baby. Poor APGAR scores (between 0 to 3) indicate that the baby needs resuscitation.

Arterial occlusion: A blockage in an artery making it difficult to impossible for blood to flow normally.

Attachment disorders: Healthy attachment between a caregiver and baby during the first two years of the infant's life does not occur. This unhealthy attachment integrates into childhood, adolescent, and adult development. Behavioral symptoms of unhealthy early-in-life attachment as a child include inappropriate expressions of anger, impulsiveness, and antisocial personality. As adults, these individuals may have difficulty establishing and maintaining healthy, trusting relationships with appropriate respect for boundaries. More information and support can be found through the Attachment Disorder Support Group (http://adsg.syix.com/adsg/index.htm).

Attention-deficit/hyperactivity disorder (ADHD): Generally speaking, ADHD is a neurophysiological disorder. In other words, a part of the brain is not reacting fast enough to manage activity level, responsiveness, and attention span. This results in three classic symptoms: hyperactivity, impulsivity, and lack of concentration. More details about ADHD and strategies to manage symptoms may be found from the State University of New York at Buffalo, Center for Children and Families (www.ccf.buffalo.edu).

Avoidant personality disorder: Avoidant personality disorder is characterized by an exaggerated fear of being rejected by other people. These individuals find it difficult to trust others, feel inadequate compared with others, have poor socialization skills, and experience low self-esteem. As a result, they avoid social environments and intimate/close relationships with others. More details about avoidant personality disorder may be found through HEALTHY PLACE (http://www.healthyplace.com/other-info/psychiatric-disorder-definitions/avoidant-personality-disorder/menu-id-71/).

Bipolar disorder: Bipolar disorder used to be referred to in the DSM as manic depression. Basically, bipolar disorder is characterized by having at least one hypomanic or manic episode and at least one major depressive episode in one's lifetime. There are several different subtypes of bipolar disorder. More information may be found through the Depression and Bipolar Support Alliance (www.dbsalliance.org).

Catecholamines: There are several types of catecholamines; the most important ones discussed in this book are norepinephrine and dopamine. Some catecholamines behave as hormones or as neurotransmitters and activate the "fight-or-flight" nervous system in the body in response to stress.

Cerebral vascular disease: A problem in the arteries in the brain that can cause a stroke or ministroke.

Cognitive distortions: A term used to describe thinking or interpretation patterns that appear inconsistent to the thinking or interpretations of others exposed to similar events, stimuli, or conversation. For example, a mother without cognitive distortions might react to the question "How is your child doing today?" as a means to initiate a conversation, whereas a mother with cognitive distortions might react to the same question by thinking that the person who initiated the question knows that she is a "bad mother" and is checking up on her parenting abilities.

Colic: A term used to describe an episode of crying, irritability, and pain that occurs during or shortly after a baby feeds. It is estimated that 10 percent of babies experience colic.

Comorbid: A term used to describe two symptoms or diagnoses occurring at the same time.

Conduct disorder: Conduct disorder is a condition where a child or adolescent behaves in aggressive and harmful ways toward others, often showing limited remorse or understanding of how her or his behavior has affected another. Common behaviors seen in these youths include bullying, fighting, using a weapon, stealing, torturing animals, setting fires, delinquency, and running away from home. More information about conduct disorder may be found through the American Academy of Child & Adolescent Psychiatry (www.aacap.org/cs/root/facts_for_families/conduct_disorder).

Congenital: A medical term describing a condition that is present at birth.

Corticosteroid: An "umbrella" term to describe several steroid hormones that are made in the adrenal gland's cortex.

Delusions: A false belief that is held by a person. The false belief is often held so strongly that, despite contrary evidence, the false belief is still held.

Dependent personality disorder: Individuals with dependent personality disorder appear naïve, clingy, self-sacrificing, and passive. These people will spend a lot of time trying to please others, with an underlying fear of abandonment. Due to these characteristics, people with dependent personality disorder do not like to be alone and excessively depend on others to take care of them. More information can be found at Psych-Central (http://psychcentral.com/disorders/sx13t.htm)

Depersonalization: A feeling of being disconnected from oneself, such as "being outside one's body."

Dissociation: A feeling of emotional numbness or disconnection that involves the absence of memory at times (usually associated to trauma).

Ectopic pregnancy: A pregnancy that occurs in a location other than the uterus, typically the fallopian tubes.

Embolism: A blockage, such as from a blood clot or air bubble, within a blood vessel.

Endometrium: The internal lining of the uterus.

Endorphins: An opioid chemical produced by the body that acts as a pain killer.

Epidural: A space that surrounds a sac filled with fluid; this sac surrounds the spine. During labor, an anesthetic is inserted into the epidural, resulting in deadening pain sensations in parts of the abdomen and legs.

Etiology: A term used to describe the search for the cause of a condition, syndrome, or disease.

Euphoria: Feeling extremely happy. When used in reference to hypomania or mania, a person feels extreme elation or happiness that is inappropriate to the situation or environment and over an abnormally, extended time.

fMRI: An acronym that stands for functional magnetic resonance imaging. This medical test takes images of the brain while monitoring blood flow to specified areas of the brain.

GABA: An acronym that stands for gamma-aminobutric acid. GABA is a neurotransmitter that helps control anxiety and sleep.

Glucocorticoid: A steroid hormone made in the adrenal gland's cortex that assists with carbohydrate, fat, and protein metabolism.

Grandiosity: A sense of greatness. When used in relation to hypomania or mania, it refers to a sense of self-importance, greatness, superiority, and feeling "larger than life."

Hallucinations: The sensory experience of something that is not real; for example, hearing voices when there is no one in the environment.

Heterosexism: Promoting heterosexuality and discriminating against individuals who are homosexual, including gays, lesbians, transsexuals, and transgenders.

Hyperammonemia: An excessive amount of ammonia in the blood.

Hyperprolactinemia: An excessive amount of prolactin in the blood.

Hyponatremia: Extremely low levels of sodium in the blood.

Hypopituitarism: Hormone deficiency due to endocrine gland dysfunction.

Individualized Education Program (IEP): A written assessment, diagnosis, and treatment protocol for students with a disability. Detailed information about IEPs may be obtained through the U.S. Department of Education (http://idea.ed.gov)

Lutenizing hormone: A hormone produced in the pituitary that tells the ovaries to release an egg (ovulation).

Marginalized: Refers to a group of people who are treated as "second-class citizens" or lower than the "majority" in a society.

Meconium: Fecal matter located in the fetus's intestines that is discharged at, during, or very shortly after delivery.

Melatonin: A serotonin-developed hormone that regulates sleep cycles.

Neurohormones: Describes hormones that are created and released by neurons.

Neurotransmitter: A chemical in charge of transmitting information from one nerve cell to the next.

Obsessive–compulsive personality disorder: A person with obsessive–compulsive personality disorder has a perfectionistic attitude; prefers order, control, and rules; but does not meet the criteria for obsessive–compulsive disorder. More information about obsessive–compulsive personality disorder can be found through OCD Online (http://www.ocdonline.com/articlephillipson6.php).

Oppositional defiant disorder: Children who have oppositional defiant disorder have many temper tantrums, frequently challenge adults, refuse to obey rules or requests, purposefully do or say things that will upset others, and fail to take responsibility for their behaviors. More information about oppositional defiant disorder can be found through the American Academy of Child & Adolescent Psychiatry (http://www.aacap.org/cs/root/facts_for_families/children_with_oppositional_defiant_disorder).

Oxytocin: A hormone released by the brain during childbirth and lactation.

Perinatal: The time during pregnancy and up to one year postpartum.

Peripartum: The time during pregnancy and up to one year postpartum.

Preeclampsia: Most often occurring during the third trimester, preeclampsia is marked by high blood pressure; high protein levels in the mother's urine; and swelling in the mother's face, hands, and feet.

Premature: Premature delivery occurs when the baby is born at 37 weeks or less.

Prenatal: Before becoming pregnant.

Primiparous: This term is used to describe women who have delivered a baby only one time.

Psychotropics: A class of medications used to help alleviate mental health symptoms.

Puerperal: The period between labor or very shortly after delivery.

Puerperium: The period immediately after delivery.

Index

Interpersonal psychotherapy, 278–280
Interpersonal relationships, 13, 14
Intracytoplasmic sperm injection, 171
Intrauterine insemination (IUI), 170
Intrusive mothers, 105–107
In vitro fertilization (IVF)
    explanation of, 172
    impact on child of, 178
    mental health issues and preparation for,
        172–174
    multiple births and, 176, 177

Kava, 251
Krebs-Henseleit disorder, 85

Lactation, 28
Legal issues, related to surrogacy, 181–182
Lesbians
    access to care by, 204–205
    children raised by, 201–203
    mental health statistics for, 199–200
    methods of having children by, 200
    postpartum mood changes and, 103–204
Levonorgestrel, 148
Life Stress Scale, 57
Light therapy, 253
Lithium, 237, 239
Loss, postpartum sense of, 16–17
Lutenizing hormone (LH), 10, 329
Lutenizing hormone releasing hormone
    (LHRH), 10

Major depression. See also Depression;
    Postpartum depression (PPD)
    in females, 8
    postpartum onset of, 31
Male infertility, 166, 171
Marginalized, 329
Marriage
    effects of infertility on, 168–169
    effects of multiple births on, 176
Massage, 252–253, 288
Maternal–child nurses, 219–220
Meconium, 329
Medical professionals
    education and assessment skills of, 301–302

family physicians, 215–216
general practitioners as, 216–217
midwives as, 217–218
nurses as, 218–220
obstetricians and gynecologists as, 217
pediatricians as, 214–215
in perinatal care agencies, 303–304
PMD specialists among, 305
psychiatrists as, 213–214
Medications, Psychotropics. See also
    Antidepressants; Antipsychotics
    to aid in spontaneous abortion, 144
    assessment and monitoring of, 245–246
    hormone replacement therapy, 246–247
    to induce abortion, 148–149
    infertility, 169–170, 172
    medical professionals prescribing, 213–214,
        216–217
    pregnancy safety categories for, 237–245
    research needs for, 313
    table of, 239–243
Melanie Stokes Postpartum Depression
    Research and Care Act (H.R.-20
    Bill), 301
Melatonim, 329
Mental health
    following abortion, 149–151
    following miscarriage, 136, 139
    infertility and, 166–167
    risk factors and, 39
Mental Health and Addiction Equity Act of
    2008, 301
Mental health care
    access to, 291
    macro level, 298–305
    mezzo level of, 295–298
    primary level of, 298–301
Mental health counselors, 221–222
Mental health professionals
    education and assessment skills of,
        295–296
    in perinatal care agencies, 297–298
    PMD specialists among, 298
    psychologists and mental health counselors
        as, 221–222
    social workers as, 221
Midwives, 217–218
Mifepristone, 144, 148
Minerals, 34–35

Public health nurses, 219
Puerperal, 330
Puerperium, 330
Purcell, Brangwynne, 17–18, 89–90, 103–104, 125–126, 139–140, 145–146, 167–168, 271–272
Pychodynamic therapy, 277–278

Race
    miscarriage and, 136, 140
    postpartum depression and, 32–33
Referral resources, 322–324
Registered Nurses Association of Ontario, Canada, 299
Relational-cultural theory (RCT), 19–20, 40
Replacement child, 142
Resiliency, in infants, 112, 113
Resperidone, 237
"Risk-Benefit Decision Making for Treatment of Depression during Pregnancy (Wisner et al.), 214
Risk factors. *See specific conditions*
Roles, conflict in, 40
Rural areas, 44

Same-sex couples, 200–203. *See also* Lesbians
Schemas, 16
Schizoaffective disorder
    explanation of, 83–84
    postpartum psychosis and, 87
Schizophrenia
    bonding and, 88
    postpartum psychosis and, 87–88
    prevalence of, 81
    symptoms of, 82, 83
Screening
    by general practitioners, 216
    tools for, 296–297
Selective serotonin reuptake inhibitors (SSRIs), 238, 240
Self-efficacy, transition to motherhood and, 13–14
Self-identity
    interactions between interpersonal relationships and, 13, 14
    relational-cultural theory and, 19–20

Serotonin
    explanation of, 10, 11
    production, release and metabolism of, 28
Serotonin/norepinephrine reuptake inhibitors (SNRIs), 238, 240
Sex-steroids, 10
Sexual abuse
    postpartum depression and, 37–38
    posttraumatic stress and, 67–68
SHARE Pregnancy and Infant Loss Support, Inc., 145
Sheehan's syndrome, 85
Shields, Brooke, 4
Sleep disturbances
    effect on fetus, 109
    interventions for, 234–236
    risk factors and, 35–36
    role of, 233–234
Social causation model, 18
Social isolation, 167
Social support system
    abortion and, 153
    culture and, 42–43
    family role in, 30
    function of, 40–41
    miscarriage and, 141, 144–145
    retention of, 41–42
    types of, 225–226
Social workers, 221, 306
Societal perspective, 20–22
Sociocultural-based theories
    myth of motherhood model, 18
    relational-cultural theory, 19–20
    societal perspective, 20–22
Socioeconomic status
    miscarriage and, 135
    postpartum depression and, 32
    risk factors and, 43–44
Spermatic cord abnormalities, 171
Spiritual support, 224–225
Spontaneous abortion. *See* Miscarriage
St. John's wort, 250–251
Stillbirth, 135, 141
Stress
    in adoptive parents, 197
    baby blues and pre-existing, 29
    financial issues and, 43–44
    HPA axis reactions to, 9
    infertility and, 166, 173

Stroke, 84, 85
Subarachnoid hemorrhage, 84, 85
Sudden infant death, 141
Sugars, risk factors and, 35
Suicide
    postpartum psychosis and, 91–92
    in pregnant and postpartum women, 31
    statistics related to, 1
Support and encouragement strategies
    education and debriefing as, 279–280
    nondirective counseling as, 280–281
    support groups as, 280
Support groups, 280
Support system. *See* Social support system
Surgery, for infertility, 171
Surgical evacuation, 142–143
Surrogacy
    ethical and legal issues related to, 181–185
    mother's emotional reaction to, 179–180
    parenting following, 180–181
    reasons for, 178
    surrogate emotional reaction to, 180
    types of, 179
Surrogacy Arrangements Act (1985) (United
        Kingdom), 181–182
Surrogate Motherhood Law (1996)
        (Israel), 182
Sweden, 309–310

Tears, 28
Temporary Assistance for Needy Families, 33
Testosterone, tearfulness and, 28
"There are Stories" (Purcell), 167–168
"There Seem Many Apologies Awaiting Trial"
        (Purcell), 125–126
Thrombophlebitis, 84

Thyroid disorders, 37
Toddlers, 112–114. *See also* Children; Infants
Traumatic delivery, 29
Trycyclic antidepressants (TCAs), 238, 241
Tryptophan, 28–29
T3 (thyroid-released hormone), 28
Twins. *See* Multiple births

United Kingdom, 181, 182, 310
"Uprising" (Purcell), 145–146
Urban areas, risk factors and residency in, 44
U.S. Public Health Service Task Force on
        Women's Health Issues, 310
Ussher, Jane, 21

Vas deferens, 171
Victoria, Australia, 302–303
Violence, domestic, 38

"When the Land Closes in Around Us"
        (Purcell), 89–90
Withdrawn mothers, 105–107
Women's Health Initiative (WHI), 246
World Health Organization (WHO), 31, 165,
        300, 304

Xiong-gui-tiao-xue-yin, 252

Yates, Andrea, 1

Zygote intrafallopian transfer (ZIFT), 170